Radiology for Medical Finals
A case-based guide

Radiology for Medical Finals
A case-based guide

Lt Col Edward Sellon

BSc (Hons), MBBS, MRCS, FRCR, PgD (SEM), Dip (ESSR), RAMC
Consultant Musculoskeletal Radiologist
Oxford University Hospitals
Oxford

and

Consultant Military Radiologist
Centre for Defence Radiology
Birmingham, UK

Professor David C Howlett

MBBS, PhD, FAcadMEd, FRCP (London), FRCP (Edinburgh), FRCR
Consultant Radiologist
Eastbourne Hospital
East Sussex Healthcare NHS Trust
Eastbourne

and

Honorary Clinical Professor
Brighton and Sussex Medical School
Brighton, UK

Preparation of the illustrations by:

Mr Nick Taylor

MIMI, RMIP, MRCR(Hon)
Honorary Teaching Fellow, Brighton and Sussex Medical School
and Medical Photographer
East Sussex Healthcare NHS Trust
Eastbourne, UK

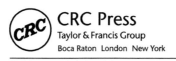

CRC Press
Taylor & Francis Group
Boca Raton London New York

CRC Press is an imprint of the
Taylor & Francis Group, an **informa** business

CRC Press
Taylor & Francis Group
6000 Broken Sound Parkway NW, Suite 300
Boca Raton, FL 33487-2742

© 2018 by Taylor & Francis Group, LLC
CRC Press is an imprint of Taylor & Francis Group, an Informa business

No claim to original U.S. Government works
Printed on acid-free paper

International Standard Book Number-13: 978-1-4987-8216-6 (Paperback)

Visit the Taylor & Francis Web site at
http://www.taylorandfrancis.com

and the CRC Press Web site at
http://www.crcpress.com

For Louise and Lottie,
for their constant love, support and belief (ES)

To my dear wife Lara and all the children, Thomas, Ella, Robert and Miles,
also to my parents, Ken and Margaret, and remembering fondly
Joanna and Christopher (DCH)

Contents

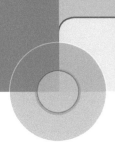

Foreword by Professor Malcolm Reed

From the initial discovery of X-rays and their application to medical imaging by Wilhelm Röntgen, imaging has been an increasingly vital part of medical practice. The modern doctor needs a strong understanding of the different modalities and their application in the diagnosis and management of a wide range of medical conditions. While in many situations images are reported by expert radiologists, the ability to understand and interpret radiological images is essential and the vast majority of medical schools will require students to demonstrate fundamental skills in this area.

More importantly, diagnostic and therapeutic imaging opens a window to the internal structure and function of the human body and links the fundamental sciences of anatomy, physiology, and pathology to the patient as a whole presenting with symptoms and signs of disease. The clues gleaned from a careful history and thorough examination lead us to select the most appropriate investigations to expedite a diagnosis, allowing us to inform the patient about their condition and commence appropriate treatment. It is the distinction between normal and abnormal structure and function, which is at the core of radiological diagnosis, that provides an illustrative basis for learning and a truly patient-orientated understanding of medical disorders. As such, the use of radiology in teaching and learning facilitates and enhances the understanding of medicine and is of enormous benefit in preparing for examinations such as medical school Finals. This textbook edited by Edward Sellon and David Howlett provides an invaluable learning resource not just for students preparing for medical school Finals but any doctor preparing for subsequent professional assessments. In addition to the well-illustrated cases and a useful introduction to OSCE-style exams, the real value in this text is in the clearly structured cases based on high-quality radiological imaging, which span the whole spectrum of medicine. The book takes a regional anatomy approach with additional chapters on the normal chest and abdominal X-rays and paediatric cases.

The contributors and editors are to be commended for producing a high-quality, comprehensive compilation of cases with clear and concise questions, answers, and explanatory notes. I would commend this text book to its target audience of final year medical students but also to doctors in training in a wide range of clinical disciplines as well as those in established practice.

Professor Malcolm Reed BMedSci, MBChB, FRCS
Dean, Brighton and Sussex Medical School
Brighton, UK

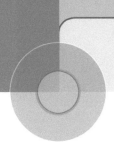

Foreword by
Dr Giles Maskell

Radiology is an unusual medical discipline in being able to trace its origin precisely to a specific event – the discovery of X-rays by Wilhelm Röntgen in 1895. The practice of medicine was transformed almost overnight by the use of X-rays in diagnosis. The development of further imaging techniques such as ultrasound, computed tomography (CT) and magnetic resonance imaging (MRI) followed in the second half of the twentieth century and has led to medical imaging occupying a central place in the management of patients with a very wide range of conditions.

Whatever branch of medicine you pursue as a career, at some stage you will find that an understanding of medical images – X-rays and scans – will be essential to your work. You will need to understand not only the principles of interpretation of tests such as the chest X-ray but also their strengths and limitations and how to make the best use of these tests to benefit your patients.

Although imaging findings can occasionally be so characteristic that they could almost be called "pathognomonic", one of the most important lessons that you will learn is that the interpretation of an imaging test depends critically on the clinical context. The classic diagnostic sequence – history, examination, tests – is as valid today as it ever has been, despite the increasing sophistication of the imaging tests. The doctor who makes a diagnosis based only on imaging findings without due regard to the clinical context is more than likely to be tripped up.

Radiology is not a discipline that can be learned in isolation from clinical medicine. In this book, David Howlett, Edward Sellon, and their colleagues, renowned educators in this field, have therefore embedded the teaching of radiology in a series of clinical cases, which illustrate not only the specific imaging findings in certain conditions but, importantly, the principles that underpin the effective use of imaging tests in clinical practice.

Although there are encouraging signs with the establishment of undergraduate radiology societies in many medical schools, the teaching of radiology to undergraduates has not always kept up with the progress in medical imaging. I believe that this book will prove invaluable, not only in preparing students for medical Finals, but also in giving them a better understanding of the central role of imaging in modern clinical management, which will serve them well in the early years of their careers as doctors. Maybe some will even be inspired to consider a future career in this most exciting and rapidly developing discipline.

Dr Giles Maskell MA, FRCP, FRCR, FRCPE
President, Royal College of Radiologists (2013–2016)
Consultant Radiologist
Royal Cornwall Hospitals NHS Trust
Truro, UK

Preface

This book has been a long time in the making and is the product of many years of both teaching and examining undergraduate medical students. Over this time there has been an exponential increase in the use of all forms of imaging in both acute and elective patient care and this has been reflected in undergraduate medical school curricula and also examinations. Radiology images feature prominently in both Finals written papers and Objective Structured Clinical Examination (OSCE), and whole OSCE stations may be based upon a chest X-ray for example. Various imaging modalities tend to feature, in particular X-rays of the chest, abdomen, and common fractures, but increasingly CT and MR images. The incorporation of radiology/imaging into Finals reflects the increasing exposure of both medical students and junior doctors to all forms of radiology and the requirement for trainees to be able to provide provisional interpretation of many forms of imaging.

This book is not intended to be an all-encompassing textbook of radiology, and the bibliography provides supplementary reading for those who wish to dig deeper. A case-based approach has been adopted and radiology images in questions have been selected in two broad categories – those that students could expect to encounter in Finals or, alternatively, to cover key learning points/educational aspects of radiology. This structure should allow students and also foundation doctors to approach both Finals and the foundation years with more confidence.

Inevitably within the book there is a strong emphasis on plain film interpretation, as these investigations are the most common form of imaging that students and junior doctors will encounter and they will also often be expected to provide a provisional interpretation. Extensive additional examples are used in case answer sections to explain and reinforce learning points throughout the book. There is widespread use also of common/important CT/MR images, again because these modalities are increasingly frontline; for example, CT head interpretation in stroke care. There is less emphasis on ultrasound and nuclear medicine, as these modalities occur less frequently in Finals, although an understanding of their use is necessary. Ultrasound does feature in some cases reflecting more widespread use of this modality on the wards and in the emergency department.

We hope you will enjoy this book and that it will stimulate and enhance your knowledge and understanding of radiology, and improve your confidence in image interpretation.

Edward Sellon
David C Howlett

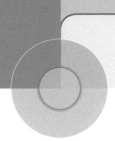

Contributors and acknowledgements

Dr Hannah Adams BSc (Hons), MBChB
Radiology Registrar
Brighton and Sussex University Hospitals
    NHS Trust, Brighton, UK

Dr Faye Cuthbert MBBS, MRCP, FRCR
Consultant Urogenital Radiologist
Brighton and Sussex University Hospitals
    NHS Trust, Brighton, UK

Dr Sarah Hancox MBBS, BSc (Hons)
Resident Medical Officer, Emergency
    Department
Townsville Hospital, Townsville
Queensland, Australia

Dr Vincent G Helyar MBBS, BSc, MSc,
FRCR, EBIR
Interventional Radiology Fellow
Guy's and St Thomas' NHS Foundation Trust
London, UK

Professor David C Howlett MBBS, PhD,
FAcadMEd, FRCP (London), FRCP
(Edinburgh), FRCR
Consultant Radiologist
Eastbourne Hospital, East Sussex Healthcare
    NHS Trust, Eastbourne
and
Honorary Clinical Professor
Brighton and Sussex Medical School
Brighton, UK

Dr Amanda Jewison BMBS, FRCR
Specialist Registrar in Radiology
Brighton and Sussex University Hospitals
    NHS Trust, Brighton, UK

Dr Thomas Kurka BSc, BMBS
Academic Foundation Doctor (Management &
    Leadership)
Brighton and Sussex University Hospitals
    NHS Trust, Brighton, UK

Dr Uday Mandalia MBBS, BSc,
MRPCH, FRCR
Consultant Radiologist
Hillingdon Hospital, Uxbridge, UK

Dr Sean Mitchell BMBS, BSc (Hons)
General Practitioner Specialty Trainee Year 2
Brighton and Sussex University Hospitals
    NHS Trust
Honorary Clinical Teaching Fellow
Brighton and Sussex Medical School
Brighton, UK

Dr Cristina Ruscanu MBBS
Foundation Year 2 Doctor
East Sussex Healthcare NHS Trust
Eastbourne, UK

Lt Col Edward Sellon BSc (Hons),
MBBS, MRCS, FRCR, PgD (SEM),
Dip (ESSR), RAMC
Consultant Musculoskeletal Radiologist
Oxford University Hospitals, Oxford
and
Consultant Military Radiologist
Centre for Defence Radiology
Birmingham, UK

Dr Lucy Shimwell MB BCh, BAO
Resident Medical Officer
Royal Perth Hospital, Perth
Western Australia, Australia

Dr Andrew Snoddon MBChB, FRCR
Specialist Registrar in Radiology
Leeds General Infirmary, Leeds, UK

Dr Olwen Westerland MBBS, BSc, FRCR
Consultant Radiologist
Guy's and St Thomas' NHS Foundation Trust
London, UK

ACKNOWLEDGEMENTS

Two people in particular have been fundamental to the successful production of this book. Nick Taylor, medical photographer, has worked tirelessly and with great skill preparing the images, which are such a vital component of any book on imaging. Also Susi Arjomand who has, with her customary patience and attention to detail, typed up the numerous editing iterations of the manuscript. Thank you both.

The editors would also like to thank Jo Koster, commissioning editor at Taylor Francis, for her support and guidance throughout the publishing process. Dr Gillian Watson and Dr Justin Harris kindly provided some of the radiological images used in the text and Kirstie Leach also helped with manuscript preparation.

Finally, we would like to gratefully acknowledge all the book's contributors for their hard work and enthusiasm, and for finding the time to prepare their cases amidst busy schedules.

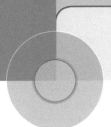

Abbreviations

AA	aortic arch
AAA	abdominal aortic aneurysm
AAFB	acid-and-alcohol fast bacilli
AAST	American Association for the Surgery of Trauma
ABCDE	airway, breathing, circulation, diaphragm, everything else
ABG	arterial blood gas
ACE	angiotensin-converting enzyme
AIDS	acquired immune deficiency syndrome
ALP	alkaline phosphatase
ALT	alanine transaminase
ALARA	as low as reasonably achievable
ANA	antinuclear antibodies
AP	anteroposterior (view)
ARB	angiotensin receptor blocker
AST	aspartate transaminase
AVN	avascular necrosis
AVPU	alert, voice, pain, unresponsive
AXR	abdominal X-ray
BCG	bacille Calmette-Guérin
BMI	body mass index
BNP	brain natriuretic peptide
BP	blood pressure
BPD	bronchopulmonary dysplasia
bpm	beats per minute/breaths per minute
CABG	coronary artery bypass graft
CBD	common bile duct
CC	craniocaudal (view)
CDH	congenital diaphragmatic hernia
CF	cystic fibrosis
CFTR	cystic fibrosis transmembrane conductance regulator (gene)
CLD	chronic lung disease of prematurity
CLL	chronic lymphoid leukemia
CMC	carpometacarpal
CNS	central nervous system

CO_2	carbon dioxide
COPD	chronic obstructive pulmonary disease
CPPD	calcium pyrophosphate deposition disease
CRP	C-reactive protein
CSF	cerebrospinal fluid
CT	computed tomography
CT IVU	computed tomography intravenous urogram
CT KUB	computed tomography kidneys ureters and bladder
CTR	cardiothoracic ratio
CTPA	computed tomography pulmonary angiogram
CXR	chest X-ray
2D	two-dimensional
3D	three-dimensional
DCIS	ductal carcinoma in situ
DEXA	dual energy X-ray absorptiometry
DHS	dynamic hip screw
DJ	duodenojejunal
DIP	distal interphalangeal
DLCO	diffusion capacity of the lung for carbon monoxide (test)
DMARD	disease modifying antirheumatic drug
DRUJ	distal radioulnar joint
DSA	digital subtraction angiography
DVT	deep vein thrombosis
DWI	diffusion-weighted imaging
ECG	electrocardiogram
ECMO	extracorporeal membrane oxygenation
ED	emergency department
eGFR	estimated glomerular filtration rate
ENT	ear, nose, and throat
ERCP	endoscopic retrograde cholangiopancreatography

ESR	erythrocyte sedimentation rate	LBO	large bowel obstruction
ESWL	extracorporeal shock wave lithotripsy	LCIS	lobular carcinoma in situ
		LDH	lactate dehydrogenase
ET	endotracheal	LFTs	liver function tests
ETT	endotracheal tube	LHB	left heart border
EVAR	endovascular aneurysm repair	LMP	last menstrual period
FAST	focused assessment with sonography for trauma	LMWH	low molecular weight heparin
		LUQ	left upper quadrant
FBC	full blood count	LV	left ventricle
FDG	fluorodeoxyglucose	LVA	left ventricular aneurysm
FEV	forced expiratory volume	MAC	*Mycobacterium avium* complex
FFDM	full field digital mammography	MAS	meconium aspiration syndrome
FLAIR	fluid-attenuated inversion recovery	MCA	middle cerebral artery
		MCP	metacarpophalangeal
FOOSH	fall on an outstretched hand	MCV	mean cell volume
GCS	Glasgow coma scale	MDT	multidisciplinary team
GFR	glomerular filtration rate	MI	myocardial infarction
GGT	gamma-glutamyl transferase	MIBG	metaiodobenzylguanidine
GH	glenohumeral	micromol/L	micromoles per litre
GI	gastrointestinal	MIP	maximum intensity projection
GORD	gastro-oesophageal reflux disease	MLO	medial lateral oblique (view)
		mmol/L	millimoles per litre
GP	general practitioner	MR	magnetic resonance
GTN	glyceryl trinitrate	MRCP	magnetic resonance cholangiopancreatography
Hb	haemoglobin		
HCG	human chorionic gonadotropin	MRI	magnetic resonance imaging
HER2	human epidermal growth factor 2	mmHg	millimetres of mercury
		MS	multiple sclerosis
HIV	human immunodeficiency virus	MSU	mid-stream urine
HLA	human leukocyte antigen	mSv	millisieverts
HR	heart rate	MTP	metatarsophalangeal
HRCT	high-resolution computed tomography	NAI	nonaccidental injury
		NEC	necrotising enterocolitis
HU	Hounsfield units	NG	nasogastric
ICD	implantable cardiac defibrillator	NHL	non-Hodgkin lymphoma
ICE	ideas, concerns, and expectations	NICU	neonatal intensive care unit
ICP	intracranial pressure	NPSA	National Patient Safety Agency
ICU	intensive care unit	NSAID	nonsteroidal anti-inflammatory drug
Ig	immunoglobulin		
INR	international normalised ratio	NYHA	New York Heart Association
IP	interphalangeal	OA	osteoarthritis
ITU	intensive therapy unit	OGD	oesophago-gastro-duodenoscopy
IUCD	intrauterine contraceptive device	ORIF	open reduction and internal fixation
IV	intravenous		
IVC	inferior vena cava	OSCE	Objective Structured Clinical Examination
kg	kilogram		
LA	left atrium	PA	posteroanterior (view)

PAOD	peripheral artery occlusive disease	SCFE	slipped capital femoral epiphysis
PCR	polymerase chain reaction	SH	Salter–Harris
PE	pulmonary embolism	SIADH	syndrome of inappropriate antidiuretic hormone (secretion)
PEFR	peak expiratory flow rate	SOBOE	short of breath on exertion
PET	positron emission tomography	SPO_2	saturation pressure of oxygen
PIC	peripherally inserted catheter	STIR	short tau inversion recovery
PIP	proximal interphalangeal	SUFE	slipped upper femoral epiphysis
PKD	polycystic kidney disease	TB	tuberculosis
PPHN	persistent pulmonary hypertension of the newborn	TFCC	triangular fibrocartilage complex
PPP	projection, personal demographics, previous CXR comparison	TFTs	thyroid function tests
		THA	total hip arthroplasty
		THR	total hip replacement
PR	per rectum	TIA	transient ischaemic attack
PTH	parathyroid hormone	TNF	tumour necrosis factor
RA	right atrium	TNM	tumour, nodes, metastases
RCC	renal cell carcinoma	UAC	umbilical arterial catheter
RDS	respiratory distress syndrome	U&Es	urea and electrolytes
RhA	rheumatoid arthritis	UGI	upper gastrointestinal
RHB	right heart border	US	ultrasound
RhF	rheumatoid factor	UVC	umbilical venous catheter
RIF	right iliac fossa	VBG	venous blood gas
RIP	rotation/inspiration/penetration	VCF	vertebral compression fracture
RLQ	right lower quadrant	VUJ	vesicoureteric junction
RR	respiration rate	V/Q	ventilation/perfusion scan
RTA	road traffic accident	WBC	white blood cell
rTPA	recombinant tissue plasminogen activator	WCC	white cell count
		WHO	World Health Organisation
RUQ	right upper quadrant	XR	X-ray
SBO	small bowel obstruction	ZN	Ziehl–Neelsen

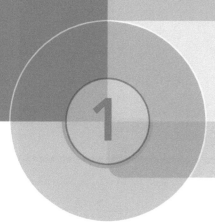

Overview of imaging modalities

1

THOMAS KURKA AND DAVID C HOWLETT

It is helpful for finals to have an understanding of the core imaging modalities you are likely to encounter and to have an idea of the relative strengths/weaknesses and indications/contraindications for each.

PLAIN FILMS: CHEST X-RAY, ABDOMINAL X-RAY, AND ORTHOPAEDIC BONE/JOINT X-RAYS

Conventional X-ray remains an important diagnostic tool in medicine and remains the most commonly used imaging modality. Plain films are commonly the chest X-ray (CXR), abdominal X-ray (AXR), and orthopaedic bone/joint X-rays (XRs). An XR is relatively inexpensive, time effective, and does not require any special preparation of the patient. There is a degree of ionising radiation associated with X-ray exposure and this radiation dose varies with body part; a lumbar spine XR entails a far higher radiation dose than a wrist XR for example owing to radiation of pelvic organs. However, generally X-ray doses are far lower than those associated with computed tomography (CT). Dose information is included in Chapters 3 and 4. As always 'justify' the exposure: does the benefit to the patient outweigh the potential risk of irradiation?

When a radiograph is taken, the X-ray beam passes through the body part onto an X-ray sensitive screen. Bones, owing to their high calcium content, absorb most of the X-rays whereas soft tissues absorb a smaller amount, depending on composition and density. As a result, X-rays from the bones do not reach the screen and appear white on the radiograph, with the soft tissue appearing darker. X-rays pass through the air without being absorbed at all, which is then detected by the screen and appears black on the radiograph.

ADVANTAGES

- Inexpensive.
- Usually quick to perform.

- Painless, noninvasive.
- Good diagnostic tool for many pathologies.

DISADVANTAGES

- Soft tissue, lung, bone resolution much reduced compared with CT/magnetic resonance imaging (MRI).
- Provides a two-dimensional (2D), single image only.
- Radiation exposure.

INDICATIONS – ARE BROAD

CXR

- Respiratory – infection, septic screen, pneumothorax, chest trauma, inhaled foreign body, pleural effusion, suspected malignancy.
- Cardiac – clinical heart failure, clinical cardiomegaly, heart murmurs.

AXR

- Abdomen – bowel obstruction, perforated viscus (erect CXR more sensitive), ingested foreign body, abdominal pain in the emergency setting.
- Pelvic – pelvic fracture, neck of femur fracture.

Soft tissue XR neck

- Inhaled foreign body.
- Retropharyngeal abscess.

Bone XR

- Limbs – trauma, fractures, skeletal survey, acutely swollen joint, osteomyelitis, septic arthritis, bone pain, tumour/metastasis.
- Skulls – skeletal survey, myeloma, dental imaging.
- Spine – trauma, scoliosis.

ULTRASOUND

Ultrasound (US) uses sound waves of high frequencies, which are emitted towards the studied tissues and are reflected/echoed back to the probe depending on the tissue density and composition. This signal is then translated into an US image. US is a 'live' imaging modality and requires interpretation while the investigation is being carried out. US colour Doppler techniques are used to assess moving blood and are used in vascular assessment, e.g. carotid stenosis.

ADVANTAGES

- No radiation, noninvasive (some US is performed using endocavity probes, e.g. transrectal, transvaginal, transoesophageal).
- Real-time assessment and interpretation of results.
- Relatively inexpensive.

- Useful for imaging of soft tissue and muscles, extremities, testes, breast, and eye, plus abdomen, pelvis, chest, and vascular colour Doppler applications.

DISADVANTAGES

- Requires a skilled practitioner with US interpretation skills, operator dependent.
- No use for bone imaging as sound is attenuated/absorbed by bone.
- Images are degraded by gas and fat, and this restricts US use in the abdomen/pelvis in some patients.

INDICATIONS

- Abdomen – trauma, malignancy, abdominal aortic aneurysm (AAA) surveillance, gallstones, suspected hydronephrosis.
- Chest – assessment of pleural spaces.
- Musculoskeletal – assessment of muscles, ligaments, and tendons.
- Scrotal – assessment of testicles, epididymis, and scrotum.
- Obstetrics – growth scans, placental sighting, anomaly scans.
- Gynaecology – transabdominal and transvaginal imaging of ovaries, uterus, and Fallopian tubes.
- Baby hips.
- Breast, eye assessment.
- Vascular applications – suspected upper/lower limb deep vein thrombosis (DVT), carotid/peripheral vascular assessment.

COMPUTED TOMOGRAPHY

CT uses X-rays, which are emitted from a rotating X-ray source around the patient with multiple detectors to produce a series of 2D axial images of the studied body part. This can then be computer-reconstructed to obtain axial, coronal, sagittal 2D, and three-dimensional (3D) images of the studied body parts. There are other imaging modalities that make use of CT imaging such as positron emission tomography (PET scan).

ADVANTAGES

- Provides 2D cross-sectional images of the body, which are rapidly acquired with the potential to reformat in multiple planes; 3D reformatting is also possible.
- Provides a detailed image of the studied body part and the surrounding tissue.
- High sensitivity and specificity in particular for assessment of the lungs, mediastinum, bones, abdomen/pelvis structures, the brain – especially acute blood.

DISADVANTAGES

- CT scanners are expensive.
- Moderate to high dose of radiation, depending on areas scanned.
- May require intravenous (IV) iodinated contrast use – risk of contrast reaction (allergy, anaphylaxis) and nephrotoxicity in those at risk.

INDICATIONS

- Head – trauma, brain imaging (ischaemic/haemorrhagic strokes, calcifications, haemorrhage, malignancy).
- Chest – detailed imaging of the lungs to detect abnormalities not seen on CXR, used in diagnosis and surveillance of malignancy, pulmonary embolism (CT pulmonary angiogram: CTPA), emphysema, fibrosis. Cardiac – CT to image coronary arteries.
- Abdomen and pelvis – diagnosis, staging, and surveillance of malignancies, bowel obstruction, AAA, pancreatitis, renal calculi (CT kidneys ureters and bladder [CT KUB] and CT IV urogram [CT IVU]).
- CT angiography and venography – for example, suspected limb or mesenteric vascular occlusion, sagittal sinus thrombosis.
- Orthopaedic – complex fractures.
- CT-guided biopsy, surgery, and radiosurgery.

MAGNETIC RESONANCE IMAGING

MRI does not use any X-rays, thus does not expose the patient to ionising radiation. It is superior to CT in obtaining detailed images of the soft tissues and also the brain. MRI uses strong magnetic fields, radio waves, and field gradients to generate the image.

In structural MRI, the images are obtained by proton alignment by an external magnet and a subsequent radiofrequency pulse disrupts the equilibrium, which gives an MRI signal. Details of MRI protocols and sequences are not needed for finals – T1- and T2-weighted are common sequences (in the brain cerebrospinal fluid [CSF] appears bright/white on T2), and IV contrast can also be used (gadolinium).

ADVANTAGES

- No ionising radiation exposure.
- Provides 2D and 3D cross-sectional images of the body.
- Superior to other imaging modalities in obtaining high-resolution images of the brain and musculoskeletal system.
- Ideal for soft tissue structures, cartilage, and ligament imaging.
- Vascular and cardiac applications.

DISADVANTAGES

- Expensive equipment – the most expensive imaging modality.
- Time consuming, requiring patient cooperation, ability to lie still, often for 30–60 minutes.
- Contraindicated in patients with ferrous metal implants – pacemakers, cochlear implants, metallic foreign bodies in the eyes.
- MRI is undertaken in a relatively enclosed space – unsuitable for patients with claustrophobia and young children (may need general anaesthesia).
- Relatively contraindicated in pregnancy, particularly first trimester.

INDICATIONS

- Head and neck – neuroimaging – clear differentiation between the grey and white matter, diagnosis of demyelinating disease, cerebrovascular disease, detailed imaging of malignancies and infectious diseases, epilepsy imaging, functional MRI brain studies. CT is more accurate in the detection of acute blood; new MRI techniques, e.g. diffusion weighting, can detect cerebral ischaemia very early (minutes) when compared with CT.
- Spine imaging – nerve compression (cord and cauda equina), malignancies, disc disease.
- Hepatobiliary – liver, pancreas, and biliary lesions, MR cholangiopancreatography (MRCP) for structural imaging of the biliary tree.
- Small bowel – Crohn's disease diagnosis.
- Knee and other joints – used in cartilage and ligament imaging.
- Angiographic, vascular protocols, cardiac MRI.
- Prostate imaging, diagnosis, and staging of prostate cancer.
- Rectal, gynaecological cancer staging.

NUCLEAR MEDICINE

Nuclear medicine uses injected (or inhaled) radioactive isotopes to diagnose or treat many conditions: endocrine, heart, and gastrointestinal (GI) diseases. It images the emission of isotope radiation from within the body and can construct a 2D/3D image of the areas of the radioactive substance uptake. It is used for functional imaging, rather than structural imaging, as contrast/spatial resolution is poor. Some nuclear medicine is combined with CT/MRI to improve anatomical detail.

IMAGING MODALITIES

- Myocardial perfusion scan – assessment of the function of myocardium for diagnosis of hypertrophic cardiomyopathy and coronary artery disease, in combination with MRI +/– CT.
- Genitourinary scan – assessment of renal blood flow and function, evaluate renovascular hypertension, and assess vesicoureteral reflux.
- Bone imaging – assessment of bone metastases, infection.
- PET – imaging of metastases, neuroimaging – imaging of brain activity in dementias, combining injection of metabolically active substances, e.g. fluorodeoxyglucose (FDG) and tomography/CT detection.

ADVANTAGES

- Provides functional information of organs and disease processes.
- Advancement of treatment options for cancer patients.
- Allows early or improved detection of metastases (PET).
- Provides detailed and accurate information in hard to reach areas.
- Radioisotopes are used to treat some cancers, e.g. radioiodine and papillary thyroid cancer.

DISADVANTAGES

- High cost.
- Exposure to radiation doses, which may be significant, e.g. PET.
- Not all techniques are widely available, e.g. PET.

FLUOROSCOPY TECHNIQUES

Fluoroscopy combines ionising radiation from X-ray exposure with administration (ingested/injected) of contrast medium, which is then imaged passing through the structures/organs of interest to assess their function and structure in real time. Examples include:

- Contrast swallow – assessment of the structure and function of the pharynx and oesophagus (largely replaced by oesophago-gastro-duodenoscopy [OGD]).
- Barium follow through – assessment of the structure and function of the small bowel (MRI small bowel replacing).
- Contrast enema – assessment of structure and function of the large bowel and rectum (colonoscopy replacing), used particularly to evaluate the integrity of postoperative bowel anastomoses.
- Tubogram (hysterosalpingography) – assessment of the shape of the uterine cavity and the shape and patency of the Fallopian tubes.
- Arteriogram, venogram (CT/MRI replacing).

ADVANTAGES

- Allow a 'live' assessment.
- Relatively inexpensive, readily available.
- Relatively noninvasive.

DISADVANTAGES

- Exposure to ionising radiation, which may be significant, e.g. barium enema.
- Poor soft tissue resolution.
- Endoscopy techniques are more accurate in bowel mucosal assessment and allow tissue biopsies.

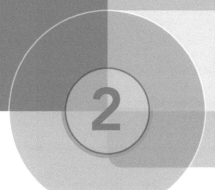

Hints and tips for finals
Objective Structured Clinical Examination

2

THOMAS KURKA

The OSCE (Objective Structured Clinical Examination) is designed to test clinical and communication skills in a structured environment in real time. Many medical schools use the 'integrated station' approach in their OSCE exams, which means that you may be asked to take a focused history, do a part of a clinical examination, and interpret a test result all in one station. This tests your knowledge, skills, and your thinking process towards reaching a working diagnosis. Remember that most people pass their OSCE and you are allowed to fail a small proportion of the stations – your medical school will be able to advise on the specific rules of the exam.

LOGISTICS OF PREPARATION AND THE DAY ITSELF

- Practice ... practice ... practice! Then practice even more. It is important to have some regular quality group study time before your OSCE. This exam is about your skills and practical experience, and you cannot pass the OSCE if you only study from books.
- You should observe other students practicing OSCE-style scenarios, give each other constructive feedback, and correct mistakes. It is important to be helpful and polite to your colleagues and friends but it is very important to be constructive with your feedback and verbalise what went wrong. Some people may not be aware of their mistakes and cannot improve unless you tell them.
- Although it may seem intimidating, do ask doctors to assess you when on the wards. Most are keen to teach and help you pass and it will give you more experience in presenting real cases.
- The OSCE is a role play, not a real-life scenario. You need to learn to play the game. Speak to previous students who passed finals OSCE at your medical school to understand the structure of the stations and the day.
- Have a good night's sleep before the OSCE day. Tiredness decreases concentration and organisational skills and hinders your ability to communicate effectively. The OSCE is a type of performance and you need to be fresh and alert to perform well.

- Read the OSCE station instructions properly and follow the script – this ensures you stay on the topic of the OSCE station and will earn you points. If the station says take a history from the patient you will not score any points on educating or advising the patient. Stay focused on the tasks specified in your station brief.
- Begin every station with a polite introduction of yourself. Knock on the door before entering and say hello with a smile on your face (even a nervous smile counts). Introduce yourself with a full name and your role, and do not forget to articulate. Most feedback from the patients from OSCE stations was that they could not understand the students' names and introduction because they spoke too fast as they were nervous. Be the one to be remembered for appearing calm, with a smile on your face and a clear introduction.
- Ask your patient's permission to take their history and/or examine them – there is a mark for gaining a verbal consent.
- Follow up with letting the patient tell you their story – this will allow you to have a minute to catch your breath and to connect with the patient.
- Finally, the staff who are examining you want you to pass and you need to give them the opportunity to give you the points!

YOUR COMMUNICATION SKILLS

- Smile and adopt an approachable body language.
- Make sure that each station is a dialogue between you and the patient. Avoid leading and closed-end questions, especially in the history of the presenting complaint.
- There is a balance between letting the patient explain their symptoms or problems, and them rumbling on for too long, which could be a distraction taking you off the path of the station – keep the conversation focused to the topic of the station but ensure you do not cut the patient off too soon, which could appear impolite and potentially damage the doctor–patient relationship. If you need to interrupt their story, apologise for doing so, acknowledge what they were saying, and offer to return to it if there is time at the end.
- Avoid all medical jargon! It is natural for medical students in the final year to be very familiar and fluent in medical jargon but most patients do not understand these terms and OSCEs will test that you can communicate using simple terms.
- Be clear and succinct when giving advice to the patients and always ensure their understanding – the best way is to ask the patient to repeat it back to you in their own words.
- Do not ever sound patronising or forceful with any advice you give to the patient! Remember, patients have a right to autonomy, which means that you should only advise and they can choose to accept or decline your advice (assuming full mental capacity).
- Many students like to repeat the history back to the patients at the end to summarise and buy some time to think about what next. This may not be recommended in finals especially if your OSCE station is only 8–10 minutes long. During a finals OSCE, you will have more than the history to get through (blood results, imaging or further questions) so do not waste time on repetition as you could run out of time by the end and lose some valuable points.
- OSCE stations are often divided into two sections, an 8-minute station has 4 minutes for history, for example, and then 4 minutes for further questions/looking at results/differential/further management. The examiner will usually prompt you at 4 minutes if needed.
- Listen to your patients and respond directly to what they are saying. The patient (or actor) is playing by the script and they will not mislead or give you any wrong information.

It is important to acknowledge their worries and concerns directly, even if you need to divert to continue gathering the essential information for your history. Sometimes patients can talk for a long time and go off the topic, and it is your job to politely interrupt them, acknowledge you will return to their point, and only then divert to what you want to talk about. You need to appear to be in control but do it politely.

- The examiner will nudge you if you start slowing down or diverge from the main topic or time is running short. Take the hint as they are trying to set you back on the right path, the path of the marking sheet.
- Avoid talking too much. It can be tempting to try to talk a lot to show you know your subject but remember this is a two-way discussion, not a monologue. This applies mainly to communication stations when you are asked to explain a procedure, counsel the patient or discuss a new treatment. It is tempting to quickly say everything you know about the subject to impress your examiner but remember this is about giving information to the patient who needs to understand it, be able to ask questions, and share their point of view with you.

COMMUNICATION STATIONS

- Communication stations are those where you are asked to discuss a certain treatment or procedure with a patient, to break bad news or to deal with a complaint.
- Practice communication stations with your friends and colleagues.
- Many medical schools use communication stations in their finals OSCE. Commonly the instructions prior to entering the communication stations will be very brief, allowing consultation for the full time of the station. This can be both an advantage and a disadvantage, as you need to be very organised to structure your discussion to fill the time and cover the most important areas.
- It is crucial to have a general structure on how to approach any station. There are a number of structures that ensure you are able to obtain and give all the necessary information about any topic and allow for a two-way discussion. Prior to entering the examining room decide which structure you are going to use. For example, when asked to explain a procedure, discuss a new treatment or counsel a patient, always start by gaining permission to discuss the topic with your patient: 'I am here to talk to you about X, would it be OK?' This is usually followed by, 'What do you know about X?' By asking this question, you gain the patient's understanding, perceptions, and concerns about the topic. This often provides the narrative you should use to elaborate on. Always ensure you pause regularly and check the patient's understanding and give time for questions. You have to address all of their concerns and answer all their questions by the end of the station. It is good practice to start winding down in the last minute of the station, recap all of the important points, and allow for final questions.
- Remember you cannot know everything and it is important to admit it. It is appropriate to say that you do not know but you would *check with your senior* and tell the patient later. By doing this, you show that you understand your limitations and that you will be a safe practitioner.
- It may happen that the station instructions ask you to discuss a topic you have absolutely no knowledge about. Do not panic! In such situations, remember that following a script could get you out of trouble. Allow the patient to tell you what they know about the topic, which may trigger some of your knowledge. Be honest and acknowledge that this is a topic you do

not know a great deal about but state that you will find out. Also, if you find yourself totally lost and have no more to talk about, remember to consider the patient's ideas, concerns, and expectations (ICE). One tip would be to discuss the patient's social support – do they have a partner, family or friends who they could talk to or get help from? Would they benefit from counselling, group sessions or further information from the Internet or leaflets? Do they have a general practitioner (GP) with whom they would feel comfortable discussing this further? This not only keeps the conversation going but it shows that you understand that difficult life situations and decisions require support from those who are closest to the patient.

- Sometimes you may encounter a difficult conversation station such as an angry patient or relative, or having to break bad news. Many students feel that they have to show knowledge of the topic to score all the points but often the main point is to be empathetic, respond to the patients' concerns, allow them to express their feelings and emotions, and remember that the use of silence in difficult conversations can be exactly what the patient needs.
- Practice breaking bad news with your friends and colleagues before your OSCE. It is often uncomfortable to be silent through a stressful or a sad discussion but it is important to use silence at the right moment. The more you practice, the easier it becomes.

HISTORY TAKING STATIONS

- Practice history taking stations with your friends and colleagues.
- You may be asked to take a full history, focused history or medical history. Whatever it is called, you should ensure that you always take a full history including past medical, drug, family, and social history.
- Before you start your station, be clear on how long you have to obtain the medical history. Sometimes you may only have 4 minutes out of an 8-minute station but this should be clearly stated in the station instructions. Pace yourself and do not forget to ask about drugs, allergies, smoking, alcohol intake, and social situation before you run out of time. You will lose valuable marks on relatively simple questions, which can be rehearsed and used in every history taking station.
- As a rule of thumb, in every adult history taking station, always ask the 'B questions' of cancer screening: 'Have you noticed any unexpected weight loss, if so how much and over how long? Have you had any fevers or night sweats?' You will never fail to score on these points if you make these questions a habit.
- If you run out of steam when asking about history of the presenting complaint, skip to the other sections of the history taking – drugs, allergies, family, and social history – and then return back to history of the presenting complaint. By doing this, you score all the important points for other sections and give yourself some time to think about other aspects of the presenting complaint.

EXAMINATION STATIONS

- Practice examination stations with your friends and colleagues.
- Always gain an informed consent from your patient.
- Never hurt your patient during a physical examination. It is important to ask about pain before your examination. Always check with the patient if you are causing them discomfort during the examination and warn the patient if you have cold hands before you touch them!

- Read your instructions clearly to understand which part of the body you are supposed to examine. If it says to examine the cardiovascular system, than start at the bottom of the bed with general inspection, moving onto the hands, face, neck, etc. If it says to examine the precordium, then you are only being asked to concentrate on the chest. If in doubt, always ask the examiner to clarify the instructions for you.
- Be systematic! You need to develop a sequence by which you can examine any body system. The general rule is to OBSERVE, PERCUSS/PALPATE, AUSCULTATE/MOVE. You can examine somebody's shoulder by following the sequence of observe, palpate, and move even if you cannot remember precisely how to do it.
- Students are never sure whether to narrate during the examination or not. Some medical schools have specific rules about this and you should follow them. A rule of thumb is to narrate only those parts of the examination that are not obvious to the examiner. For example, when you are inspecting the hands during an abdominal examination, you should comment on nicotine tar staining, clubbing, palmar erythema, etc. If you did not narrate this part and the examiner had a separate point for each of these findings on their scoring sheet, it would be difficult to award you all the points. On the other hand, if you were auscultating the heart, the examiner can see the areas that you are auscultating and you would not need to state this. However, you would need to state your findings with regard to heart sounds.

- Avoid saying, 'I am looking for...' because this does not inform the examiner whether you found it or not. You should always say, 'There is no pitting oedema of the legs' rather than, 'I am looking for leg oedema.'

- Practice summarising your examination findings in three succinct sentences. You do not need to state everything. Unless you found any peripheral signs of a disease, it is perfectly acceptable to say that there were no peripheral signs of disease. You have to mention all your positive findings. For example: 'I performed a full cardiovascular examination on Mr X, a 35-year-old male who had no peripheral signs of cardiovascular disease. His blood pressure was 135/70 mmHg with a regular pulse of 70 bpm, heart sounds one and two were audible with no additional sounds, and his lung bases were clear. I would conclude this to be a normal cardiovascular examination.'
- Practice using instruments. It is easy to spot a student who has never held a patellar hammer or ophthalmoscope in their hand. When practicing for your OSCE, make sure you have all the required equipment and you practice using it.
- Use alcohol gel when practicing examination stations with your colleagues. It is an easy point on the mark scheme to gain and many students forget to use it because of stress. Use it in your practice time to ensure it becomes second nature. You should gel your hands before examining your patient and again after, just before leaving the room.
- If you find something abnormal during your OSCE examination and you cannot remember what it is, what it is called or what sign of disease it represents, describe it to the examiner in your own words and say that you recognise this as abnormal but you cannot remember what it signifies. Also offer to seek advice from senior colleagues; this will demonstrate that you are safe, and there are usually OSCE points for stating this.
- Do not forget to look around the bedside. Some patients may have a walking stick, inhaler, glyceryl trinitrate (GTN) spray, glasses or hearing aids on the table. These are there to give you a hint; take it!

- Often, if there is something on the patent's table in the OSCE station, it is there to be used. If you were asked to examine the thyroid gland, make sure you use the glass of water on their table to assess swallowing. If you were to examine someone's hands, make sure you use the 50p coin on the table to observe grip and dexterity.
- Always thank the patient afterwards. In many stations the examiner will ask for the opinion of the actor with regard to how you treated them and your general demeanour. Patient opinion does not usually attract marks but will add to the overall impression of the examiner. Often patients are volunteering their services, especially if they are real patients, and although you are only doing the station once they will be repeating it with nervous students multiple times. A kind word and a smile will go a long way.

IMAGING, BLOOD RESULTS, AND OTHER TEST RESULTS IN OSCE

- You will encounter imaging and test results in many stations of your finals OSCE.
- They are often incorporated into the station but can be the main focus of the station as well. You may be asked to take a history from the patient, be asked what investigation you would want to do, and then be presented with the results of these to interpret.
- If you are asked to take a medical history or examine the patient, you should have a good grasp of the presenting problems or signs and therefore be able to interpret the test results. You should be almost able to predict what the blood results or CXR would show even before you see it.
- Be systematic when approaching test interpretation and take into account any medical history or examination findings.
- Remember that test results can be normal! Do not be scared to say that a CXR is normal if that is what you think.
- At the end of a medical history or examination you may be asked what investigations you would like to do. Always start with the easiest/noninvasive investigations first and build it up. First, you should mention bedside tests – general observations, bloods (FBC, U&Es, CRP, LFTs, TFTs, ESR, amylase, group and save, cross-match, Ca^{2+}, Mg^{2+}, PO_4^{3-}, and glucose). Often not all of those are required; be guided by your differential diagnosis. Also consider blood cultures, urine dip/MSU, capillary blood glucose, ECG, arterial/venous blood gas, wound swab, etc. Then move onto imaging tests, starting with the least invasive appropriate test first (e.g. US, CXR, AXR). Then, if appropriate, add more complex diagnostic tests at the end if indicated (CT, MRI, diagnostic laparoscopy, etc.).
- It is important to emphasise that listing these key and baseline tests is essential to pick up easy marks in the exam. Do not assume the examiner knows which tests you would request; you need to specifically go through the lists of investigations and mention them to the examiner.
- Many OSCEs will have imaging incorporated into the stations. This will most likely be displayed on a computer screen, anonymised, and with an obvious pathology. You may only have a minute or two to comment on the imaging results during the station so have a clear system of reporting CXR, AXR, CT, and MRI. Do not forget to state that you would check that the image is from the correct patient and is the most recent. Then continue describing the abnormality on the film and correlate it with the history and examination.

- Imaging in the exam is covered in detail throughout the book and may occur in the OSCE or the written papers. Imaging pathology will be clearly apparent and the image is usually nonadjustable on the computer screen. Having a clear method and approach to image presentation is essential and will reassure the examiner that you have seen/presented imaging many times in the past.

FINAL WORDS

- Practice ... practice ... practice: be systematic, practice more, and remember to be seen to wash your hands as needed. Do not panic because by the time you undergo your OSCE exams you should have a system to tackle any problem, practice again, smile, and be kind to your patients.
- Do not rely on books only to prepare for OSCE. You must get involved in regular group revision.
- Eat healthily, keep hydrated, exercise, and get some quality sleep during your revision period.
- Allow yourself some downtime to relax. Watch some television, visit friends, play your favourite sport, go for walks or anything else you used to do before you started this revision. Do not allow it to completely take over your life but at the same time make it your priority.
- Remember, there is light at the end of the tunnel and the skills you are learning now are genuinely useful for the future.
- Most people pass!

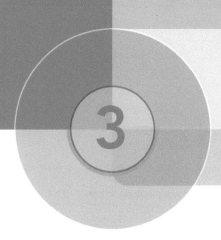

The normal chest X-ray

THOMAS KURKA

The CXR is the most common radiological investigation performed. Interpretation can be difficult and often falls initially to those with relatively limited experience. It is important to have a systematic approach to interpretation to ensure that the correct diagnosis is made and nothing is missed. This will help both in the examination situation and in real life.

This chapter provides a step-by-step approach to reviewing the CXR. It provides a comprehensive problem-solving technique, which encourages a set format involving an introduction, a detailed assessment of the key abnormality, and a systematic review of the rest of the film. It is this systematic review that students have most difficulty with and we provide two different techniques for dealing with it. We then illustrate these techniques with example cases.

INDICATIONS FOR REQUESTING A CXR

Even though a CXR may not be the diagnostic investigation of choice for pulmonary embolism (PE), lung cancer or heart failure, for example, it can provide some very useful information and as such is frequently used as the first-line investigation when cardiorespiratory patients present to the hospital. Additionally, the radiation dose of a CXR is low (0.015 mSv) – around 440 times less than a chest CT scan– making it the least invasive investigation of choice. A summary of the main indications for CXR is shown in *Table 3.1*.

MEDICAL IONISING RADIATION EXPOSURE

X-rays and gamma rays damage DNA. Some of this damage is predictable and dose dependent. There are dose-related and predictable effects, such as radiation sickness and alopecia, which occur at set doses of radiation. Other effects, such as the development of cancer, are not dose dependent and a safe level of radiation cannot be predicted. The chance of these events occurring increases with dose but does not have a known safe threshold.

Table 3.1 Common indications for requesting a CXR

	Diagnoses	Symptoms
Respiratory	Malignancy (primary or secondary)	Haemoptysis
	Infection – pneumonia, TB	Dyspnoea
	Pulmonary embolism	Chest pain
	Pleural effusion	Productive cough
	Inhaled foreign body	Severe abdominal pain
	Chest trauma	
	Pneumothorax	
	Acute exacerbation of asthma	
	Acute exacerbation of COPD	
Cardiac	Heart failure	
	Heart murmurs	
Surgical	Pneumoperitoneum	
Other	NG tube position	
	Central venous catheter position	

The lifetime risk of developing cancer is influenced by the dose and cumulative exposure to radiation. According to the Royal College of Radiologists, exposures of less than 1 mSv (equivalent to 70 CXR or 6 months of background radiation) confer a cancer development risk of less than 1:20,000. This rises to about 1:4,000 for 5 mSv and 1:2,000 for 10 mSv exposures. The risk ratio, however, is heavily influenced by age and sex, with infants and females at the greatest risk. The risk of a medical exposure, however, should always be put into the context of the population cancer risk (currently 1 in 3 in the UK) and be balanced against the investigation benefits.

Each of us is exposed daily to background radiation from the earth and space. The background radiation in the UK is around 2.2 mSv per year with a regional variation of as much as 1.5–7.5 mSv per year depending largely on rock type (notably granite in the Aberdeen area and the rocks of Cornwall). In addition, we expose ourselves to further radiation during air flight. A return flight from London, UK to New York, USA adds approximately 0.1 mSv radiation exposure, which is equivalent to seven CXRs.

ALARA (as low as reasonably achievable) is an American safety principle and regulatory requirement, which sets standards for a reasonable level of radiation exposure. The main principles are time (minimising the time of direct exposure), distance (double the distance, quarter the dose), and shielding (using absorbent materials to reduce radiation exposure). *Table 3.2* illustrates the associated radiation dose of some common imaging tests with the equivalent dose in CXR or background radiation.

CXR REPORTING TECHNIQUE

Much of this section refers to real-life CXR review and most is also applicable to the exam scenario. Remember X-rays in the exam will appear on a computer screen or an examination question sheet – they will be anonymised and pathology should be obvious. Image manipulation on the screen is not usually allowed or needed.

Table 3.2 Radiation doses for the main imaging modalities

Modality	DOSE (mSv)	Equivalent in CXRs	Equivalent period of background radiation
CXR	0.015	1	2.5 days
AXR	0.4	30	2 months
XR pelvis	0.3	20	1.5 months
XR skull	0.07	5	12 days
XR hip	0.8	60	4 months
XR hand/foot	<0.001	<1	<2 days
XR cervical spine	0.05	3	7.5 days
XR thoracic spine	0.4	30	2 months
XR lumbar spine	0.6	40	3 months
CT head	1.4	90	7.5 months
CT chest	6.6	440	3 years
CT abdomen	5.6	370	2.5 years
CT abdomen/pelvis	6.7	450	3 years
CT chest/abdomen/pelvis	10	670	4.5 years
CT KUB	5.5	370	2.5 years
CT colonography	10	670	4.5 years
Barium swallow	1.5	100	8 months
Barium meal	2.0	130	11 months
Barium enema	2.2	150	1 year
Bone (Tc-99m) scan	3.0	200	1.4 years
DEXA scan	0.0004	<1	<2 days
Mammogram	0.5	35	3 months
PET scan	18	1200	8.1 years

LEARNING POINTS: REPORTING TECHNIQUE

- Introduction:
  - 'PPP' (projection, personal demographics, previous CXR comparison).
  - Technical factors: 'RIP' (rotation/inspiration/penetration).
- Describe the obvious abnormality: what and where.
- Systematic review: ABCDE (*Table 3.4*) or anatomical approach.

First, you need to *introduce* the CXR by checking the projection of the image and mentioning any available personal demographic information (i.e. 'This is a PA CXR of an adult female.'). It is really important to check you are reviewing the correct CXR for the correct patient, and from the correct date and time. In the exam you will not be able to do this as the XR should be anonymised but mention to the examiner that you would wish to do this as part of your usual practice. Then consider its technical quality (i.e. 'There is no rotation, and inspiration and penetration are adequate.'). This ensures that any visible abnormality is likely to be related to pathology rather than an artefact of the film. Exam XRs should not have any technical issues.

Second, *describe* any obvious abnormality in terms of what and where.

Third, a *systematic review* of the entire CXR is required to make sure that you have not missed anything. Two different approaches to this (ABCDE or anatomical) are discussed below. Finally, summarise your findings, give a diagnosis or differential diagnosis, and recommend further management.

These three stages of reporting will now be discussed in greater detail.

INTRODUCTION

A number of factors should be considered for PPP.

PPP

Projection

- Pay attention to letters PA (posteroanterior) or AP (anteroposterior) on the CXR and also the words *erect* or *supine* (**Figure 3.1**).
- A standard CXR is taken in a PA, erect position (i.e. the patient is standing up with shoulders internally rotated, hands on hips, which moves the scapulae laterally so they are less visible on the film). If it is not labelled, this is the default position.
- AP films are taken for patients that are difficult to mobilise and/or very unwell and may be labelled *portable* where the patient is sat up in bed with the film cassette tucked behind them.
- AP films have more of the scapulae projected over the chest. They also have a more prominent cardiac silhouette, which can be misinterpreted as cardiomegaly. Only assess heart size on a PA projection (**Figure 3.1**).

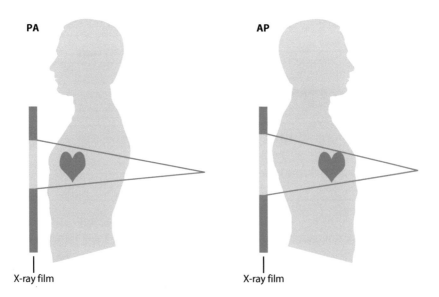

Fig. 3.1 The size of the heart on the PA and AP CXR. Note on PA projection that the heart is closer to the X-ray film and thus less magnified by the divergent beam than on the AP view.

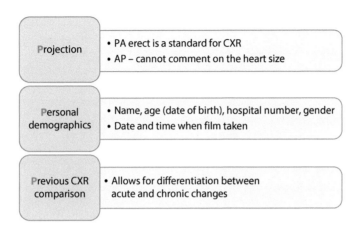

Projection	• PA erect is a standard for CXR • AP – cannot comment on the heart size
Personal demographics	• Name, age (date of birth), hospital number, gender • Date and time when film taken
Previous CXR comparison	• Allows for differentiation between acute and chronic changes

Fig. 3.2 PPP (projection/personal demographics/previous CXR comparison).

- Other projections are available (i.e. lateral, lordotic, apical, rotated, and oblique) but they have been almost entirely replaced by the use of CT. You will not see these projections in medical school exams.

Personal demographics (Figure 3.2)

- Always ensure you present the full name, date of birth (age), and hospital number of the patient (more applicable to ward rounds, rather than the exam).
- The CXR will be anonymised in the exam but you should offer to check the personal demographics at this stage. You may be able to tell if they are adult or paediatric by the presence of growth plates, also male or female by the breast shadows.
- If there is a date and time on the image remember to mention it.

Previous CXR comparison

- Offer to compare the current CXR with any previous films available. This helps to differentiate between acute and chronic changes.
- It is also important to check you are reviewing the correct CXR for the correct patient from the correct date and time.

RIP

Rotation

- To assess for rotation, find the medial heads of the clavicles and compare their distances away from the spinous process of the adjacent vertebral body (**Figures 3.3** and **3.4**).
- If the spinous process of the vertebral body is equidistant between both clavicle heads then there is no rotation.
- If the gap is less on the right then the patient is rotated to the right, and vice versa.

Inspiration

- Patients are asked to breathe in and hold their breath when a CXR is taken so that the lungs are optimally visualised.
- Poor inspiratory effort may be caused by pain, confusion or respiratory distress.

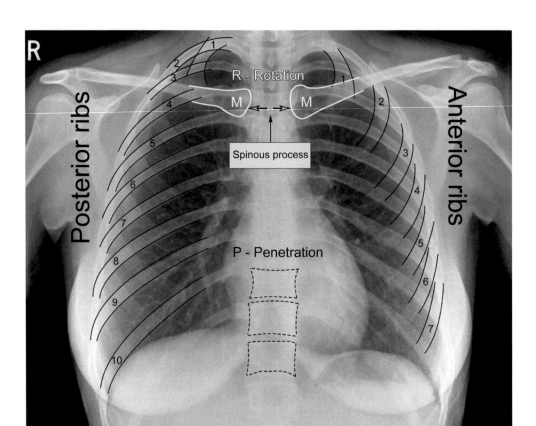

R

Posterior ribs

Anterior ribs

1
2
3
4
5
6
7
8
9
10

R - Rotation

M ←→ M

Spinous process

P - Penetration

1
2
3
4
5
6
7

Fig. 3.3 Assessing the technical quality of CXR (M = medial clavicle).

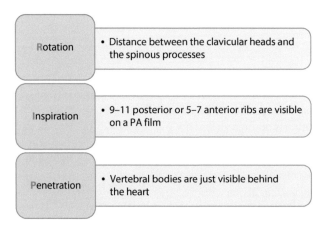

Rotation	• Distance between the clavicular heads and the spinous processes
Inspiration	• 9–11 posterior or 5–7 anterior ribs are visible on a PA film
Penetration	• Vertebral bodies are just visible behind the heart

Fig. 3.4 Technical factors: RIP (rotation/inspiration/penetration).

- Hyperexpanded lungs may be seen in COPD patients with obstructive airway disease. The diaphragms will appear flattened.
- Inspiratory effort is described as adequate when 9–11 posterior or 5–7 anterior ribs are seen.

Penetration

- The vertebral bodies should just be visible behind the heart for adequate penetration.
- If the CXR is either over- or underpenetrated, then you will not be able to fully assess all the structures and compare their densities accurately.
- An underpenetrated XR appears overly opaque/dense/white.
- An overpenetrated XR appears too lucent/dark/black.

DESCRIBE THE OBVIOUS ABNORMALITY: WHAT AND WHERE

Sit back and look over the whole CXR to spot any obvious abnormality. If you see something abnormal, describe this in terms of *what and where* before proceeding with the systematic review. Practice using the correct terminology to describe the common pathologies as outlined below.

WHAT

- *Shape:* describe the shape of the abnormality (round, diffuse, well/poorly demarcated).
- *Size:* describe size of lesion.
- *Density:* say if it is hypo- (dark) or hyperdense (bright) compared with the surrounding soft tissues, also if it is homogeneous (same density throughout) or heterogeneous (various densities). Cavitating lesions have a soft tissue rim with a hypodense core and may contain an air/fluid level. Is there calcium or fat density associated?
- *Associated factors:* presence of lung oedema, fluid level or air bronchogram. For pleural effusions, describe which side is affected, comment on the presence of a meniscus and how high the fluid level extends.

WHERE

- *Site:* say which lung is affected.
- *Site:* describe whether it is in the upper, middle or lower *zone* of the lung. This is much easier than trying to assess which *lobe* is involved, this may be difficult to evaluate on the frontal XR.

Common descriptions include:

- *Pneumonia:* mostly unilateral, patchy, soft tissue consolidation. Look for air bronchograms.
- *Pulmonary oedema:* mostly bilateral, patchy, soft tissue consolidation with associated cardiomegaly and pleural effusions (*Table 3.3*).
- *Pleural effusion:* mostly unilateral, homogeneous, soft tissue opacification. Blunting of costo- and cardiophrenic angles with a meniscus at the air–fluid level.
- *Pneumothora:* loss of lung markings in the lateral aspect of the thorax with a visible pleural line.
- *Tension pneumothorax:* as above with mediastinal and/or tracheal shift away from the pneumothorax and flattening of the ipsilateral hemidiaphragm.
- *Lobar collapse:* mediastinal and/or tracheal shift towards the collapse, raised ipsilateral diaphragm, displaced hilum, and rib space narrowing.

Table 3.3 ABCDEF of pulmonary oedema

A	Alveolar and interstitial shadowing
B	Kerley B lines
C	Cardiomegaly
D	Upper lobe Diversion
E	Effusion
F	Fluid in the horizontal fissure

SYSTEMATIC REVIEW: ABCDE OR ANATOMICAL APPROACH

There are two different systematic approaches to reviewing the CXR. One follows the familiar ABCDE approach to assessing the acutely unwell patient (*Table 3.4* and **Figure 3.5**). The second approach is used primarily by radiologists and follows the anatomical landmarks of the film. These are just two examples of how to do it and in time you will establish your own approach. Make sure before you start your systematic review that you have considered the nature of the film and its technical qualities, as described above.

ABCDE APPROACH

Airway

- *Trachea* should be central. Deviation to the right may be related to ipsilateral lung volume loss (lung or lobar collapse) or contralateral volume expansion (pneumothorax, haemothorax, pleural effusion or large lung mass). It may also be deviated by a mediastinal mass (thyroid goitre).
- *Free gas* in the soft tissues (surgical emphysema) secondary to penetrating trauma or severe asthma.
- *Neck masses,* such as an enlarged thyroid goitre or calcified vascular calcification (subclavian aneurysm), may be visible.

Breathing

- *Lung apices* should be compared. They should be symmetrical and have a similar density – take care here as pathology in the apices can easily be missed!
- *Upper, middle, and lower zones.* Follow the lateral borders down to the bases and then up towards the hila. Compare both sides (**Figure 3.5**).
- *Pneumothorax.* Close inspection of the lateral borders of each lung for a visible pleural line and rim of absent lung markings. If you are shown a pneumothorax in the exam it will usually be large and clearly demonstrated – small, subtle lesions will not be used.

Table 3.4 ABCDE of CXR

A	Airway
B	Breathing
C	Circulation
D	Diaphragm
E	'Everything else'

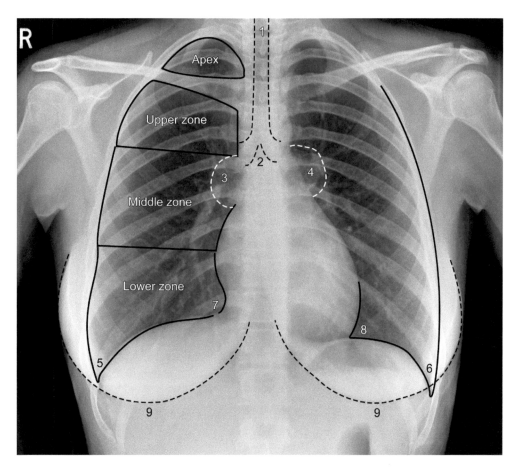

Fig. 3.5 Airway and breathing structures on CXR. Trachea (1), carina (2), right hilum (3), left hilum (4), right costophrenic angle (5), left costophrenic angle (6), right cardiophrenic angle (7), left cardiophrenic angle (8). Note bilateral, normal, symmetrical breast outlines (9).

- *Pleural angles.* The costophrenic and cardiophrenic angles are checked for blunting and increased density, as seen with consolidation (pneumonia), pleural effusion or chronic pleural thickening.
- *Hilar position, shape, and density.* The left should sit at the same level or slightly higher than the right. The hila are made up of pulmonary arteries, veins, bronchi, and lymph nodes. They should be equal in size, shape, and density. A displaced hilum may suggest lung volume loss. A dense or enlarged hilum may be caused by lymphadenopathy (due to infection, malignancy or sarcoidosis) or pulmonary hypertension (due to COPD or heart disease).
- *Nodules and masses* may be dense and well defined (calcified) or soft tissue density and poorly defined: the latter are more concerning for malignancy. They may be single or multiple. Remember to check behind the heart for a subtle mass in the left lower lobe and also to assess the basal segments of the lower lobes through the upper abdomen/diaphragm.
- *Fissures.* Check the normal appearance and position of the fissures, as these will be distorted in lobar collapse.

Circulation

- *Heart size* (if it is a PA film). If you compare the width of the heart with that of the thorax, the cardiothoracic ratio should be less than 50% in adults (**Figure 3.6**). Cardiomegaly may be caused by heart failure.
- *Mediastinal shift.* If the heart no longer appears in the centre of the thorax the film may be rotated, there may be volume loss pulling structures towards the pathology (lung or lobar collapse) or volume increase pushing structures away from the pathology (tension pneumothorax, haemothorax or large mass).
- *Aortic arch (AA).* This should be on the left. If small, there could be an atrial septal defect. If enlarged, there may be hypertension, aortic stenosis or aortic dissection.
- *Left heart border (LHB).* The left atrium (LA) or left atrial appendage may be enlarged in mitral valve disease (now rarely seen as rheumatic heart disease is less prevalent).

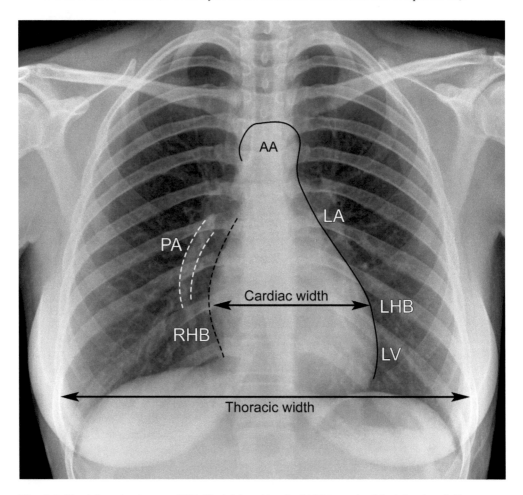

Fig. 3.6 Circulation structures on CXR. The left heart border (LHB) is made of the left atrium (LA) superiorly and left ventricle (LV). The right heart border (RHB) is made up of the right atrium (dotted line) only, as the right ventricle lies posteriorly. Aortic arch (AA), descending right pulmonary artery (PA). The CTR (cardiothoracic ratio) is the greatest cardiac width ÷ the intrathoracic width at its widest point (inner rib → inner rib), <50% in adults.

The left ventricle (LV) may be enlarged in volume overload due to aortic or mitral regurgitation, ischaemia or cardiomyopathy causing primary left ventricular disease, or pericardial effusion. If the LA enlarges (e.g. mitral stenosis) this may widen the carina (LA sits in the subcarinal region) and extend across to the right heart border (RHB) causing an apparent 'double' heart border.

- *RHB*. The right atrium (RA) may be enlarged in tricuspid regurgitation.
- *Pericardium*. Gas shadows around the cardiac silhouette into the mediastinum may indicate pneumomediastinum.

Diaphragm

- *Position*. The right hemidiaphragm should be slightly higher than the left due to the mass effect of the liver. There should be curvature in both.
- *Pneumoperitoneum* is characterised by free subdiaphragmatic gas on an erect CXR. This is usually caused by bowel perforation and would warrant urgent surgical review.

'Everything else'

- *Lines and tubes* must all be commented upon. State whether they are adequately positioned or need replacing [i.e. nasogastric (NG) tube, endotracheal (ET) tube, central venous line, and pleural drain].
- *Cardiac device*. If present, describe its position, how many leads leave the device and where they terminate, and is there lead fracture?
- *Bone fractures*. Check the clavicles and ribs. Make sure the acromioclavicular and glenohumeral joints of the shoulders are intact. Look for rib metastases.
- *Breast contours* in female patients. Note any asymmetry or evidence of previous mastectomy. There may be surgical clips.

THE RADIOLOGIST'S ANATOMICAL APPROACH

This alternative method is preferred by radiologists as it follows the usual format of a written report. The detail of what to look for under each section is the same as above.

Like the ABCDE approach, it is always preceded by a note on the projection, patient demographics, and previous films for comparison (PPP). The technical quality is also checked in terms of rotation, inspiration, and penetration (RIP). The radiologist will usually also check the lines and tubes, and review the breast shadows at the outset.

Having described any immediately obvious abnormality, the following systematic review is conducted.

Heart

- Heart size and contour.
- Mediastinal and hilar size and contour.

Lungs

- Lungs apices, upper, middle, and lower zones.

Bones

- All visible bones are checked for fractures and focal lesions.

Review areas (where abnormalities are most likely to be missed)

- Peripheral soft tissues (soft tissue mass or injury).
- Behind the heart (left lower lobe collapse or a lung nodule).
- Costophrenic angles (lung nodule, consolidation, effusion).
- Below and behind the diaphragm (lower lobe lung nodules and subdiaphragmatic gas).

SUMMARY OF REPORTING TECHNIQUE – HOW TO PRESENT IN THE EXAMS AND IN REAL LIFE

- Your summary should be succinct and straight to the point (2–3 sentences only). This is of particular importance in the exam where time is tight.
- Summarise all positive findings and correlate these with the history and examination findings.
- Offer a differential diagnosis and a sentence about further management. This might be a recommendation for a further investigation or for urgent senior medical or surgical input.

EXAMPLE OSCE STATIONS WITH CXR INTERPRETATION

CASE 1

A 45-year-old female attends the emergency department (ED) with difficulty breathing and sharp pleuritic chest pain. She has a past medical history of anxiety, depression, and hypertension. She is a nonsmoker. Her respiratory rate is 26 bpm, oxygen saturation is 98% on air and she is tachycardic at 100 bpm. A CXR is taken and you are asked to review it systematically (**Figure 3.7**).

Introduction (PPP RIP)

- *Projection.* PA erect chest radiograph (by default, as the image is not labelled).
- *Personal demographics.* Offer to check patient's details as the film is anonymised.
- *Previous films for comparison.* Ask if there are previous CXRs available for comparison.
- *Technical quality (RIP).* The film is not rotated. There is adequate inspiratory effort and penetration.

Describe the abnormality

- This is not immediately obvious so follow your systematic approach.

Systematic review

- *Airway.* The trachea is central. No evidence of free air in the soft tissue of the neck.
- *Breathing:*
  - *Right side.* The apex is clear, the lateral thoracic border has no abnormality, the costophrenic and cardiophrenic angles are visible, and the hilum is of normal size and is positioned slightly lower than the left.
  - *Left side.* The apex is clear, the lateral thoracic border has no abnormality, the costophrenic and cardiophrenic angles are visible, and the hilum is of normal size and is positioned slightly higher than the right.
- *Circulation.* The heart size is normal, the AA is visible, the left and right heart borders are normal, and there is no mediastinal shift.

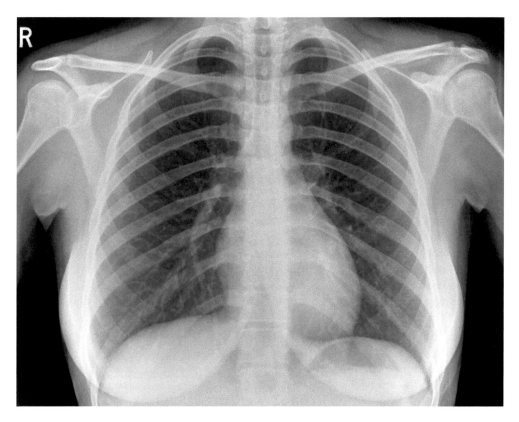

Fig. 3.7 Case 1: CXR, patient in the ED.

- *Diaphragm.* The hemidiaphragms are dome shaped, with the right slightly higher than the left. There is no visible free gas under the diaphragm. The normal gastric bubble is seen on the left.
- *'Everything else'.* There are no lines or tubes projected on the film. The breast contours are present and symmetrical, and there is no evidence of previous surgery. There are no visible fractures or bone lesions.

Summary

- This is a chest radiograph of a 45-year-old female who presents with dyspnoea and sharp chest pain. The CXR is normal with no pathology identified. Additional investigations would be advised to establish the nature of her presenting symptoms.

ALTERNATIVE 'RADIOLOGIST-REVIEW' APPROACH (WARD ROUND EXAMPLE WITH AVAILABLE PATIENT DEMOGRAPHICS)

- *Type of film and projection:*
  'This is a PA chest radiograph of ...'
- *Name:*
  'Mrs Jane Smith ...'

- *Hospital number:*
  'Hospital number 123456789 ...'
- *Date of birth:*
  'Date of birth 22nd February 19XX ...'
- *Date:*
  'Taken on 12th January 20XX ...'
- *Technical quality:*
  'It is not rotated, and there is satisfactory inspiratory effort and penetration...'
- *Lines, tubes, breast shadows:*
  'There are no visible lines or tubes, and the breast shadows are symmetrical...'
- *Check old films:*
  'I would like to compare this image with any previous images to identify any changes and to review previous history ...'
- *Heart, then lungs, then bones:*
  'The heart is normal in size, both the left and right heart borders are normal, and both hila are normal with the right hilum sitting slightly lower than the left. Both right and left lung apices, upper, middle and lower zones are clear. There are no visible bone fractures or focal bone lesions ...'
- *Review areas:*
  'The peripheral soft tissues appear normal, both right and left costophrenic and cardiophrenic angles are fully visible and clear, there is no evidence of left lower lobe collapse or mass behind the heart. Both hemidiaphragms are dome shaped with the right slightly higher than the left. No free subdiaphragmatic gas ...'
- *Summary:*
  'In summary, this is a normal chest film with no gross pathology. If pulmonary embolus is suspected urgent CT pulmonary angiogram would be recommended.'

CASE 2

A 64-year-old male was referred to the respiratory department with a 1-year history of progressive dyspnoea and unintentional weight loss of 12 kg. He has no past medical history but is a smoker with 35 pack-years. His respiratory rate is 16 bpm, oxygen saturation 98% on air, heart rate 85 bpm, and BP 135/78 mmHg. A CXR is performed and you are asked to interpret it systematically (**Figure 3.8**).

Introduction (PPP RIP)

- *Projection.* PA erect chest radiograph (by default as the image is not labelled).
- *Personal demographics.* Offer to check patient's details as the film is anonymised.
- *Previous films for comparison.* Ask if there are previous CXRs available for comparison.
- *Technical quality (RIP).* The patient is mildly rotated. There is adequate inspiratory effort and penetration.

Describe the abnormality

- *Where.* There is a rounded lesion in the left lung located in the upper zone, projected partially over the clavicle.

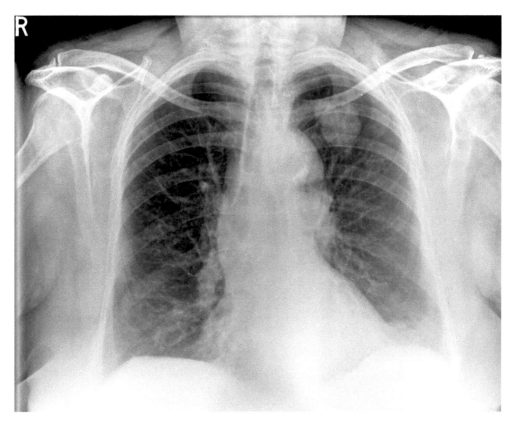

Fig. 3.8 Case 2: CXR, patient in the respiratory department.

- *What.* The lesion is round and well demarcated. It is soft tissue density, homogeneous and noncavitating. There is no consolidation around the lesion and no other lesions are visible. There is no calcification within the lesion.

Systematic review

- *Airway.* The distal trachea is not significantly deviated allowing for patient rotation.
- *Breathing:*
  - *Right side.* The apex is clear, the lateral border has no abnormality, the costophrenic and cardiophrenic angles are visible, the hilum is of normal size and is positioned slightly lower than the left.
  - *Left side.* The apex is clear, the lateral border has no abnormality, the costophrenic and cardiophrenic angles are visible, the hilum is of normal size and is positioned slightly higher than the right. The left upper zone mass is the only lung abnormality.
- *Circulation.* The heart size is normal, the AA is visible and normal, the left and right heart borders are normal, and there is no mediastinal shift.
- *Diaphragm.* The hemidiaphragms are dome shaped, with the right slightly higher than the left. There is no visible free gas under the diaphragm. The normal gastric bubble is seen on the left.
- *'Everything-else'.* There are no lines or tubes projected on the film. There is no evidence of previous surgery. There are no visible fractures or bone lesions.

Summary

- This is a chest radiograph of a 64-year-old male who presented with dyspnoea and unintentional weight loss for over 1 year. There is a soft tissue, rounded, and well-demarcated mass in the left upper zone with no associated consolidation. The appearance is suspicious for lung malignancy. Further investigation with CT of the chest and abdomen is recommended along with urgent thoracic multidisciplinary team (MDT) review.

ALTERNATIVE 'RADIOLOGIST-REVIEW' APPROACH

- *Type of film and projection:*
  'This is a PA chest radiograph of ...'

- *Name:*
  'Mr John Smith...'

- *Hospital number:*
  'Hospital number 123456789 ...'

- *Date of birth:*
  'Date of birth 22nd February 19XX ...'

- *Date:*
  'Taken on 12th January 20XX ...'

- *Technical quality:*
  'It is not rotated, and there is satisfactory inspiratory effort and penetration...'

- *Lines, tubes, breast shadows:*
  'There are no visible lines or tubes ...'

- *Check old films:*
  'I would like to compare this image with any previous images to identify any changes and to review previous history ...'

- *Heart, lungs, bones:*
  'The heart is of normal size, both the left and right heart borders are normal, and both hila are normal. There is a solitary round, well-demarcated, soft tissue, homogeneous lesion in the left upper zone. It is partially projected over the left clavicle. There is no visible cavitation. The right upper zone is clear, both right and left lung apices, middle and lower zones are clear. There are no visible bone fractures or focal bone lesions.'

- *Review areas:*
  'The peripheral soft tissues appear normal, both right and left costophrenic and cardiophrenic angles are fully visible and clear, there is no evidence of left lower lobe collapse or mass behind the heart. Both hemidiaphragms are dome shaped with the right slightly higher than the left. No free subdiaphragmatic gas ...'

- *Summary:*
  'In summary, there is a round, well-demarcated, noncavitating, homogeneous lesion in the left upper zone, lung malignancy to be excluded. Further investigation with CT of the chest and abdomen is recommended along with urgent MDT review. '

CASE 3

An 84-year-old female presented to the ED with sudden-onset right-sided chest pain and dyspnoea. She has a past medical history of asthma, for which she uses only a salbutamol inhaler, and bilateral shoulder surgery joint replacement for rheumatoid arthritis. Her respiratory rate is 26 bpm, oxygen saturation 85% on air, heart rate 112 bpm, and blood pressure 135/78 mmHg. As part of her work-up, a CXR is taken and you are asked to interpret it systematically (**Figure 3.9**).

Introduction (PPP RIP)

- *Projection.* PA erect chest radiograph (by default as the image is not labelled).
- *Personal demographics.* Offer to check patient's details as the film is anonymised.
- *Previous films for comparison.* Ask if there are previous CXRs available for comparison.
- *Technical quality (RIP).* The patient is rotated. There is adequate inspiratory effort and penetration.

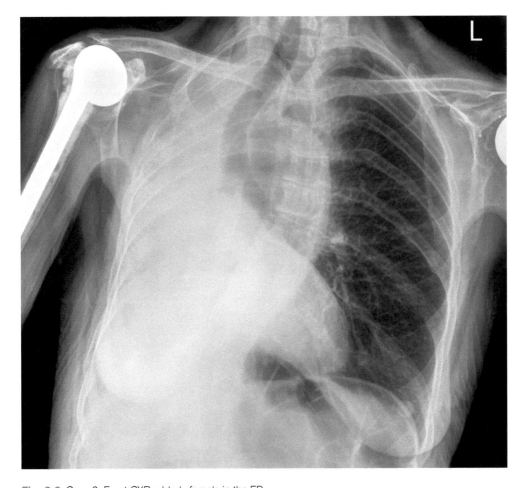

Fig. 3.9 Case 3: Erect CXR, elderly female in the ED.

Describe the abnormality

- *What and where.* The patient is markedly rotated with a pronounced thoracic scoliosis concave to the right. There is tracheal and mediastinal shift to the right, associated with complete opacification (homogeneous soft tissue shadowing /'whiteout') of the right hemi-thorax. Also on the right there is rib space narrowing in keeping with volume loss.

Systematic review

- *Airway.* The trachea is deviated to the right. Also there is apparent amputation seen at the origin of the right main bronchus suspicious for bronchial occlusion.
- *Breathing.* Aerated right lung is not visible, there is complete opacification of the right hemi-thorax, and the mediastinal structures are deviated to the right consistent with volume loss in the right hemithorax. The left apex, upper, middle and lower lung zones, the costo-phrenic and cardiophrenic angles, and the hilum are normal.
- *Circulation.* Heart size cannot be assessed as the heart borders are not fully visible. There is mediastinal shift to the right. The AA and right heart border are not visible.
- *Diaphragm.* The right hemidiaphragm is not visible due to the underlying abnormality. The left hemidiaphragm is normal. Normal air-filled bowel loops are seen beneath the left hemidiaphragm. No free intraperitoneal air.
- *'Everything else'.* There are no lines or tubes projected on the film. The breast contours are symmetrical. There are no visible fractures or bone lesions. There is evidence of bilateral shoulder joint replacement.

Summary

- This is a chest radiograph of an 84-year-old female who attended the ED with a sudden onset right-sided chest pain and dyspnoea. The CXR shows severe tracheal deviation and mediastinal shift to the right, and complete opacification of the right hemithorax. There is likely right bronchial occlusion. The appearances are consistent with right lung collapse. A possible cause for this is bronchogenic malignancy. An urgent respiratory team review is advised regarding further investigation and likely bronchoscopy.

ALTERNATIVE 'RADIOLOGIST-REVIEW' APPROACH

- *Type of film and projection:*
  'This is a PA chest radiograph of ...'
- *Name:*
  'Mrs Jane Smith ...'
- *Hospital number:*
  'Hospital number 123456789 ...'
- *Date of birth:*
  'Date of birth 22nd February 19XX ...'
- *Date:*
  'Taken on 12th January 20XX.'
- *Technical quality:*
  'The patient is markedly rotated with a thoracic scoliosis concave to the right, with good inspiratory effort and adequate penetration.'

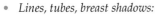

- *Lines, tubes, breast shadows:*
  'There are no visible lines or tubes, and the breast shadows are present …'
- *Check old films:*
  'I would like to compare this image with any previous images to identify any changes and to review previous history …'
- *Heart, lungs, bones:*
  'There is a significant tracheal deviation to the right with right mediastinal shift and a complete loss of normal aerated right lung. There is likely occlusion at the origin of the right main bronchus. There is right rib space narrowing. The heart size cannot be assessed as the right heart border is obliterated by the abnormality. The left lung appears normal. There are no bony lesions or fractures.'
- *Review areas:*
  'The peripheral soft tissues appear normal, the left costophrenic and cardiophrenic angles are fully visible and clear, there is no evidence of left lobar collapse or mass behind the heart. The left hemidiaphragm is dome shaped with some visible air in the bowel loops below.'
- *Summary:*
  'In summary, there is a severe right tracheal deviation with mediastinal shift and complete collapse of the right lung. A possible cause for this is a central obstructing lung malignancy and the patient should be reviewed urgently by the respiratory team with a view to further investigation and bronchoscopy.'

Note: This is an instructive case and should be compared with other causes of hemithoracic complete opacification later in the book. With lung volume loss as a cause, the mediastinum will move towards the affected lung. If a large pleural effusion is the aetiology this will have mass effect and push the mediastinum away from the affected side. Consolidated lung may opacify the hemithorax but will usually not displace the mediastinum, unless there is associated effusion or collapse. US will readily differentiate effusion from collapse.

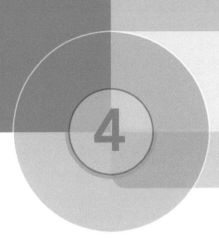

The normal abdominal X-ray

4

SEAN MITCHELL

The AXR is still commonly undertaken in the acute abdomen where perforation or acute bowel obstruction is suspected, particularly in the elderly where acute abdominal signs and symptoms are often nonspecific. You will also find that along with the CXR the AXR is one of the more common images that you will be expected to be able to interpret during your foundation years and as part of your final year OSCE/written examinations.

Example indications for AXR include:

- Abdominal pain where there is a suspicion of perforation or obstruction.
- Renal calculi – however, CT KUB is becoming the imaging technique of choice.
- Inflammatory bowel disease, particularly where toxic dilatation is suspected (CT increasingly being used).
- Foreign body ingestion.
- Postoperatively where there is a suspicion of ileus.

CONTRAINDICATIONS

An AXR is relatively contraindicated in the pregnant patient. If you are unsure, or if the woman is of childbearing age, a pregnancy test should be undertaken. If the patient is certain she is not pregnant then it is best practice to ask her to sign a disclaimer before proceeding. If in doubt discuss with the radiologist as alternative imaging methods may be more appropriate.

AXR is not usually indicated for the investigation of gallstones [right upper quadrant (RUQ) pain] or in diagnosing constipation.

LIMITATIONS

The AXR is far less sensitive than CT for identifying intraperitoneal free air, ischaemic bowel, the retroperitoneum, abscesses, and calcifications – particularly gallstones where only 10% at best will be seen on AXR. However, it is worth remembering that CT exposes the patient to a far higher dose of radiation.

RADIATION EXPOSURE

- ALARA (as low as reasonably achievable)– keep dose down!!

You should always consider the amount of radiation that the patient will be exposed to and try to minimise this where practicable. The exact amount of exposure will vary between individuals, dependent on body habitus and type of imaging being undertaken (*Table 4.1*).

Before requesting an AXR it is worth considering if a nonionising imaging modality (that uses no ionising radiation) would be more beneficial such as US or MRI. However, you need to consider the benefits and risks to the patient. For example, if a patient presents with suspected renal colic an AXR would not be of some benefit, whereas a CT KUB, despite exposing the patient to a higher dose of radiation, would lead to a more accurate and rapid diagnosis. In cases such as these you need to be able to justify a higher radiation exposure, i.e. ensuring that the clinical benefit to the patient outweighs the risk.

- Remember – if in doubt, discuss with a senior colleague or radiologist.

Table 4.1 Modality dose comparisons

Imaging	Dose mSv	Equivalent in CXR
CXR	0.015	1
AXR	0.4	30
CT abdomen	5.6	370
CT abdomen and pelvis	6.7	450

See Chapter 3 for a full table of imaging modalities and associated doses.

TECHNIQUE

The AXR is taken AP with the patient in the supine position. This is often combined with an erect CXR where perforation is suspected, especially in the elderly as the erect CXR is far more sensitive for free intraperitoneal air than an AXR and perforated viscus is in the differential for many acute abdominal presentations, especially in older patients.

TOP TIPS

The patient should ideally be sat upright for 5–10 minutes prior to the erect CXR being taken, to allow any free air to rise and collect under the diaphragm where it can be visualised. Check with the radiographer that this has occurred if in doubt.

Erect or decubitus AXRs, although still mentioned in many textbooks, are no longer under-taken in clinical practice. If the patient is unable to lie supine it is always worth discussing with the radiologist beforehand, as they will be able to advise you on how to best further investigate.

AXR INTERPRETATION AND PRESENTATION

When interpreting an AXR remember that because of the varying densities of the tissues within the abdominal cavity, the amount of anatomy that can be identified may vary from individual to individual dependent on factors such as the amount of fat surrounding the abdominal contents and gas within the digestive tract. Therefore, prior to interpreting the AXR consider the underlying anatomy; a sound understanding of this and those aspects that can usefully be visualised will aid in identifying any abnormalities (**Figure 4.1**).

When presenting a radiographic image, particularly in an OSCE, it is worth remembering that time is tight and you will not have the luxury of being able to go through everything in too much detail, so be succinct and briefly explain what you would normally do. Examiners want to see that you have presented and reviewed radiology images before and may allow/encourage you to move on to the image abnormalities once they see you have a good technique. Some medical schools base the whole OSCE case around one XR – which may be normal – just to examine technique, although this is unusual. Start by identifying the type of film and projection, making note of the orientation markers (L, R). Then check the patient demographics and image details to ensure you have the right patient with the right image on the right date at the right time. In an OSCE this information will be anonymised, but you should still ensure that you mention these aspects. Having done this you should then ensure the film is adequate before systematically interpreting the image.

An adequately exposed film is one that includes the entire abdomen from diaphragm to pubic symphysis and the lateral abdominal walls. This is vital to be able to accurately interpret the image. In an adequately penetrated film you should also be able to identify the vertebrae but they should not be so exposed that everything is too overexposed (excessively black) or underexposed (excessively white). Not all cases in exams will be perfect and do not go into too much detail on this – any abnormalities on the XR should be readily apparent.

Having ensured that you have the correct film and that it is adequate for diagnostic purposes you then need to have a systematic approach to identifying any clinical abnormalities that may aid you in your diagnosis, for example:

* Gases.
* Masses.
* Stones.
* Bones.
* Artefacts.

Some people find it useful to check artefacts first (tubes, lines, surgical clips) as this can give a clue as to the patient's presentation. However, the important thing is to have a system that suits you and to stick to it.

Learning to interpret an XR in a systematic way is not just a skill for OSCEs but one that will stand you in good stead throughout your career. Although it may seem pedantic to go through all these steps, it ensures the appropriate image is being studied and that nothing is missed, which can be easy to do when under pressure on a busy ward or in a busy medical/surgical assessment unit.

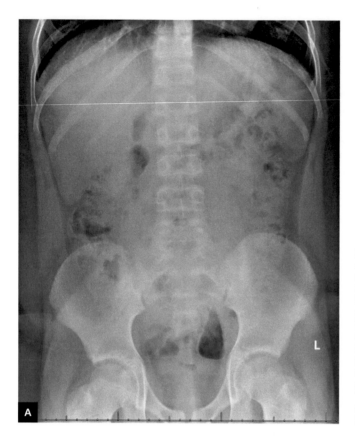

Figs. 4.1A, B Nonlabelled AXR (**4.1A**). Labelled AXR (**4.1B**) showing normal abdominal anatomy. Depending on body habitus and bowel gas pattern, you may be able to identify the liver, spleen, kidneys, stomach, small bowel, large bowel, and bladder (not the ureters). In this patient the tips of the right lobe of liver and spleen can be seen and the collapsed stomach. The renal outlines are largely obscured by faecal residue/bowel gas.

GASES

It is worth starting with a systematic review of the gas-filled GI tract, as this is often the most prominent anatomy visible. Start with a general overview and ask yourself if it looks normal or abnormal. As a general rule, if you are not sure or if it looks borderline it is often normal, as the most common sign of abdominal pathology is dilated bowel, which is usually obvious and if used in an OSCE will stand out clearly on a computer screen.

Then identify the small and large bowel (**Figure 4.2**).

The small bowel can usually be identified by its central location and the valvulae conniventes that form complete bands across the bowel, often described as 'stacks of coins'.

The large bowel is usually located at the peripheries. As it contains a mixture of gas and faeces the pattern will vary between individuals and over time. You should be able to identify the ascending, transverse, descending, and sigmoid colon as well as the rectum.

If the bowel is very dilated (>7 cm) it is most likely to be large bowel as small bowel does not get this large before perforating. Note the '3-6-9 rule' for size (*Table 4.2*). This topic is covered in more detail in later chapters.

The stomach lies across the midline towards the left upper quadrant (LUQ) and may be identified by an air–fluid level formed by gastric body fluid and air in the fundus. The gas-filled pylorus and duodenum may also be visible.

The rectum lies at the distal end of the GI tract and may contain gas or faeces.

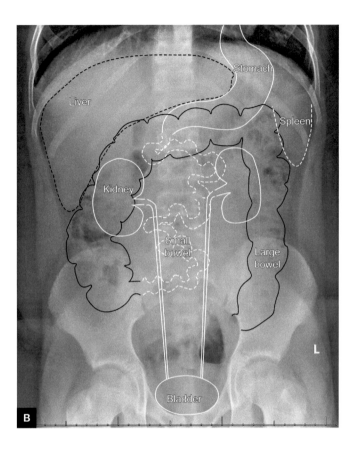

Fig. 4.1B

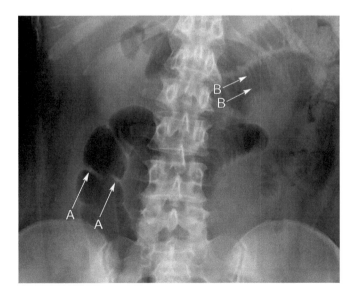

Fig. 4.2 AXR showing normal loops of small and large bowel. Note the differing appearances of valvulae conniventes (B) and haustra (A).

Table 4.2 AXR features of small and large bowel

	Small bowel	Large bowel
Position	Central	Peripheral
Features	Valvulae conniventes	Haustra
Size	<3 cm	<6 cm or <9 cm in the caecum
Content	Liquid and air	Solid faeces, liquid, and air

MASSES (SOLID VISCERA)

The solid organs (liver, spleen, kidneys) are not always identifiable due to overlying bowel gas but may become more conspicuous if there is an abnormality (**Figure 4.3**).

The liver fills the RUQ and may have a smooth well-defined inferior border visible just below the right costal margin. Extension of the liver tip below this level raises suspicion of hepatomegaly. An exception to this is the presence of a Riedel's lobe, which is a common normal anatomical variant with inferior projection of the right lobe of liver, and this can project below the inferior costal cartilage and simulate pathology. The normal gallbladder and pancreas are not visible.

The spleen tip may be seen in the LUQ, just superior to the left kidney, inferior to the 9th–11th ribs.

The kidneys are located between T12 and L2 with the right kidney 2–3 cm lower than the left owing to the position of the liver, and clear renal outlines are often difficult to see.

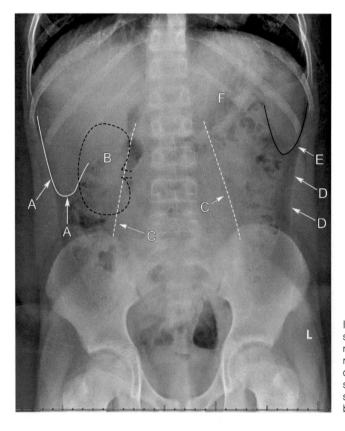

Fig. 4.3 AXR with annotated structures. Tip of Riedel's lobe right liver (A), expected outline of right kidney (B), iliopsoas muscle outlines (C), left paracolic fat stripe (D), spleen tip (E), collapsed stomach (F). Left kidney obscured by faecal matter.

STONES (CALCIFICATIONS)

Identify structures that can become calcified or contain stones, particularly the kidneys and urinary tract. Remember that 90% of kidney stones are radiopaque owing to their high calcium content. Conversely, only 10% of gallstones are radiopaque and, therefore, are much less likely to be visible. Calcium deposition can also be seen within the liver, spleen, pancreas, and arterial walls and it may, for example, delineate the wall of an AAA.

To identify urinary tract calcification, start by identifying the course of the urinary tract (**Figure 4.4**). The kidneys are not always seen but the path of the ureters can be traced from the level of the renal pelvis, down the lateral borders of the lumbar transverse processes, over the iliac vessels and sacroiliac joint and into the bladder at the vesicoureteric junction. The normal bladder is located low in the pelvis and has the density of soft tissue on AXR. It may or may not be visible depending on the degree of distension. Renal calculi may be visible anywhere along this tract and if suspected may warrant further investigation with CT.

The aorta, iliac, and femoral arteries may be visualised if calcified, suggesting atherosclerosis. An incidental AAA may be identified and warrant further investigation with CT.

Phleboliths are small calcifications located within veins, and are commonly found within the pelvic veins of women. They can easily be mistaken for distal ureteric calculi and may require CT to help tell them apart. Typically, however, phleboliths have a relatively lucent centre and look a bit like a tiny polo mint when seen 'en face' (**Figure 4.5**).

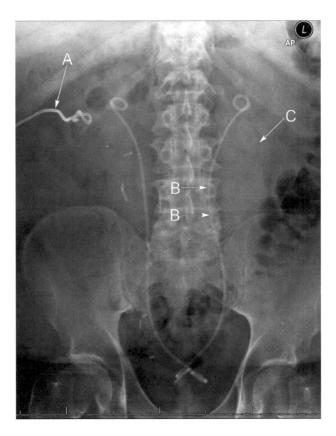

Fig. 4.4 AXR with bilateral ureteric stents and a right-sided nephrostomy tube (arrow A). The right stent demonstrates the normal position of the renal pelvis, ureter, and bladder. Note the mid left stent is medially deviated (B) by a retroperitoneal soft tissue mass (C).

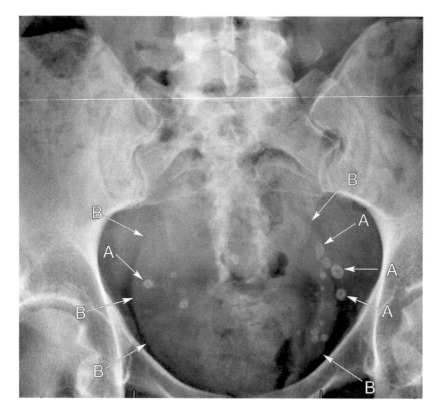

Fig. 4.5 Cropped pelvic XR showing multiple phleboliths (A) with central lucency, projected over the distended urinary bladder (B).

Gallstones may also be visible in the gallbladder if they are radiopaque. Pancreatic calcification (chronic pancreatitis) may be visible on AXR, although CT is far more sensitive.

BONES, ASSOCIATED STRUCTURES, AND OTHER ARTEFACTS

Having reviewed the abdominal organs, you should move on to the bones, associated structures and artefacts.

At the superior border of the film the lower ribs should be visible along with both hemidiaphragms. The normal AXR should not have any air under the hemidiaphragms; however, remember that the normal AXR is taken with the patient supine and therefore, even in the case of a perforation, you are unlikely to see air under the diaphragm, hence the need for an erect CXR if you have any suspicion of a visceral perforation.

The lower thoracic and lumbar vertebrae should also be clearly visible; if not the film may be underpenetrated. The outline of the lumbar vertebrae should be traced to assess for any abnormalities such as a fracture. While assessing the lumbar spine you may also be able to identify the outline of the iliopsoas muscles (these may enlarge in cases of retroperitoneal tumour, abscess or bleed).

To complete the examination of the bones you should check the pelvis, sacroiliac joints, symphysis pubis, and hip joints for any deformity.

ARTEFACTS

Artefacts, such as surgical clips, drains, tubes, body piercings, and foreign bodies, may be visible on the AXR and provide useful clues about the patient's history (**Figures 4.6** and **4.7**). For example, surgical clips in the RUQ may represent previous cholecystectomy or, in the female pelvis, may suggest previous sterilisation. In female patients you may also see a ring pessary or an intrauterine coil.

Findings such as these may warrant further investigation into the patient's past surgical history.

- Remember, postsurgical adhesions represent the major cause of small bowel obstruction (in over 90% of cases). A past surgical history is essential, as is examining the abdomen carefully for scars.

Medical devices, such as ECG leads and oxygen tubing, may also be visible. In an OSCE you should endeavour to point these out as they give a clue to the patient's clinical condition.

Finally, take the opportunity to review content on the AXR that is unrelated to the abdomen, such as the lung bases (pneumonia, mass), the peripheral abdominal wall soft tissues,

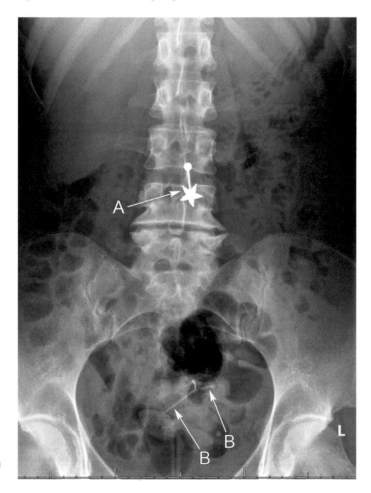

Fig. 4.6 AXR showing metal artefacts from umbilical jewellery (A) and an intrauterine coil (B).

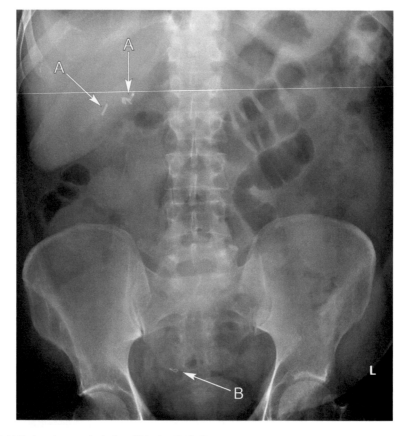

Fig. 4.7 AXR showing surgical clips (A) in the RUQ, likely to relate to previous cholecystectomy. There is a further clip visible in the pelvis (B), which could relate to a migrated cholecystectomy clip or, possibly a sterilisation clip.

and the groins. This may reveal findings such as hernias or consolidation, which can add to the overall clinical picture.

Review areas:

- Ribs.
- Lung bases.
- Hernial orifices.
- Abdominal wall.

EXAM TECHNIQUE

When preparing for your OSCE exam you should consider the context in which the AXR is likely to be presented. The examiners will be looking for a systematic approach, a reasonable differential diagnosis, and a management plan.

Cases in exams will be common and radiology findings will not be subtle/equivocal. Images will have obvious pathology that can be clearly seen, usually on a computer screen. Imaging in exams is usually presented on a personal computer screen (often a laptop) and will not be adjustable, while images are also increasingly being used in written papers. The imaging should be anonymised but do not let this distract you into forgetting to mention the importance of noting patient details as these are easy marks in an OSCE. You need to clearly state to the examiner right from the outset that you would normally check the patient demographics. Radiology in OSCEs usually features in the second half of the case where further discussion around the case occurs. Occasionally a radiology image will form the basis of the whole case, and rarely a normal AXR may be used for discussion.

Common OSCE AXR radiological presentations may include:

- Bowel perforation with free intraperitoneal air (more usually erect CXR utilised).
- Small or large bowel obstruction.
- Sigmoid volvulus.
- Foreign body (e.g. swallowed coin or migrated intrauterine coil).
- Inflammatory bowel disease with 'thumbprinting' or 'toxic megacolon'.
- Pancreatic calcification (chronic pancreatitis).

Remember that although in real life we do not always know the answer, in the exam you need to describe your findings with confidence. Likewise, in any exam you can still pass without getting the correct diagnosis so long as you are confident and systematic.

TOP TIPS

- In an exam you will not have time to make a full presentation but will need to indicate how you would normally approach an AXR. Therefore, demonstrate a systematic approach.
- Ask to review previous imaging – always compare with previous imaging if available.
- Normal/abnormal – clearly state whether the bowel gas pattern is normal or abnormal.
- Offer the examiner an initial management plan to include bedside tests and bloods.
- Escalation – say who you would discuss this with and why. Remember that if you are unsure it is never wrong to seek advice.
- If you suspect bowel perforation you should review an erect CXR.
- If undertaking an erect CXR the patient must be allowed to sit upright beforehand to allow any free air to rise up below the diaphragm.
- If you are considering requesting an AXR for a diagnosis other than bowel perforation or obstruction, consider whether another imaging modality may be more appropriate.

HOW TO PRESENT YOUR FINDINGS

- Practice ... practice ... practice.

This will build confidence. You are not expected to know everything so, if you do not know the answer, say you do not know but suggest how you might find out or who you would seek advice from – be safe. Use the example cases below to get started (**Figures 4.8–4.10**). Consider the different ways you might structure your presentation along the lines described in Chapter 2.

CASE 1

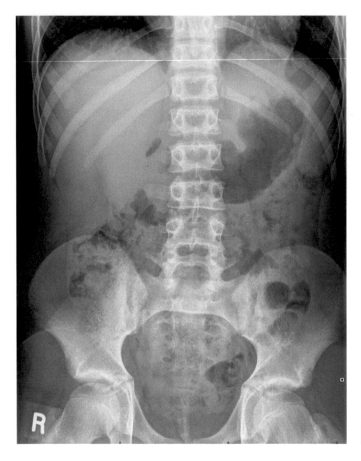

Fig. 4.8 Case 1: AXR, young female with abdominal pain.

- *Type of film and projection:*
  'This is a supine abdominal radiograph of ...'

- *Name:*
  'Miss Jo Smith ...'

- *Hospital number:*
  'Hospital number 123456789 ...'

- *Date of birth:*
  'Date of birth 22nd February 1992 ...'

- *Date:*
  'Taken on 12th January 2016 ...'

- *Exposure + rotation:*
  'It is adequately exposed ...'

- *Penetration:*
  'There is adequate penetration...'

- *Gases, masses, stones, bones:*
  'The bowel gas pattern is within normal limits. No dilated loops of small or large bowel are seen. No intraperitoneal free gas. No organomegaly. No abnormal calcifications. The bones appear normal. The review areas are clear.'
- *Check old films:*
  'I would like to compare this image with any previous images to identify any changes and to review the previous history.'
- *Summary and plan:*
  'In summary, this is a normal abdominal radiograph with no gross pathology. I would like to review any blood tests, bedside observations, and urinalysis, and correlate with the clinical presentation.'

CASE 2

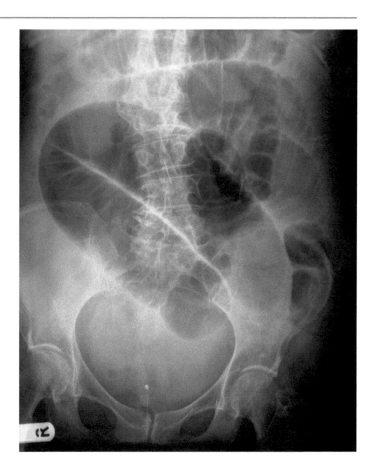

Fig. 4.9 Case 2: AXR of an elderly female with increasing abdominal pain and distension.

- *Type of film and projection:*
  'This is a supine abdominal radiograph of …'
- *Name:*
  'Mrs Edwina Bloggs …'

- *Hospital number:*
  'Hospital number 123456789 ...'
- *Date of birth:*
  'Date of birth 17th February 1949 ...'
- *Date:*
  'Taken on 2nd August 2015 ...'
- *Exposure + rotation:*
  'It is adequately exposed and not rotated. The upper abdomen and right lateral border of the abdomen and iliac crest are not included in the field of view as the image is not central ...'
- *Penetration:*
  'There is adequate penetration ...'
- *Gases, masses, stones, bones:*
  'There is marked dilatation of several centrally located loops of bowel with valvulae conniventes evident, in keeping with small bowel. The large bowel is not clearly visible. The liver, spleen, and kidneys are not visible. There are no obvious calcifications within the renal tract, or visible phleboliths. The lumbar spine is scoliotic, concave to the left, with degenerative change between L4 and S1. There is the tip of a urinary catheter present, no surgical clips are seen.'
- *Check old films:*
  'I would like to compare this image with any previous images to identify any changes and to review previous history and clinical presentation.'
- *Summary and plan:*
  'In summary, this is an abnormal abdominal radiograph with signs of small bowel dilatation. The appearances would be consistent with small bowel obstruction, although ileus could have a similar radiological appearance. Correlation with clinical findings and previous surgical history is essential. She will also need an erect CXR to exclude perforation. This patient will need to be admitted have an NG tube inserted and started on IV fluids. I would like to review any blood tests, bedside observations and urinalysis, and then refer her to the surgical team for further management.'

CASE 3

- *Type of film and projection:*
  'This is a supine abdominal radiograph of ...'
- *Name:*
  'Mrs Alice Jones ...'
- *Hospital number:*
  'Hospital number 123456789 ...'
- *Date of birth:*
  'Date of birth 15th March 1948 ...'
- *Date:*
  'Taken on 30th January 2016 ...'
- *Exposure + rotation:*
  'The upper abdomen is not fully included in the field of view, otherwise the coverage and exposure are adequate. The radiograph is not rotated.'

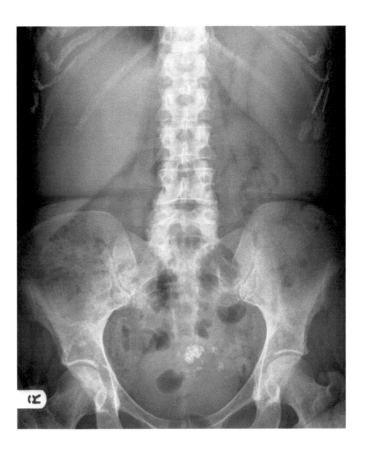

Fig. 4.10 Case 3: elderly female with abdominal pain, distension, and weight loss.

- *Penetration:*
  'There is adequate penetration …'

- *Gases, masses, stones, bones:*
  'The bowel gas pattern is within normal limits. No dilated loops of small or large bowel are seen. There is abnormal punctate calcification within the pelvis, which likely relates to uterine fibroid calcification. There is pronounced smooth enlargement of the liver and spleen, no calcification is seen. The bones are normal. In the left upper quadrant I can see two ports suggestive of a PIC line.'

- *Check old films:*
  'I would like to compare this image with any previous images to identify any changes and to review previous history and the clinical presentation.'

- *Summary and plan:*
  'In summary, this is an abnormal abdominal radiograph with hepatosplenomegaly in a patient with a likely underlying chronic disease as indicated by the PIC line. This suggests a myeloproliferative disorder such as chronic myeloid leukaemia or myelofibrosis. There is calcification within the pelvis that is likely to be longstanding. I would like to undertake a full physical examination including a set of bedside observations and urinalysis. I would also like to take a set of bloods to include FBC, U&Es, and LFTs. The patient is likely to need a CT scan of chest, abdomen, and pelvis, and I would refer her to haematology as she may already be known to them.'

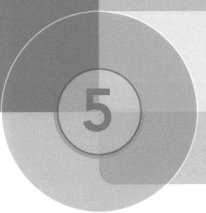

Thoracic cases

HANNAH ADAMS, SARAH HANCOX,
CRISTINA RUSCANU, AND
DAVID C HOWLETT

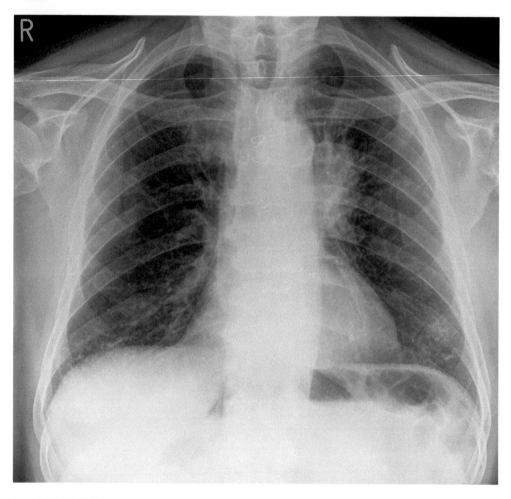

Fig. 5.1A PA CXR.

A 69-year-old male presents to his GP with an ongoing cough for 8 weeks. He also reports feeling tired all the time and has noticed some weight loss, which he associates with his poor appetite. He gave up smoking 5 years ago after undergoing a coronary artery bypass graft (CABG). Prior to this he smoked 20 cigarettes per day for 40 years.

On examination he has normal vital observations. A 1 cm hard supraclavicular lymph node is palpated on the left and clubbing of his nails is noted. Cardiorespiratory examination is normal with no added sounds on auscultation.

The GP arranges for an urgent CXR (**Figure 5.1A**). Routine blood tests are also requested, which show:

FBC	Normal	Urea	2.4 mmol/L (1.7–8.3 mmol/L)
Sodium	120 mmol/L (135–146 mmol/L)	Creatinine	74 micromol/L (62–106 micromol/L)
Potassium	3.1 mmol/L (3.2–5.1 mmol/L)	LFTs	Normal

CASE 5.1: QUESTIONS

1 What does the CXR show?
2 What is the most likely diagnosis?
3 What is the likely explanation for this patient's hyponatraemia?
4 What further investigations should be arranged?
5 What are the treatment options for this condition?

CASE 5.1: ANSWERS

1 What does the CXR show?

The PA view CXR shows a spiculated opacity in the left hilum (M) (**Figure 5.1B**). The mass is clearly separate from the aortic knuckle (A). This is an example of the silhouette sign; the left pulmonary artery/hilar structures are obscured, confirming that the origin of the hilar density is at the hilum rather than in front or behind the hilum when the hilar outline would then be clearly seen. The mass is also separate from the aortic knuckle, which can be clearly seen. Sternotomy wires confirm the history of previous cardiothoracic surgery.

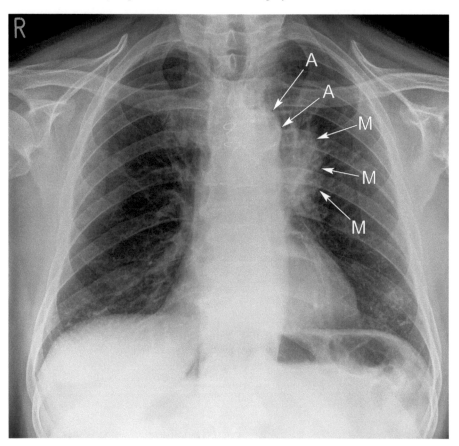

Fig. 5.1B CXR showing a spiculated mass in the left hilum (M), separate from the aortic knuckle (A). Note: obscuration of normal left hilar structures and also sternotomy clips.

2 What is the most likely diagnosis?

The most likely diagnosis is primary lung carcinoma. The combined features of persistent cough, weight loss, lymphadenopathy, and appearance on CXR are highly suggestive of malignancy. Bronchogenic cancer accounts for 95% of primary lung tumours and is now the commonest cancer in the UK. It has an extremely poor prognosis with 25% of patients surviving 1 year and only 7% surviving 5 years.

Risk factors for developing lung cancer can be divided into modifiable and nonmodifiable:

- Modifiable.
  - Smoking.
  - Asbestos exposure.
  - Air pollution.
  - Ionising radiation (radon gas).
- Nonmodifiable.
  - Family history/genetic factors.
  - Male gender.

There are four main histological types of lung cancer (*Table 5.1*):

- Small cell carcinoma.
- Non-small cell carcinoma.
  - Squamous cell carcinoma.
  - Adenocarcinoma (previously bronchioalveolar carcinoma).
  - Large cell carcinoma.

Table 5.1 Lung cancer histological types and features

	Small cell carcinoma	Squamous cell carcinoma	Adenocarcinoma	Large cell carcinoma
Incidence (%)	15	40	30	15
Tissue type	Endocrine (Kulchitsky cells)	Squamous epithelium	Glandular (goblet cells/clara cells)	Undifferentiated cells
Location	Hilar	Hilar	Peripheral	Peripheral/central
Treatment	Chemotherapy	Surgery	Surgery	Surgery
Metastatic spread	Early	Late	Intermediate	Early

3 What is the likely explanation for this patient's hyponatraemia?

The most likely cause for hyponatraemia in a patient with lung cancer is paraneoplastic syndrome. These syndromes arise at distant sites from the primary tumour and result from the production of hormones, antibodies, peptides or prostaglandins by the carcinoma. Syndrome of inappropriate antidiuretic hormone (SIADH) secretion is often seen in patients with small cell carcinoma, resulting in hyponatraemia, hypokalaemia, and hypouricaemia, confirmed with low serum and raised urine osmolarity. Treatment consists of fluid restriction (<1.5 L/day) and prescription of a vasopressin receptor antagonist.

This patient underwent investigation and was found to have SIADH secondary to his small cell lung cancer.

4 What further investigations should be arranged?

Investigations required in the diagnosis and staging of lung cancer include:

- CT chest (**Figure 5.1C**) and abdomen with contrast.
- PET.

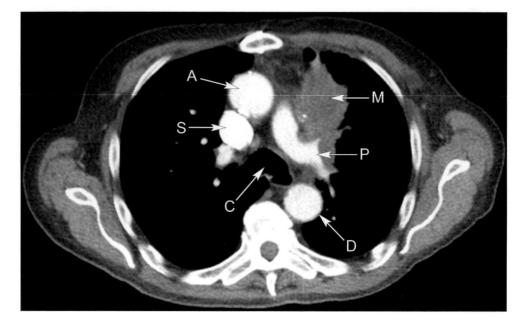

Fig. 5.1C Axial thoracic CT with contrast demonstrating a large mediastinal/hilar mass (M). Normal ascending aorta (A), carina (C), descending aorta (D), left pulmonary artery (P), and superior vena cava (S).

- Bronchoscopy +/− biopsy or washings.
- Transthoracic fine needle aspiration biopsy (dependent on tumour location).
- Sampling of pleural fluid in the presence of a pleural effusion.

Staging of non-small cell lung cancer uses the tumour, nodes, metastasis (TNM) classification. Small cell lung cancers are, however, described simply as being limited or extensive.

5 What are the treatment options for this condition?

There is a variation in treatment regimens dependent on the histological classification of the lung cancer:

- Surgical intervention.
  - Considered in non-small cell lung cancers.
  - Majority of cases are inoperable at the time of presentation.
  - Must undergo full staging investigations to ensure the tumour has not metastasised and lung function tests to demonstrate sufficient respiratory reserve.
- Radiotherapy.
  - Used for inoperable cancers.
  - Radiation pneumonitis and fibrosis are recognised complications.
  - Used for relief of symptoms such as superior vena cava obstruction and chest wall pain.
- Chemotherapy.
  - Generally reserved for small cell lung cancer.
  - Not a curative intervention, improves prognosis by months only.

- Palliation.
  - Symptom control – transbronchial stenting.
  - Opioid analgesia and laxatives.
  - Steroids can be used to improve appetite.

LEARNING POINTS: LUNG CANCER

- Lung cancer is the most common cause of cancer deaths per annum.
- Cigarette smoking is the major risk factor for developing lung cancer.
- Small cell lung cancers are rapidly growing, aggressive, and have usually metastasised at the time of presentation.
- Chemotherapy and radiotherapy improve quality of life when surgical resection is not a valid treatment option.
- Paraneoplastic syndromes are most common with small cell lung cancer.

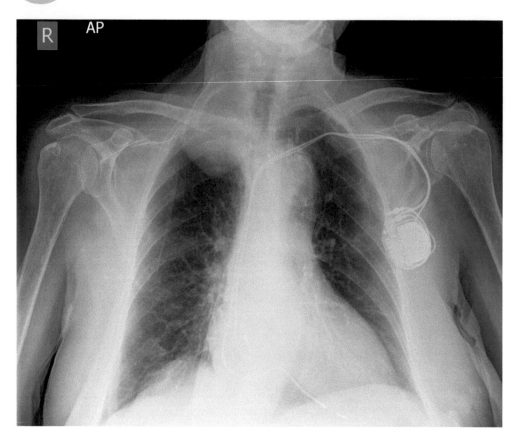

Fig. 5.2A PA CXR.

A 76-year-old female presents to Respiratory Outpatients with a persistent dry cough, poor appetite, and weight loss. She reports a 4–5-month history of worsening right shoulder pain radiating into her axilla, described as an aching sensation from which she has little relief. She is a current smoker and has smoked 10 cigarettes a day for 40 years.

On examination she has normal vital observations but appears cachectic. No lymphadenopathy is present and examination of the shoulder joint is unremarkable. Respiratory examination reveals equal expansion and air entry, normal percussion sounds, and normal breath sounds throughout. A CXR has been performed (**Figure 5.2A**).

CASE 5.2: QUESTIONS

1 What radiological findings are demonstrated on this CXR?
2 What is the most likely diagnosis?
3 What is the syndrome often associated with this condition?
4 What further investigations should be undertaken?
5 What are the treatment options available?
6 What is 'pack-year history' and how is it calculated?

CASE 5.2: ANSWERS

1 What radiological findings are demonstrated on this CXR?

The CXR demonstrates (**Figure 5.2B**):

- A right apical lung opacity within the superior sulcus (A).
- Destruction of the posterior aspect of the right second rib (expected course of rib marked with dashed line).
- Presence of a permanent dual chamber pacemaker.

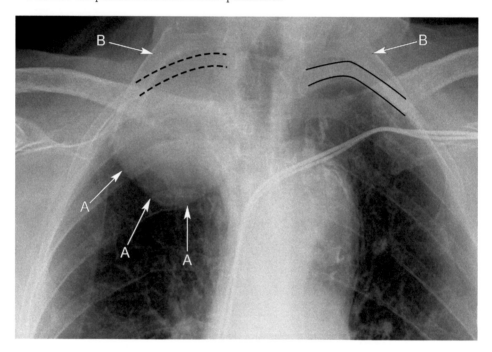

Fig. 5.2B CXR demonstrating a large right apical opacity (A) with destruction of the posterior aspect of the right second rib (dashed line shows expected position of the rib). The normal posterior aspect of the left second rib is shown by the solid lines, first ribs arrowed (B).

2 What is the most likely diagnosis?

Right apical opacity with rib destruction is indicative of a Pancoast (superior sulcus) tumour. The opacity alone could be a pleural tumour (fibroma, lipoma, metastasis), a neural tumour such as neurofibroma, possibly TB or fungus ball (mycetoma), or an aneurysm.

3 What is the syndrome often associated with this condition?

The history, examination, and CXR are suggestive of a Pancoast tumour. This is the description given to a malignant neoplasm at the extreme lung apex; involvement of the brachial plexus and sympathetic chain by the tumour results in Pancoast syndrome. This syndrome is represented by:

- Shoulder pain (chest wall invasion).
- Ipsilateral C8–T2 radicular pain.
- Horner's syndrome resulting from infiltration of the tumour into the thorax involving the sympathetic chain causing ptosis, miosis, enophthalmos, and anhydrosis.

- Only 25% of patients with Pancoast tumour are diagnosed with Pancoast syndrome as the majority do not exhibit complete signs of Horner's syndrome.

Patients report pain in the shoulder and axilla due to erosion of the ribs. Anhydrosis occurs secondary to involvement of the stellate ganglion, a collection of sympathetic nerves anterior to the sixth and seventh cervical vertebrae. Invasion of the tumour into the brachial plexus results in wasting of the small muscles of the hand and neuropathic pain, while invasion of the vertebral foramen can lead to spinal cord compression, a medical emergency.

There is often a delayed diagnosis of Pancoast syndrome as the apical lung cancer can be slow growing and insidious, and may not be visualised on initial CXRs. Once the patient presents with worsening symptoms the cancer has often already invaded nearby structures. Delayed diagnosis can also occur due to prominence of musculoskeletal symptoms, which are incorrectly interpreted, such as shoulder symptoms and radicular pain.

4 What further investigations should be undertaken?

CT provides vital information on the extent and spread of the suspected lesion, and can be used to plan the most appropriate approach to obtain a sample for histological diagnosis.

The majority of Pancoast tumours are squamous cell carcinomas but samples should be obtained for diagnostic purposes. Adenocarcinomas may also occur in old areas of scarring (history of TB). Sputum samples may be beneficial in patients who cannot tolerate invasive investigations. Bronchoscopy or CT-guided biopsy is used to obtain histology, as these are peripheral lesions usually and more amenable to CT access.

MR scanning is particularly useful in providing multiplanar visualisation of the chest wall and the brachial plexus.

PET scans can provide further detail regarding the extent of the disease and location of metastases. This information can be used in a multidisciplinary meeting to determine the best course of treatment for each patient.

5 What are the treatment options available?

Surgery is indicated in patients with early disease, which is only seen in a minority of patients. Contraindications to surgery include metastatic spread, nodal mediastinal extension, and invasion into the neck, brachial plexus, and vertebrae.

Medical management is suitable for most patients, providing a degree of palliation, such as radiotherapy for relief of associated symptoms. Chemotherapy can be considered but is often more appropriate in preoperative patients.

6 What is 'pack-year history' and how is it calculated?

Pack-year history is a measurement of a smoking history. It is calculated by multiplying the number of packs of 20 cigarettes smoked per day by the number of years the person has smoked. For example, 20 cigarettes/day for 1 year = 1 pack-year history, or in the case of this patient 10 cigarettes/day for 40 years = 20 pack-year history.

LEARNING POINTS: PANCOAST TUMOUR

- Pancoast tumour is a malignant neoplasm at the extreme lung apex.
- Pancoast syndrome is a triad of shoulder pain, C8–T2 radicular pain, and Horner's syndrome.
- Investigations include CT chest and liver, sputum samples, bronchoscopy +/– biopsy, MRI, and PET scan.
- Treatment is often limited to radiotherapy due to the late presentation.
- Pack-year history = number of cigarettes (day) × number of years.

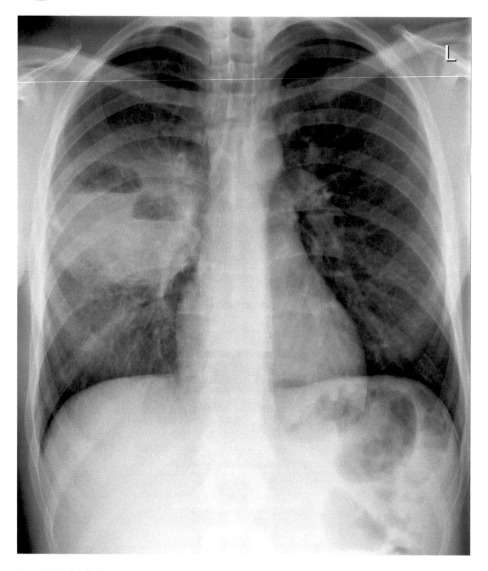

Fig. 5.3A PA CXR.

A 52-year-old male presents to the ED with a 3-week history of feeling generally unwell, fatigue and coughing up purulent green sputum. He has lost his appetite but does not report any weight loss. He has no fixed abode, drinks over 60 units of alcohol per week, and is a nonsmoker.

On examination he has a temperature of 38.4°C, blood pressure 129/78 mmHg, pulse rate of 90 bpm, respiratory rate 20 bpm, and oxygen saturations 95% breathing room air. He looks generally unwell, pale, and clammy. Respiratory examination reveals some dullness to percussion and decreased breath sounds in the right middle zone.

An urgent CXR is requested (**Figure 5.3A**) and bloods are performed:

Hb	132 g/L (130–180 g/L)	U&Es	Normal
WCC	17.8 × 10⁹/L (4.0–11.0 × 10⁹/L)	LFTs	Normal
Neutrophils	15.2 × 10⁹/L (2.0–7.5 × 10⁹/L)	CRP	246 mg/L (<5 mg/L)
Platelets	288 × 10⁹/L (150–450 × 10⁹/L)		

CASE 5.3: QUESTIONS

1 What key radiological findings are demonstrated?
2 What is the most likely diagnosis?
3 What are the possible causes for this appearance?
4 What investigations and management are required?
5 What are the complications that may occur with this condition?

CASE 5.3: ANSWERS

1 What key radiological findings are demonstrated?

There is a large ill-defined opacity in the right lung containing two lucent areas, with an air–fluid level (**Figure 5.3B**).

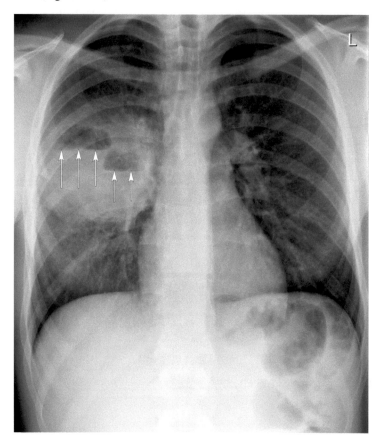

Fig. 5.3B Frontal CXR with arrows delineating air–fluid levels within a large ill-defined area of opacification in the right middle zone.

2 What is the most likely diagnosis?

The most likely diagnosis is a cavitating abscess of the right lung (causative organisms are given in *Table 5.3*). Pulmonary cavities are gas-filled areas within a mass or area of consolidation. They are referred to as a lung abscess when they contain areas of infected parenchyma with necrosis and suppuration, and are typically thick walled.

Table 5.3 Causative organisms

Anaerobes	Aerobes	Other
Bacteroides spp.	*Staphylococcus aureus*	Mycobacterial infection
Peptostreptococcus spp.	*Streptococcus pyogenes*	Fungus – *Aspergillus* spp.
Fusobacterium spp.	*Pseudomonas auriginosa*	Parasites – *Entamoeba* spp.
	Klebsiella pneumoniae	

Risk factors for lung abscesses include:

- Immunosuppression (human immunodeficiency virus, chemotherapy).
- Alcoholism and drug use.
- Lung disease (cystic fibrosis).
- Aspiration (cerebral palsy, cerebrovascular accident).

3 What are the possible causes for this appearance?

Possible causes for lung cavitation include (mnemonic CAVITY):

- **C**ancer (primary – squamous cell; secondary – head and neck, oesophagus).
- **A**utoimmune (Wegener's granulomatosis, rheumatoid nodules).
- **V**ascular (septic pulmonary emboli).
- **I**nfection (TB, abscess).
- **T**rauma (pneumatocoeles).
- **Y**outh (bronchogenic cyst).

4 What investigations and management are required?

Management follows an initial ABCDE assessment and stabilisation of the patient. Blood cultures and sputum samples provide crucial information about correct antibiotic therapy. Further imaging with CT will help to determine the exact cause of the cavity prior to starting treatment (**Figure 5.3C**). CT-guided aspiration and drainage may also be required to obtain a sample of the organism and relieve the collection.

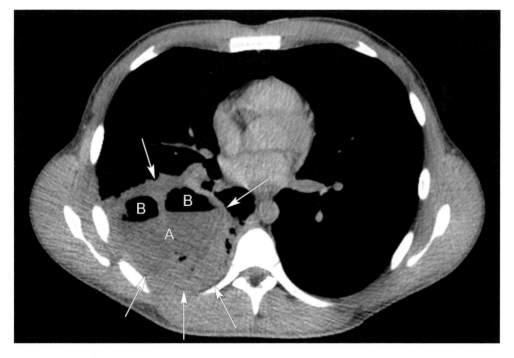

Fig. 5.3C Axial postcontrast CT section through right posterior lung lesion demonstrating a large thick-walled mass in the right lower lobe (arrows), with necrotic fluid centre (A) and areas of internal cavitation (B).

Prompt broad-spectrum IV antibiotic therapy to include anaerobe cover is recommended in the first instance.

Resolution is normally rapid following the commencement of suitable antibiotics. Patients must be followed up with CT scans to ensure complete resolution and that there is no underlying malignancy.

5 What are the complications that may occur with this condition?

With the correct treatment, lung abscesses should heal completely to leave a small fibrous scar. However, complications can occur such as:

- Empyema (needing CT/surgical drainage).
- Haemorrhage (caused by erosion into nearby vessels).
- Septicaemia.
- Pyopneumothorax.

LEARNING POINTS: CAVITATING LUNG ABSCESS

- Pulmonary cavities are gas-filled areas within a mass or area of consolidation.
- Mnemonic 'CAVITY' can be used to remember the causes of cavitating lesions.
- Immediate broad-spectrum IV antibiotic therapy to include anaerobes is essential.
- Follow-up using CT is an indicator of treatment progress.
- Complications include empyema and haemorrhage.

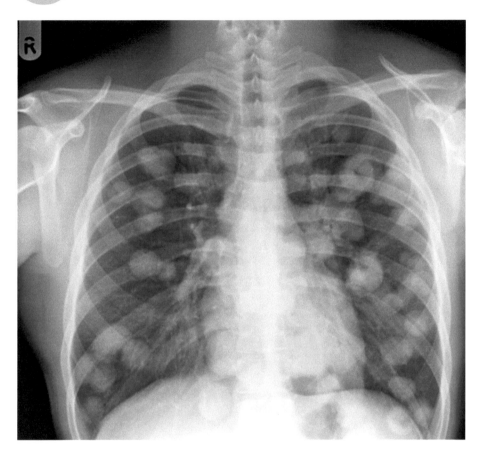

Fig. 5.4A PA CXR.

A 59-year-old male presents to his GP with a 3-week history of persistent painless macroscopic haematuria. Prior to this he thinks he lost approximately 10 kg in weight over 5–6 months. His wife reports she has noticed he is recently short of breath when he climbs the stairs.

On examination he is apyrexial with a blood pressure of 134/85 mmHg, heart rate 78 bpm, respiratory rate of 16 bpm, and oxygen saturations 96% breathing room air. Examination reveals a soft abdomen with some tenderness in the left loin but no palpable mass. Auscultation of his chest is normal.

Urine dipstick confirms 3+ blood but nil else. A CXR is requested for his shortness of breath (**Figure 5.4A**) and he is referred urgently to the haematuria clinic at the local hospital.

CASE 5.4: QUESTIONS

1 What radiological findings are demonstrated?
2 What is the most likely diagnosis?
3 Is there a differential for this appearance?
4 How should this patient be investigated?

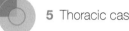

CASE 5.4: ANSWERS

1 What radiological findings are demonstrated?

Radiological features include (**Figure 5.4B**):

- Multiple large, bilateral, well-circumscribed round pulmonary lesions.
- No calcification in lesions, early cavitation in some lesions.
- No obvious pleural effusion.
- No bone lesions.
- No mediastinal lymphadenopathy.
- Heart size normal.

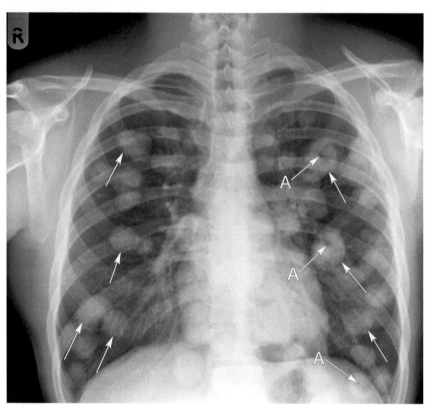

Fig. 5.4B CXR showing multiple large, bilateral, well-circumscribed round pulmonary lesions (arrows). Note small areas of lucency in some lesions consistent with early cavitation (A).

2 What is the most likely diagnosis?

The most likely diagnosis based on the patient's history is renal (or urinary tract) carcinoma with pulmonary 'cannonball' metastases. Metastases spread to the lung via the following routes:

- Haematogenous – tumours that have direct venous drainage to the lungs, such as breast, kidney, melanoma, testes, and head and neck squamous carcinoma.
- Lymphatic – tumour cells deposited in mediastinal lymph nodes, which spread along the lymphatics into the lung, such as stomach, colon, and breast.
- Direct invasion – e.g. malignant melanoma directly through the chest wall.

Pulmonary metastases are seen in up to 50% of extrathoracic malignancies, with the lungs being the second most common site of metastatic spread. Pulmonary metastasis indicates a poor prognosis as a result of the late stage of disease.

Appearances of lung metastases on CXR include (see *Table 5.4*):

- Cannonball appearance.
- Ill-defined 'snowstorm' appearance (**Figure 5.4C**).
- Solitary lung nodule (+/– cavity).
- Multiple lung nodules (+/– cavities, **Figure 5.4D**, page 70).
- Miliary nodularity (military = seed = fine and small, 1–3 mm).
- Lymphangitis carcinomatosa.

Table 5.4 Lung metastases appearance and tumour origin

Cannonball appearance	Snowstorm appearance	Solitary nodules
Kidney	Kidney	Kidney
Bladder	Bladder	Bowel
Uterus	Breast	Breast
Testes	Prostate	
Bowel	Thyroid	
Melanoma		

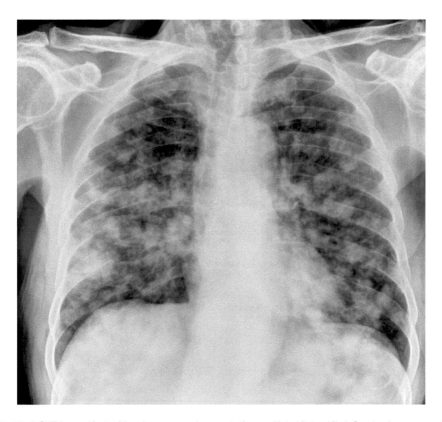

Fig. 5.4C A CXR in a patient with colon cancer demonstrating multiple bilateral ill-defined pulmonary nodules.

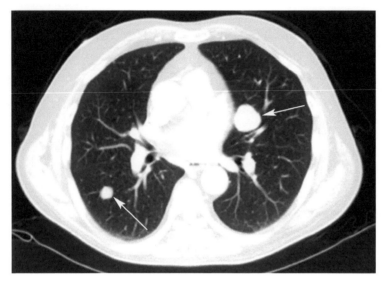

Fig. 5.4D CT thorax (lung window settings) image in a patient being staged for testicular cancer demonstrating circumscribed lung metastases (arrows).

Complications associated with pulmonary metastases include:

- Pleural effusion.
- Pericardial effusion.
- Lobar collapse.

3 Is there a differential for this appearance?

Differential diagnoses for multiple lung nodules:

- Metastases.
- Sarcoidosis.
- TB.
- Pulmonary lymphoma.
- Kaposi sarcoma.
- Rheumatoid nodules.
- Pulmonary/septic infarcts (tend to be ill-defined +/− cavitate).

4 How should this patient be investigated?

This patient should be investigated urgently in the haematuria clinic with the following investigations:

- Bloods, including renal function, FBC, bone profile, LFTs.
- CT chest, abdomen, pelvis (**Figure 5.4D**).
- Cystoscopy.

LEARNING POINTS: PULMONARY METASTASES

- Metastases can spread via haematogenous and lymphatic routes or by direct invasion.
- Lung metastases can be solitary or multiple with a cannonball or snowstorm appearance.
- Common primary sites include breast, melanoma, GI tract, and kidney.
- Complications of lung metastases include pleural effusion and lobar collapse.

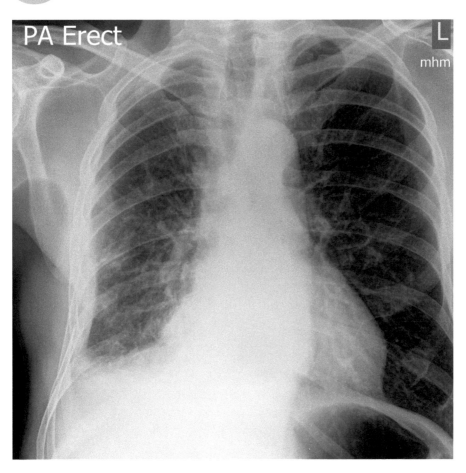

Fig. 5.5A PA CXR.

A 64-year-old male presents to his GP with a 4-month history of shortness of breath and a dull ache in the right side of his chest. He has not noticed any weight loss and reports having a good appetite. He denies a smoking history. He has recently retired but prior to this worked as a self-employed plumber for 45 years.

On examination his respiratory rate is 18 bpm and oxygen saturations are 93% breathing room air. He has decreased lung expansion on the right side with dullness to percussion but no pain on palpation of his chest wall. He does, however, have bibasal crackles on auscultation. An urgent CXR is performed (**Figure 5.5A**).

CASE 5.5: QUESTIONS

1 What are the radiological findings?
2 What is the most likely diagnosis?
3 What occupational exposure might be to blame?

CASE 5.5: ANSWERS

1 What are the radiological findings?

Radiological features include (**Figure 5.5B**):

- Decreased lung volume in the right hemithorax.
- Mediastinal shift to the right.
- Lobulated pleural thickening encasing the right hemithorax (arrows).
- Pleural opacity at the right costophrenic angle, indicating a pleural effusion or further pleural thickening.
- Some increased reticular density in the right mid/lower zone, possibly relating to an inflammatory process.

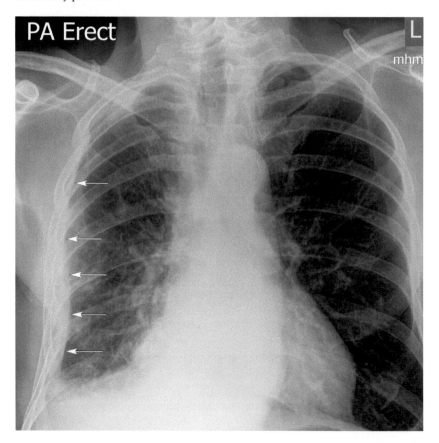

Fig. 5.5B CXR showing increased reticular density in the right mid/lower zone with lobulated pleural thickening (arrows) and right hemithoracic volume loss.

2 What is the most likely diagnosis?

Mesothelioma, in the context of his symptoms, occupational history, pleural plaques, and irregular pleural thickening on CXR. CT is the technique of choice for further assessment of the lungs and pleura and in cases of suspected malignancy (**Figure 5.5C**).

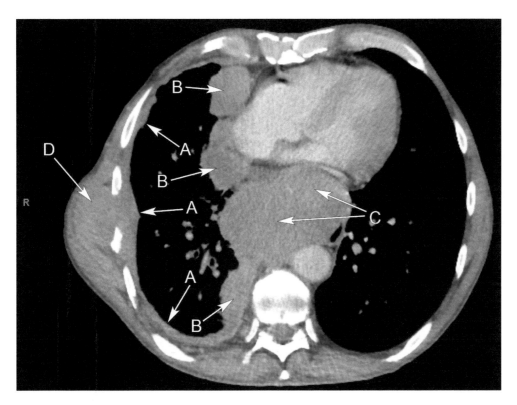

Fig. 5.5C An axial postcontrast CT section at the level of the left ventricle in another patient with mesothelioma, demonstrating pleural thickening (A) around the right hemithorax, with pleural masses (B) and enlarged subcarinal nodes (C). There is also extension of a large right pleural mass into the right chest wall (D).

Asbestos-related pleural disease can be benign or malignant:

- Benign pleural disease.
  - Pleural effusion: early sign of asbestos exposure (need to exclude underlying malignancy).
  - Diffuse pleural thickening: owing to irritation of the pleura.
  - Pleural plaques (calcified, noncalcified or hairy): following longstanding asbestos exposure (>20 years).
  - Rounded atelectasis: atypical, peripheral lung collapse adjacent to pleural plaque.
  - Asbestosis-related pulmonary fibrosis (asbestosis, predilection for lower zones).
- Malignant pleural disease.
  - Pleural mesothelioma: irregular pleural thickening owing to a primary tumour, following asbestos exposure.
  - Bronchogenic carcinoma: increased risk in smokers with history of asbestos exposure.

Pleural plaques (**Figure 5.5D**) are often reported as an incidental finding on CXR, and may calcify. They are an indication of possible asbestos exposure and in themselves do not cause any lung function impairment. Extensive pleural thickening, however, can lead to a restrictive picture causing shortness of breath. A diagnosis of pleural plaques is important as it allows patients to apply for compensation following exposure to asbestos.

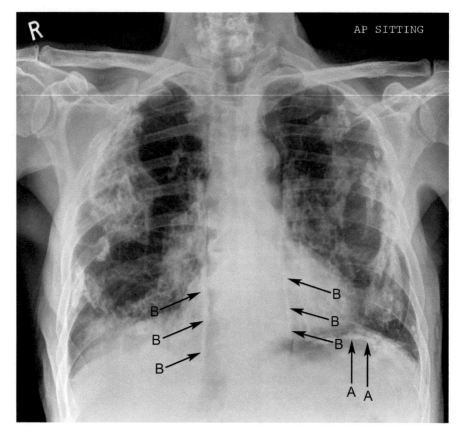

Fig. 5.5D CXR in a different patient showing widespread bilateral and symmetric calcified pleural plaques with a 'holly leaf' effect. Diaphragmatic (A) and mediastinal (B) calcified plaques are also shown.

Mesothelioma is a malignancy arising from the pleura and has a strong association with asbestos exposure (90% of cases). The lag interval from exposure to diagnosis is approximately 30–40 years and, as precautionary measures were not introduced until the 1970s, it is predicted that the prevalence of mesothelioma is likely to continue to rise for another 5–10 years.

Mesothelioma exhibits an aggressive disease progression (as indicated in **Figure 5.5C**), encasing the lung, pericardium or peritoneum depending on the tumour location. The mass infiltrates the chest wall, resulting in chest pain, despite there often being little or no bony destruction. Mesothelioma regularly metastasises through haematogenous spread. Although treatment options such as radical pneumonectomy, radiotherapy, and chemotherapy are available, the response rate is generally poor and most patients die within 2 years of diagnosis.

3 What occupational exposure might be to blame?

The most hazardous occupational exposure is contact with asbestos. Asbestos is the collective term given to a number of naturally occurring mineral silicates, which were previously used in construction for their insulating and fire resistant properties. The two main categories are:

- Serpentine asbestos fibres (white asbestos). Long flexible fibres, which are more difficult to inhale.

- Amphibole asbestos fibres (blue or brown asbestos). Short straight, brittle fibres, which penetrate deeply into lung tissues on inhalation, these are considered more hazardous to the body, and result in pleural disease.

Occupations associated with asbestos exposure include:

- Miners.
- Plumbers.
- Builders/demolition workers.
- Fire fighters.
- Dock workers.

In the 1970s, precautionary measures were introduced to limit the exposure to asbestos through the use of personal protective equipment such as respiration masks. However, owing to the long interval between asbestos exposure and development of disease, asbestos-related lung conditions are still commonly diagnosed.

LEARNING POINTS: MESOTHELIOMA AND PLEURAL PLAQUES

- Mesothelioma is a malignancy of the pleura caused by inhalation of asbestos.
- Blue and brown asbestos have been identified as the most hazardous forms.
- A diagnosis of mesothelioma should be considered in patients presenting with pleural thickening and chest discomfort.
- Mesothelioma has a poor prognosis.

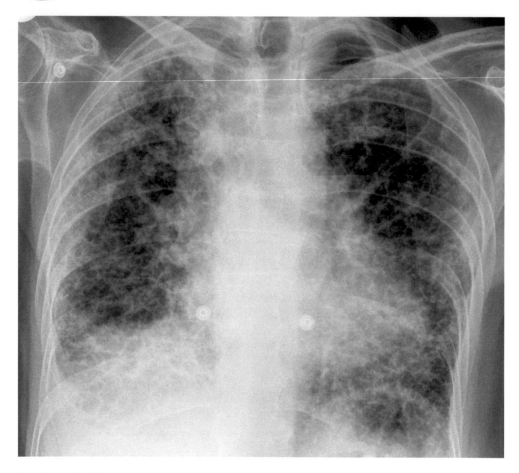

Fig. 5.6A PA CXR.

A 67-year-old male presents to his GP with ongoing shortness of breath on exertion for several months. He does not report having a cough, ankle swelling or chest pain. His past medical history is unremarkable and he does not take any regular medications. He is a retired farmer and denies having a smoking history.

On examination he is apyrexial, BP 129/72 mmHg, pulse rate 67 bpm, respiratory rate 17 bpm, and oxygen saturations 92% breathing room air. He has noticeable clubbing of his nails, jugular venous pressure is within normal limits, and heart sounds are normal. Respiratory examination reveals equal expansion of the chest wall, normal percussion, and bibasal end-inspiratory crepitations. A CXR is performed (**Figure 5.6A**).

CASE 5.6: QUESTIONS

1 What are the key radiological findings?
2 What are the possible causes for this condition?
3 What further investigations would be helpful?
4 How should this patient be further managed?

CASE 5.6: ANSWERS

1 What are the key radiological findings?

These include (**Figures 5.6B** and **5.6C**):

- Irregular reticular density throughout both lung fields.
- 'Shaggy' ill-defined cardiac borders.
- Loss of costophrenic angles bilaterally.
- Decreased lung volumes.

Reticular = 'net-like', also called interstitial, and this increase in density is caused by pathology that involves and thickens the lung interstitium (borders the air space). These appearances with history and examination findings would be consistent with interstitial pulmonary fibrosis.

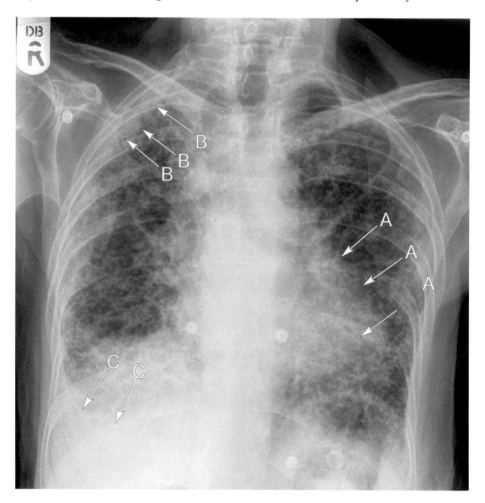

Fig. 5.6B CXR demonstrates reduced volume lungs with diffuse reticular, interstitial increase in lung density. Note the 'shaggy' irregular left heart border (A). There is additional pleural thickening in the right hemithorax (B) with right basal pleural opacity (C), which may relate to thickening or effusion.

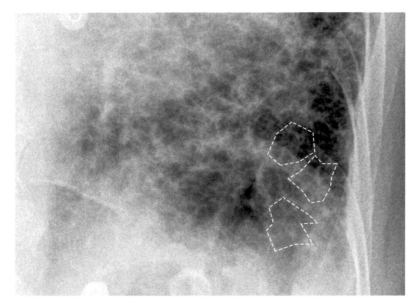

Fig. 5.6C
A magnified view of a section of lung better demonstrating the interstitial, reticular 'net-like' pattern of interstitial fibrosis (see areas highlighted).

2 What are the possible causes for this condition?

There are a large number of possible aetiologies for lung fibrosis, although often patients will present with advanced disease and the cause is unknown (idiopathic). Some diseases may involve certain parts of the lung.

Upper zones	Lower zones
Bronchopulmonary aspergillosis	**C**onnective tissue disease
Radiation	**A**sbestosis
Extrinsic allergic alveolitis	**R**heumatoid arthritis
Ankylosing spondylitis	**D**rugs (methotrexate, amiodarone)
Sarcoidosis	**AS**piration
TB	
Silicosis	

Note: Mnemonic BREASTS.   Note: Mnemonic CARDS.

Neurofibromatosis, histocytosis, and tuberose sclerosis can present with advanced disease, the so-called 'honeycomb' lung.

3 What further investigations would be helpful?

When considering a diagnosis of pulmonary fibrosis, these should include:

- Blood profile: FBC, rheumatoid factor, antinuclear antibodies, and avian precipitins.
- LFTs: a restrictive pattern will be demonstrated.
- High-resolution CT: may indicate the presence of acute inflammation ('ground-glass density'), which may indicate a potential for response to steroid treatment. CT can also be used to guide diagnostic lung biopsy in difficult cases (**Figure 5.6D**).
- Bronchoscopy with washings: lymphocytic picture is indicative of sarcoidosis.

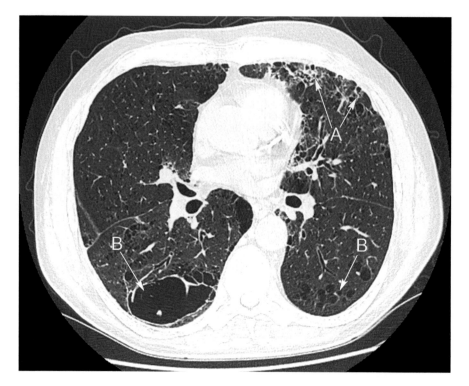

Fig. 5.6D A high-resolution CT, lung window setting, in another patient, demonstrating subpleural interstitial fibrotic changes in the left upper lobe (A) and posterior emphysematous/bullous changes (B).

4 How should this patient be further managed?

Pulmonary fibrosis is the overarching term given to a number of conditions that result in inflammation and scarring of the alveoli, distal airways, and interstitium of the lung, thus causing impaired gas diffusion and shortness of breath. It most commonly affects older men in their seventh decade of life who have been exposed to environmental dusts such as metal and wood dust. Idiopathic pulmonary fibrosis is the commonest subtype.

Treatment is dependent on the cause but steroids and other immunosuppressants, such as pirfenidone, can often be used to reduce inflammation and relieve symptoms. If the cause is a drug reaction it is important to stop the offending drug. Pulmonary fibrosis patients have an increased risk of developing lung cancer if they have a smoking background, and cessation advice should be provided.

> **LEARNING POINTS: PULMONARY FIBROSIS**
>
> - Pulmonary fibrosis is the term given to inflammation and scarring of the alveoli, distal airways and interstitium of the lung.
> - Causes of upper zone pulmonary fibrosis can be remembered using the mnemonic 'BREASTS'; lower zone 'CARDS'.
> - Investigations include lung function tests and high-resolution CT.
> - Idiopathic pulmonary fibrosis is the most common subtype.
> - Steroids and immunosuppressive agents can be used to relieve symptoms.

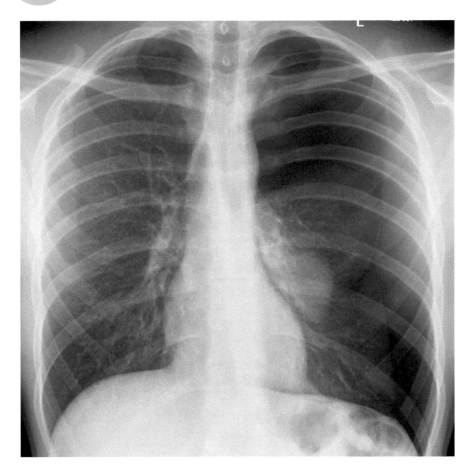

Fig. 5.7A PA CXR.

A 26-year-old male presents to the ED complaining of sudden onset of left-sided chest pain, which is worse on deep inspiration and is associated with shortness of breath. He is usually fit and well, and does not report a cough.

On examination he is not distressed but is mildly short of breath. He is apyrexial, has a BP of 108/76 mmHg, heart rate of 89 bpm, respiratory rate of 19 bpm, and oxygen saturations of 94% breathing room air. He has a central trachea, reduced expansion, and increased resonance on percussion of the left side. There is also reduced air entry on auscultation and reduced vocal resonance on the left. A CXR has been performed portably in the department (**Figure 5.7A**).

CASE 5.7: QUESTIONS

1 What key radiological findings are demonstrated?
2 What is the likely diagnosis?
3 How should this patient be managed?
4 What information should this patient be provided with on discharge?

CASE 5.7: ANSWERS

1 What key radiological findings are demonstrated?

Key findings are (**Figure 5.7B**):

- Large left-sided pneumothorax with a large air-filled pleural space and loss of lung markings in the left hemithorax.
- Collapse of the left lung with a visible 'pleural line' (arrows).
- Mild mediastinal shift to the right suggesting the pneumothorax is under tension.

A pneumothorax is the presence of air in the pleural space. Air enters the pleural space through a hole in the soft tissues and causes pressure to build in the intrapleural space, resulting in progressive collapse of the lung.

Young patients are often able to compensate for a large pneumothorax for a long period of time before becoming unwell quickly, requiring urgent intervention.

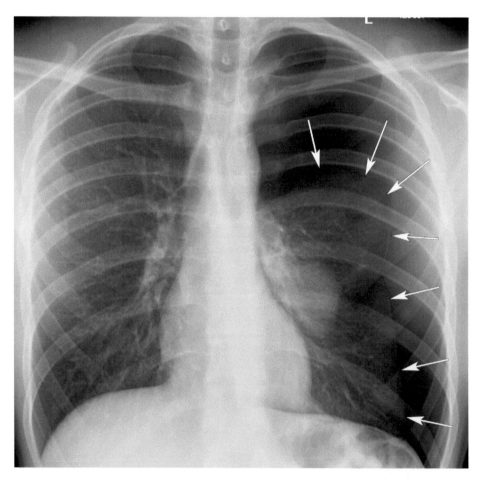

Fig. 5.7B CXR showing a left-sided pneumothorax; the margin of the collapsed left lung is shown (arrows).

2 What is the likely diagnosis?

A spontaneous primary pneumothorax with an element of tension. Pneumothoraces are classified as:

- Spontaneous.
  - Primary: in the absence of lung disease.
  - Secondary: in the presence of lung disease, such as COPD or cystic fibrosis.
- Tension.
  - Medical emergency.
  - Air enters the pleural space during each inspiration but is unable to leave as the pleural tear acts as a one-way valve.
  - Intrapleural pressure increases causing the lung to collapse and venous return to be impaired.
  - Commonest causes include thoracic trauma (rib fractures, stab wounds) and positive pressure ventilation.
- Iatrogenic: following central line insertion or biopsy.

3 How should this patient be managed?

The initial management of this patient should involve an ABCDE assessment to ensure resuscitation and stabilisation of the patient with administration of oxygen.

Tension pneumothorax is a medical emergency, and patients should be assessed immediately. If a tension pneumothorax is apparent clinically and the patient is showing signs of distress, they should undergo aspiration of the pneumothorax under senior guidance, before proceeding to chest drain insertion. Do not wait for a CXR in these cases: if unsure ask for an urgent portable radiograph in A/E so the patient can be observed.

Following these initial steps the management should be according to local/national guidelines:
- Primary pneumothorax.
  - >2 cm* and/or respiratory distress → aspirate with large bore cannula and review.
  - <2 cm and/or no respiratory distress → no intervention, consider discharge and review in 2–4 weeks.
- Secondary pneumothorax.
  - >2 cm and/or respiratory distress → admit for insertion of a chest drain.
  - 1–2 cm → aspirate with large bore cannula and review.
  - <1 cm → admit for high-flow oxygen (unless contraindicated) and observation for 24 hours.
- Tension pneumothorax.
  - If suspected do not wait for a CXR, it is a clinical diagnosis.
  - Immediate aspiration with a large bore cannula.
  - Definitive management by inserting a chest drain.

Note: 2 cm* refers to the measurement of the intrapleural distance at the level of the hilum.

If there is no improvement in the pneumothorax following aspiration then a chest drain should be inserted.

A chest drain is inserted into the pleural cavity to allow drainage of air in the context of a pneumothorax. Effective drainage requires adequate positioning of the drain with an air-tight, one-way seal to maintain subatmospheric pressure, allowing re-expansion of the lung. An aseptic technique should be used within a sterile field. Local anaesthetic must be infiltrated with sufficient time for good effect. Chest drains can be inserted using the Seldinger technique, which incorporates the use of a guide wire and dilator system over which the chest drain is passed, or via an open surgical incision (thoracostomy). Chest drains should be inserted into the 'safe triangle'.

Borders of the 'safe triangle':

- Medially – lateral border of pectoralis major.
- Laterally – anterior axillary line.
- Inferiorly – 4th to 5th intercostal space.

Once the drain is positioned adequately it should be connected to a closed drainage system using an underwater seal acting as a one-way valve to prevent re-entry of air into the pleural space during inspiration. Application of an airtight dressing follows this.

Post drain insertion:

- Monitor for oscillation/swinging of the underwater seal during inspiration to ensure the drain is patent.
- Repeat CXR to confirm the position of the drain and determine re-expansion of the lung (**Figure 5.7C**).

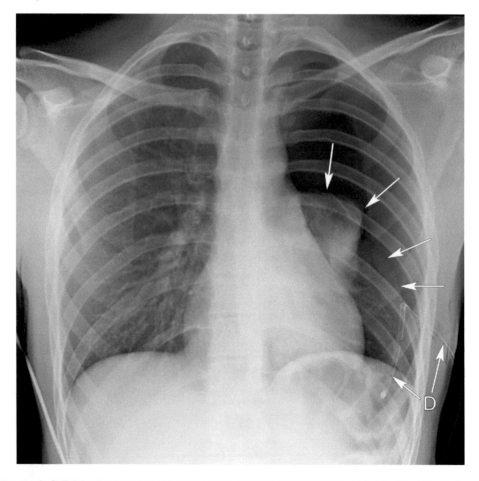

Fig. 5.7C CXR following insertion of a small-calibre drain (D) into the left pleural space. The left-sided pneumothorax remains (lung edge, arrows), the mediastinal shift has resolved.

4 What information should this patient be provided with on discharge?

The patient should be advised of the following:

- To return to hospital immediately if their symptoms deteriorate ('safety netting').
- The chance of a recurrent pneumothorax on the same side is 50%.
- Smoking increases the risk of further pneumothoraces.
- Air travel should not be undertaken until 1 week following resolution of the pneumothorax on CXR.
- Underwater diving cannot be undertaken unless preventative surgery has been performed.

LEARNING POINTS: PNEUMOTHORAX

- A pneumothorax is defined as the presence of air in the pleural space.
- Primary pneumothorax (absence of lung disease), secondary pneumothorax (presence of underlying lung disease).
- Tension pneumothorax is a medical emergency, diagnosed clinically, CXR should not delay aspiration.
- Treatment is based on the 2 cm rule, using aspiration +/– chest drain insertion.
- Chest drains should be inserted into the 'safe triangle'.

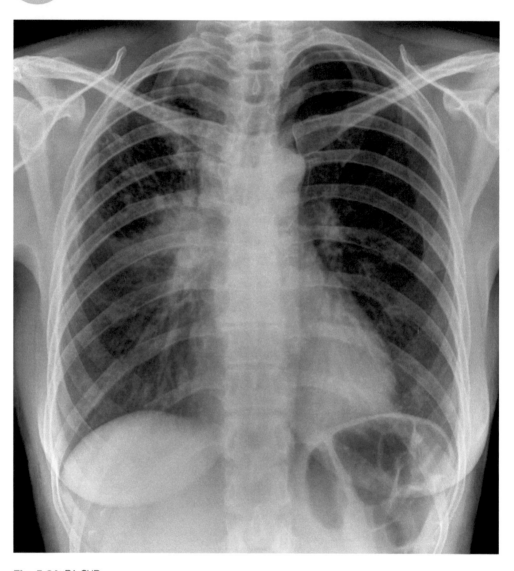

Fig. 5.8A PA CXR.

A 28-year-old female migrant from Somalia who has been resident in the UK for 2 months is referred to the respiratory clinic by her GP. She has a 4-month history of a cough, which is associated with purulent sputum and is occasionally streaked with blood. She reports some shortness of breath when she climbs the stairs but no chest pain, fevers or night sweats. Over the last 2 weeks she also reports feeling more tired than usual and has been experiencing a loss of appetite.

On examination she appears well and is apyrexial, with a normal BP and pulse rate. Respiratory rate is 16 bpm and oxygen saturations are 97% breathing room air; there is no palpable lymph-adenopathy. Respiratory examination reveals equal expansion and air entry, normal percussion sounds, and some coarse crepitations anteriorly on the right. A CXR has been performed (**Figure 5.8A**).

CASE 5.8: QUESTIONS

1 What radiological features are demonstrated?
2 What is the most likely diagnosis?
3 What investigations should be performed?
4 What is the management of this patient?
5 What are the extrathoracic manifestations of this condition?
6 Is there a facility in place to prevent this condition?

CASE 5.8: ANSWERS

1 What radiological features are demonstrated?

Radiological features (**Figure 5.8B**):

- Nodular infiltrates in the right upper zone.
- Right hilar mass.
- Right paratracheal nodes.
- Apical consolidation.

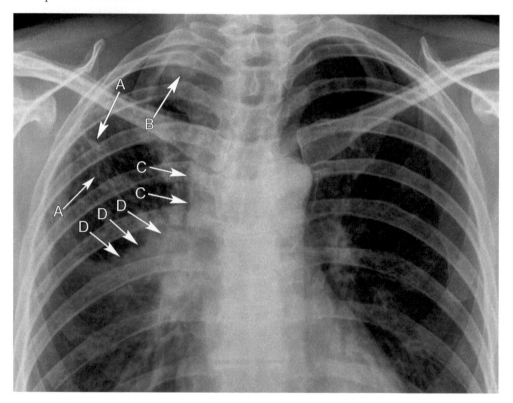

Fig. 5.8B Magnified CXR demonstrating nodular infiltrates in the right upper zone (A) with apical consolidation (B), right paratracheal nodes (C), and right hilar nodes (D).

2 What is the most likely diagnosis?

Primary tuberculosis (TB) is most likely. TB is a notifiable disease and its prevalence in the UK is increasing. The causative agent is *Mycobacterium tuberculosis*; however, atypical mycobacteria should be considered in immunosuppressed patients or those with pre-existing lung conditions. Atypical mycobacteria include *Mycobacterium avium* complex (MAC) and *Mycobacterium kansaii*.

Stages of TB are defined as:

- Primary TB.
  - Initial lesion, which is normally solitary, located in the upper or middle zones of the lung.
  - The focus of the primary infection is called the Ghon focus.

- Secondary TB (postprimary TB).
  - Reactivation of primary TB or reinfection.
  - Usually bilateral cavitating lung lesions.
- Miliary tuberculosis (**Figure 5.8C**).
  - Acute, diffuse dissemination of tubercle bacilli ('millet seed' size) via haematogenous spread.
  - Formation of small granulomas in other organs.
  - A result of either primary or secondary TB, usually fatal without treatment.

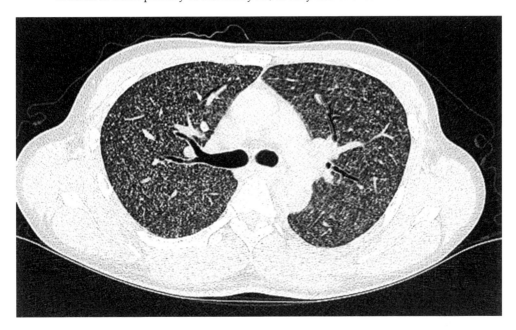

Fig. 5.8C Axial CT image at the level of the carina using lung window setting, demonstrating multiple tiny lung nodules, consistent with miliary TB. Differential diagnoses include sarcoid and metastases.

3 What investigations should be performed?

Patients suspected of having TB who require admission to hospital must be treated in an isolated environment. Those who can be treated at home must be advised to wear a mask to ensure protection for others coming into contact with the patient.

A CXR must be performed in those suspected of having TB. Cavitating apical lung lesions are characteristic of TB but are not diagnostic as other conditions may demonstrate a similar appearance, such as lung malignancy, Wegener's granulomatosis, and rheumatoid nodules. In this patient the combination of upper lobe infiltrates with mediastinal lymphadenopathy is highly suggestive of TB.

Sequential sputum samples should be obtained over at least 3 consecutive days and sent to the microbiology laboratory for Ziehl–Neelsen (ZN) staining, a method used to identify acid-and-alcohol fast bacilli (AAFB). Cultures have a higher sensitivity than staining sputum; however, it may take up to 8 weeks for a positive culture and a further 2 weeks for antibiotic sensitivity testing. If sputum samples cannot be obtained, alternatives such as bronchial washings or biopsies, can be used. Pleural fluid aspiration is also appropriate if a pleural effusion is present.

DNA techniques using polymerase chain reaction (PCR) are available in some specialist centres. These techniques have a similar sensitivity rate to culture and results are available within days; however, this technique is much more expensive.

4 What is the management of this patient?

The majority of patients are treated in an outpatient setting using a combination therapy (mnemonic RIPE) outlined below. All four antibacterial drugs are given for the first 2 months of initial therapy and two are given for a further 4 months in the continuation phase. All drugs are given once daily:

- **R**ifampicin (6 months).
- **I**soniazid (6 months).
- **P**yrazinamide (2 months).
- **E**thambutol (2 months).

Supervision of treatment is essential and patients should be reviewed on a monthly basis to ensure they are compliant. Poor compliance is a major cause of treatment failure and directly observed therapy should be considered in patients who are likely to have difficulty adhering to the treatment regime. This can also help in the prevention of drug-resistant TB.

5 What are the extrathoracic manifestations of this condition?

TB can occur in most organs, including the skin, kidney, adrenal glands, and bone. In the brain, TB can lead to meningitis or tuberculoma formation (a space-occupying lesion). In the adrenal glands, TB can cause primary adrenocortical insufficiency and must be considered as an underlying cause in a new diagnosis of Addison's disease.

6 Is there a facility in place to prevent this condition?

Prevention of TB is facilitated by the Bacille Calmette–Guérin (BCG) vaccine, prepared using attenuated live *Mycobacterium bovis*. The vaccine was previously offered to schoolchildren aged 12–13 years in the UK; however, this vaccination programme has now ceased. The vaccine is now given to individuals and neonates from high-risk groups, such as migrants and those with a family history of TB. Immunisation has been shown to decrease the risk of developing TB by 60–80%. Effectiveness of the vaccine varies and is dependent on genetic differences in the population, environmental factors, and exposure to other infections.

LEARNING POINTS: TUBERCULOSIS

- Causative agent is *Mycobacterium tuberculosis*.
- Stages of TB: primary, secondary, and miliary.
- Investigations include CXR, ZN staining, and sputum cultures.
- Treatment is with 'RIPE'.
- Extrapleural manifestations of TB can cause other disease processes, such as meningitis and Addison's disease.

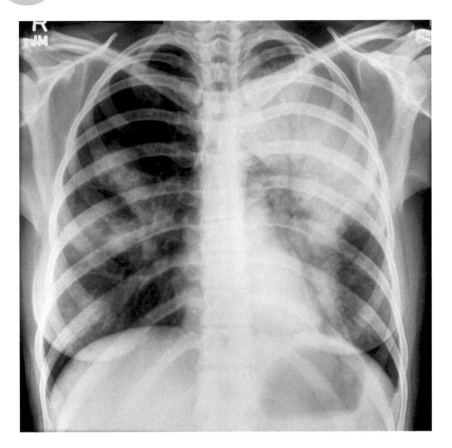

Fig. 5.9A PA CXR.

A 35-year-old female presents to the ED with a 2-week history of a productive cough with green purulent sputum, shortness of breath, and fever. She is a nonsmoker with a past medical history of asthma, which is well controlled with both short- and long-acting bronchodilators and a steroid inhaler.

On examination she appears clammy, has cold peripheries, and a capillary refill time of 4 seconds. She has a temperature of 38.3°C, BP 102/65 mmHg, pulse rate of 105 bpm, respiratory rate 24 bpm, and oxygen saturations 91% breathing room air. Respiratory examination reveals a central trachea with reduced expansion on the left, dullness to percussion in the left upper zone with reduced air entry and crepitations on auscultation. An urgent CXR is performed (**Figure 5.9A**).

CASE 5.9: QUESTIONS

1 What are the key radiological findings?
2 What is the most likely diagnosis?
3 What are the possible causes for this condition?
4 Name a scoring system used to determine the severity of this condition.

CASE 5.9: ANSWERS

1 What are the key radiological findings?

Key radiological findings include (**Figure 5.9B**):

- Extensive consolidation in the upper lobe of the left lung.
- Infiltrates in the middle zone of the right lung.
- Air bronchograms on the left.

Mnemonic for remembering the features of consolidation (A2BC2):

- **A**ir bronchograms – air-filled bronchi made visible by the opacification of surrounding alveoli.
- **A**cinar rosettes.
- **B**at wing appearance (bilateral, symmetrical changes, more common in pulmonary oedema, **Figure 5.9C**).
- **C**onsolidation (diffuse, segmental/lobar).
- **C**onfluent ill-defined (fluffy) appearance.

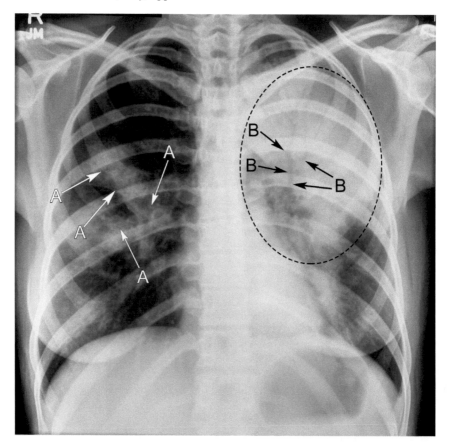

Fig. 5.9B CXR showing a large area of consolidation in the left upper lobe (dashed circle), containing air bronchograms (B) and right-sided infiltrates (A).

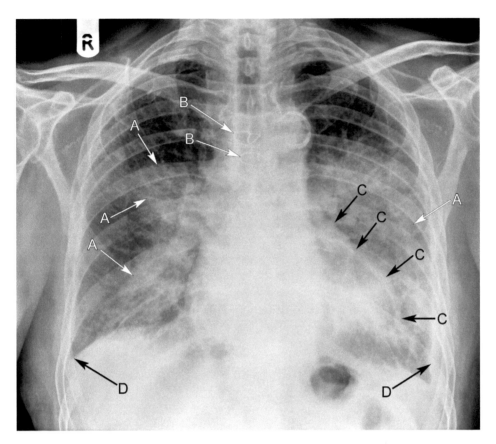

Fig. 5.9C CXR of a different patient demonstrating symmetrical, bilateral, and perihilar consolidation (A) suggestive of pulmonary oedema. Note the sternotomy wires (B) and ill-defined left heart border (C) and small bilateral basal pleural effusions (D).

2 What is the most likely diagnosis?

Consolidation is a nonspecific radiological sign, therefore the history, examination, and review of previous CXRs are very important. The most likely diagnosis given the history of purulent sputum, pyrexia, and large area of consolidation on CXR is a lobar pneumonia of the left upper lobe, with focal changes seen in the right lung also.

Causes for a consolidated appearance include:

- Pus (infection), as in this case.
- Blood (trauma, bleeding diathesis).
- Tumour (lung cancer).
- Water (pulmonary oedema) **(Figure 5.9C)**.

3 What are the possible causes for this condition?

The most common organism seen in community-acquired pneumonia is *Streptococcus pneumoniae*; however, pneumonia can be caused by other typical and atypical organisms shown in *Table 5.9A*.

Table 5.9A Organisms associated with pneumonia

Typical organisms	Atypical organisms
Streptococcus pneumoniae	Mycoplasma pneumoniae
Haemophilus infuenzae	Legionella pneumophila
Moraxella catarrhalis	Chlamydia spp. (C. pneumoniae)
Influenza A	Coxiella burnetii

4 Name a scoring system used to determine the severity of this condition.

CURB-65 score (*Table 5.9B*) can be used to determine the severity of pneumonia and the most appropriate setting for treatment, scoring 1 point for each positive category:

- **C**onfusion: new onset mini mental test score <8.
- **U**rea >7 mmol/L.
- **R**espiratory rate ≥30 bpm.
- **B**lood pressure ≤90 mmHg systolic and/or ≤60 mmHg diastolic.
- Age ≥**65** years.

Table 5.9B CURB-65 score used to determine the severity of pneumonia

CURB-65 Score	Severity	Appropriate treatment location
0 or 1	Mild	Community
2	Moderate	Hospital – short stay
3 or more	Severe	Hospital – consider ITU

Other features that should be taken into consideration when determining the most appropriate location for treatment include:

- Co-morbidities: particularly lung conditions (COPD, asthma, cystic fibrosis).
- Involvement of more than one lobe or a bilateral picture.
- Hypoxia requiring oxygen therapy (P_aO_2 <8 kPa or Sats <92%).

Treatment for moderate and severe pneumonia is with IV antibiotics, usually a penicillin and macrolide combination to cover typical and atypical organisms. Less severe pneumonia is treated with oral antibiotics according to local hospital protocol.

Patients require a follow-up CXR after 6 weeks to ensure there is substantial resolution of the consolidation. If signs of consolidation remain, further investigations may be warranted to ensure there is not an underlying malignancy.

LEARNING POINTS: PNEUMONIC CONSOLIDATION

- Features of consolidation can be remembered with mnemonic A2BC2.
- Differential diagnoses include infection, pleural effusion, and congestive cardiac failure.
- Most likely organism causing community-acquired pneumonia is *Streptococcus pneumoniae*.
- Consider atypical organisms or alternative diagnosis if not responding to treatment.
- Repeat CXR after 6 weeks to ensure resolution.

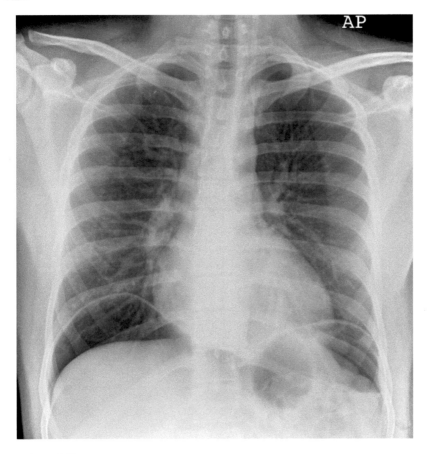

AP

Fig. 5.10A Erect CXR.

A 54-year-old male presents to the ED with abdominal pain, nausea, and having vomited once. He has had recent epigastric discomfort for which he has been taking over-the-counter medication but is otherwise fit and well. He has a history of abdominal surgery following a road traffic accident 30 years ago.

On examination, he is lying still on his back, in pain but alert and orientated. He is tachycardic at 110 bpm and hypotensive at 110/76 mmHg but apyrexial at 36.4°C. His abdomen is mildly distended and rigid with generalised tenderness with rebound tenderness and guarding throughout. Bowel sounds are quiet.

A supine AXR and erect CXR (**Figure 5.10A**) are arranged. The AXR (not shown) demonstrates no acute abnormality.

CASE 5.10: QUESTIONS

1 What is the key radiological finding demonstrated on the CXR?

2 What is the likely diagnosis?

3 Is further imaging required?

4 How would you manage this patient?

CASE 5.10: ANSWERS

1 What is the key radiological finding demonstrated on the CXR?

The key abnormality on the erect CXR is presence of free air beneath the diaphragm (**Figure 5.10B**). This is indicative of free intraperitoneal gas, otherwise known as pneumoperitoneum. An erect CXR is the most sensitive XR method of detecting free intraperitoneal air, as air rises to lie beneath the diaphragm. It is important that patients sit up for several minutes prior to the erect CXR to allow time for the air to migrate. A good quality erect CXR can detect as little as 1 cc of free air, with AXR being relatively insensitive. Occasionally 'Rigler's sign' can be seen on AXR; this is also known as the double wall sign and indicates air on both sides of the intestinal wall. Common causes of free intraperitoneal air are shown in *Table 5.10A*.

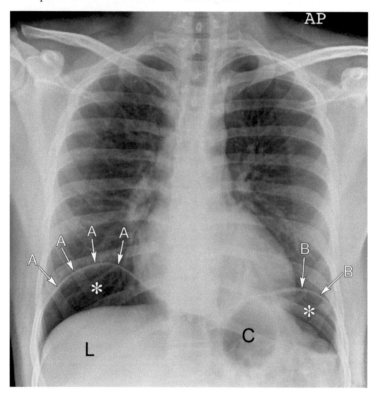

Fig. 5.10B Erect CXR showing a large amount of free subdiaphragmatic air (*). This is seen overlying the liver on the right (L) beneath the right hemidiaphragm (A) and beneath the left hemidiaphragm (B) in the LUQ where it is distinguishable from the gastric bubble (C). Note absent splenic density in the LUQ likely to relate to previous splenectomy.

Table 5.10A Common causes of free intraperitoneal air

- Perforated peptic ulcer
- Perforation following bowel obstruction
- Perforated diverticulitis/appendicitis
- Recent abdominal surgery
- Peritoneal dialysis

TOP TIPS

- When asked in a practical exam a question such as 'What are the causes of free intraperitoneal air?' use a surgical sieve (with a mnemonic such as VITAMIN D) to ensure that you do not forget anything.
- VITAMIN D: **V**ascular, **I**nfection/**I**nflammatory, **T**rauma, **A**utoimmune, **M**etabolic, **I**atrogenic/**I**diopathic, **N**eoplastic, **D**egenerative.
- Alternatively, remember the most common causes and list them in order with the ability to talk a little about each.
- You do not have to have a cause in each of the categories, just use it as an aide memoire for causes when under pressure.

2 What is the likely diagnosis?

The clinical and XR findings indicate a perforated viscus, most likely a gastric or duodenal ulcer in this patient (note: history of epigastric discomfort). Other causes of perforated viscus include diverticulitis, bowel obstruction, and ischaemic bowel, although the clinical findings in this case are not suggestive of these entities. A nonpathological finding of free subdiaphragmatic gas is also sometimes seen following recent laparoscopic surgery or peritoneal dialysis. A more subtle case of subdiaphragmatic free air is shown in **Figure 5.10C**. A mimic of subdiaphragmatic free air is shown in **Figure 5.10D.**

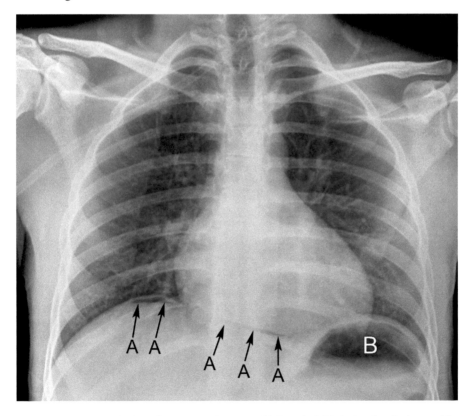

Fig. 5.10C A more subtle finding of pneumoperitoneum with free air visible below the diaphragm (A). Normal gastric bubble (B).

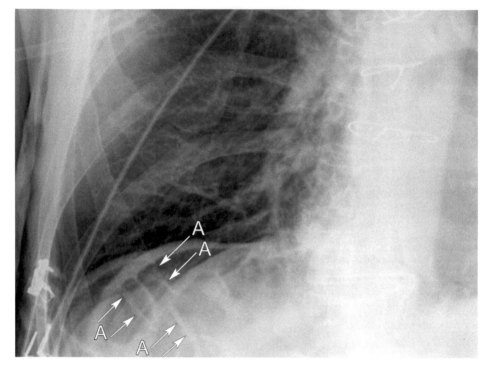

Fig. 5.10D Magnified X-ray of the chest right lower zone shows small bowel loops interposed between the right hemidiaphragm and the liver. Bowel loops are distinguishable from free intraperitoneal air by the presence of valvulae conniventes (A). This is 'Chilaiditi's sign' and an important mimic of free air.

TOP TIPS

Know a little about each major cause of free intraperitoneal air and be able to talk for 2 minutes about each.

For example, peptic ulcers are associated with the use of nonsteroidal anti-inflammatory drugs (NSAIDs), steroids, aspirin, and gastro-oesophageal reflux disease. Perforation occurs when the ulcer erodes through the full thickness of the gut wall and the gastric contents spill into the peritoneum causing peritonitis and free intraperitoneal air. The most frequent site of perforation is the anterior wall of the first part of the duodenum. Posterior duodenal perforation is more likely to result in haematemesis owing to gastroduodenal artery involvement. Longstanding peptic ulcers can result in obstruction due to fibrosis or oedema.

---

3 Is further imaging required?

In cases where the diagnosis is uncertain and where patient condition allows, a CT scan may be helpful. This will/can confirm the diagnosis and help guide surgical management. CT is highly accurate and extremely sensitive in the detection of free intraperitoneal air and also in demonstrating the likely aetiology. It is particularly useful in elderly patients who often have relatively nonspecific symptoms and signs.

In patients with clear clinical findings and free intraperitoneal air on erect CXR, urgent senior surgical opinion should be requested.

4 How would you manage this patient?

Initial management follows an ABCDE approach (*Table 5.10B*) as these patients are often particularly unwell and in severe pain. Early senior support should be sought in each case (this is very important to mention in the exam situation). Resuscitation with IV fluids to maintain blood pressure and cardiac monitoring is necessary. Pain control is usually by IV opiates. The definitive management is surgical once the diagnosis is confirmed by a senior surgeon.

Table 5.10B Initial management of patient with free intraperitoneal air

Be able to discuss the ABCDE approach to initial management

Airway (is the patient talking? Use of adjuncts if necessary)

Breathing (central trachea, RR, O_2 sats, listen, percuss, equal expansion?)

Circulation (HR, BP, IV access, bloods, ABG, fluids, ECG)

Disability (AVPU: alert, voice, pain, unresponsive, GCS, pupils)

Exposure (abdomen, genitalia, legs, sacral/peripheral oedema, glucose)

In an OSCE scenario, a CXR will be given that shows obvious free intraperitoneal air. Once you have recognised this, the examiner will want to know how you will manage the patient. Depending on how unwell the patient is, always start with ABCDE then say you would take a full history and examine the patient. Following on from this, bloods are necessary (say which bloods you need and why – ensure to include clotting and group, and save as this is a patient likely to need surgery). An ABG or VBG is often very helpful in these situations as it is an indicator of how unwell a patient is and whether senior ITU support is necessary. You will ALWAYS need to inform a senior colleague and ask for their advice/support.

TOP TIPS

ALWAYS ask for senior support and mention this in the OSCE.

It may be helpful to know a little about the type of surgery to be performed (open or laparoscopic gastrectomy or vagotomy) but the examiners will not expect you to go into any detail. It is most important to recognise from the history, examination, and test results that this patient is unwell and to discuss the immediate management.

LEARNING POINTS: FREE INTRAPERITONEAL AIR

- When examining a peritonitic abdomen it is important to obtain an erect CXR to look for signs of bowel perforation, usually in combination with a supine AXR.
- Erect CXR is the most sensitive type of radiograph in the detection of free intra-abdominal air.
- Pneumoperitoneum can be subtle on CXR and therefore a CT scan may be indicated for definitive diagnosis but always ask for senior advice at an early stage.
- The most common causes of pathological pneumoperitoneum are perforation of bowel (i.e. secondary to a peptic ulcer, diverticulitis or appendicitis) or it can be a normal finding up to 10 days following laparoscopic surgery.

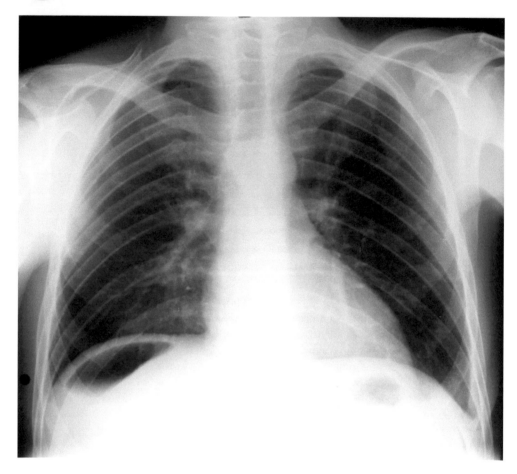

Fig. 5.11A Erect CXR.

A 25-year-old male is readmitted through the ED 2 weeks following a laparoscopic appendicectomy for a perforated appendix. He has severe RUQ and shoulder tip pain, has vomited, and is feeling feverish.

On examination he looks flushed but is alert and orientated. He has RUQ tenderness but his abdomen is soft and not distended. Per rectum (PR) exam reveals soft brown stool. He is hypotensive at 90/63 mmHg, tachycardic at 110bpm, tachypnoeic at 25 bpm, and febrile at 38.8°C. An erect CXR is arranged initially (**Figure 5.11A**). Bloods are perfomed:

Hb	106 g/L (130–180 g/L)	K+	3.7 mmol/L (3.2–5.1 mmol/L)
WBC	22 × 10⁹/L (4.0–11.0 × 10⁹/L)	Urea	6.2 mmol/L (1.7–8.3 mmol/L)
CRP	266 mg/L (<5 mg/L)	Creatinine	90 mmol/L (62–106 mmol/L)
Na+	138 mmol/L (135–146 mmol/L)	Lactate	4.2 mmol/L (0.5–2.2 mmol/L)

CASE 5.11: QUESTIONS

1 What is the main radiological finding?
2 What are your differential diagnoses?
3 How would you confirm the diagnosis?
4 How would you manage this patient?

CASE 5.11: ANSWERS

1 What is the main radiological finding?

The CXR shows a large loculation of gas under the right hemidiaphragm (**Figure 5.11B**). The loculation outlines a thickened hemidiaphragm and overlies a hazy looking superior liver edge indicating free fluid. There appears to be an air–fluid level within the collection. There are no bowel wall markings or signs elsewhere of pneumoperitoneum. The appearances are therefore consistent with a large subphrenic abscess.

- The difficulty here lies with differentiating this from free intraperitoneal air. The hemidiaphragm thickening and air–fluid level are the most useful signs.
- Other signs that may be visible on CXR in a patient with a subphrenic abscess include a raised hemidiaphragm, fluid within the ipsilateral costophrenic angle, and collapse or consolidation at the lung base.
- Additionally, the raised inflammatory markers and high lactate indicate that the patient is septic and has likely developed a postoperative abdominal infection.

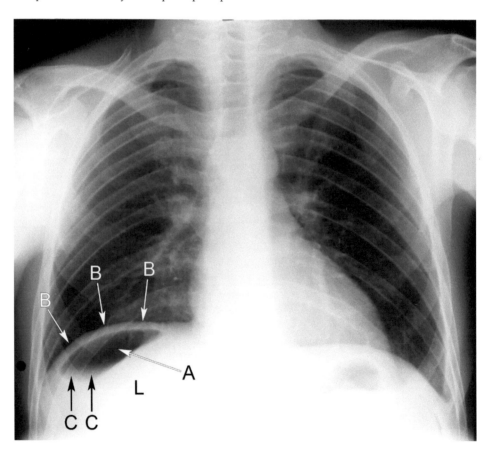

Fig. 5.11B Erect CXR showing a large gas loculation (A) under the thickened right hemidiaphragm (B) overlying the liver (L). There is an air–fluid level within the collection (C). Note the lack of valvulae conniventes (small bowel) or haustral (large bowel) markings.

2 What are your differential diagnoses?

The history suggests either postoperative perforation or infection causing an abscess and diaphragmatic irritation with referred pain to the shoulder. Normal postlaparoscopic intraperitoneal air would be unlikely at 2 weeks post surgery.

Knowing a few key points about abscess formation within the abdomen will get you marks in an exam situation:

- A subphrenic abscess develops due to accumulation of fluid between the diaphragm and the liver or spleen, which becomes infected.
- The abscess can be simple or complex (multiloculated).
- Abdominal abscesses are most common in the subphrenic, subhepatic, pelvic, and paracolic gutter locations.
- The symptoms and signs are location dependent but usually include fever, pain, and diarrhoea or ileus.
- Subphrenic abscesses can cause diaphragmatic irritation and referred shoulder tip pain.
- They may complicate abdominal surgery, often originally associated with peritonitis, and usually present 2–3 weeks following surgery.

3 How would you confirm the diagnosis?

Further imaging would be necessary to confirm the diagnosis of a subphrenic abscess. In an emergency setting, US can identify large collections or the presence of fluid or air within the peritoneal cavity; however, a CT scan is more sensitive (**Figure 5.11C**). CT is also useful in guiding percutaneous drainage.

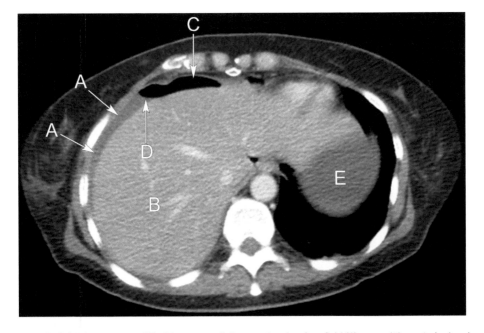

Fig. 5.11C Axial postcontrast CT of the upper abdomen showing free fluid (A) around the anterior border of the liver (B). A pocket of free gas (C) has risen to the superior antidependent aspect of the peritoneal cavity (the patient is lying on his back) and an air–fluid level is seen (D). This is a subphrenic fluid and gas collection. Stomach (E).

4 How would you manage this patient?

Initial management would be via an ABCDE approach as the patient is clinically septic. It would be necessary to start analgesia, IV fluid resuscitation, and IV antibiotics following blood cultures. Antibiotic choice should follow the local trust guidelines but should include broad-spectrum enteric and anaerobic cover.

Calling for senior help at an early point is important and clearly mention this in the exam. The on-call surgical team should be informed and it is also good practice to inform the surgeon who performed the original operation.

Definitive management may be conservative, interventional or surgical:

- If the patient is not septic or particularly unwell, antibiotic therapy may be sufficient to clear the abscess.
- If the abscess needs draining then an interventional radiologist may be able to do this percutaneously.
- If the patient is too unwell or the abscess unsuitable for percutaneous drainage, then the patient may need a full abdominal washout and surgical drainage.

The important point in cases like this is to recognise that the patient is unwell. Remember to mention the following points in management:

- ABCDE, bloods, blood cultures, monitoring, analgesia, antibiotics, and resuscitation. If bloods are not included in the exam case history then inform the examiner what blood tests you would perform and why.
- Full history and examination.
- Inform a senior colleague.
- Further imaging to confirm diagnosis.
- Definitive management is surgery or radiological drainage in some cases.

LEARNING POINTS: SUBPHRENIC ABSCESS

- Subphrenic abscess on CXR: look for a well-defined collection with an air–fluid level beneath a thickened hemidiaphragm.
- Be able to differentiate this from pneumoperitoneum and bowel loops.
- A subphrenic abscess can develop following peritonitis and complicated abdominal surgery. It is an important consideration in a patient who improves postoperatively but deteriorates 2–3 weeks later.
- A CT scan is useful for confirming the diagnosis and for treatment planning.

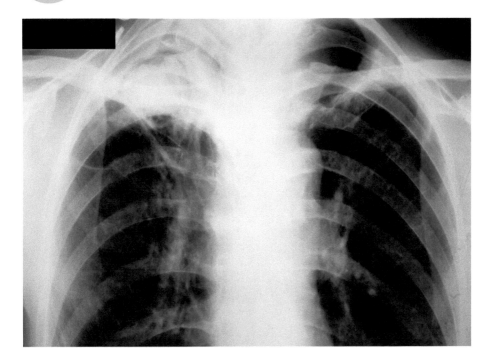

Fig. 5.12A Magnified CXR view of the upper lung zones.

An 82-year-old male presents to the ED with a 6-week history of productive cough with yellow sputum, occasionally bloodstained, associated with wheeze and shortness of breath. He is an ex-smoker, with a past medical history of asthma for which he takes a short-acting bronchodilator. He is a keen gardener in his spare time.

On examination he is apyrexial, BP 132/76 mmHg, pulse rate 87 bpm, respiratory rate 19 bpm, and oxygen saturation 94% breathing room air. Respiratory examination reveals equal expansion of the chest wall, dullness to percussion in the right apex with associated coarse crepitations anteriorly on the right.

A CXR is requested (**Figure 5.12A**) and bloods are performed:

Hb	139 g/L (130–180 g/L)	Platelets	328 × 10⁹/L (150–450 × 10⁹/L)
WCC	12.8 × 10⁹/L (4.0–11.0 × 10⁹/L)	U&Es	Normal
Neutrophils	8.4 × 10⁹/L (2.0–7.5 × 10⁹/L)	LFTs	Normal
Eosinophils	2.8 × 10⁹/L (0–0.4 × 10⁹/L)	CRP	106 mg/L (<5 mg/L)

CASE 5.12: QUESTIONS

1 What are the key radiological findings?
2 What are the differential diagnoses in this case?
3 What treatment should be initiated for this gentleman?
4 Discuss the spectrum of lung involvement that may be associated with this condition.

CASE 5.12: ANSWERS

1 What are the key radiological findings?

Key findings (**Figure 5.12B**) include:

- Scarring of the left apex.
- Opacity in the right apex and volume loss, with elevated right hilum.
- There is a curvilinear lucent halo present within the right apical opacity.
- Note also calcified lung granulomata indicative of likely previous tuberculous infection.

This is the pathognomonic appearance of cavitation around a fungus ball that has formed in an old area of right upper lobe lung scarring, usually due to previous TB. The main differential diagnosis is malignancy. Another example is given in **Figure 5.12C**.

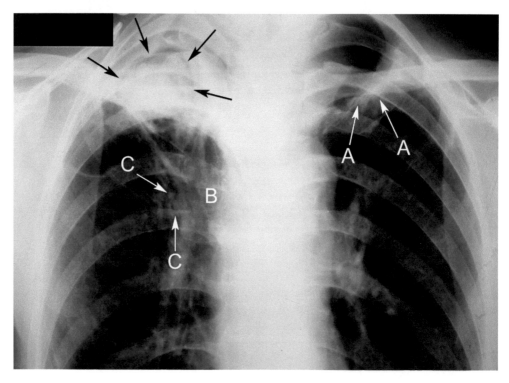

Fig. 5.12B Magnified CXR view of the upper lung zones with arrows delineating a lucent halo within the right apical lung mass. Left apical scarring (A), right hilum (B), which is elevated indicative of right upper lobe volume loss and scarring, calcified granulomata (C).

2 What are the differential diagnoses in this case?

The following differential diagnoses should be considered in this case:

- Mycetoma or pulmonary aspergilloma.
- Lung malignancy.
- Possibly cavitating infection (reactivation TB).

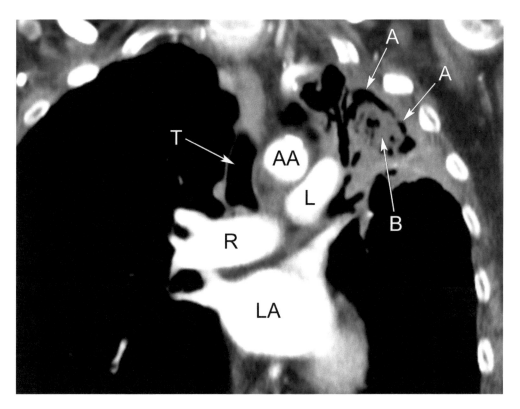

Fig. 5.12C Coronal postcontrast CT through the lung apices of another patient with mycetoma. A lucency (A) surrounds the central fungus ball (B) in an old area of TB scarring. Normal anatomical features include aortic arch (AA), left main pulmonary artery (L), left atrium (LA), right main pulmonary artery (R), and trachea (T).

Mycetoma is a mass caused by a fungal infection, predominantly *Aspergillus* spp. The fungus grows in a previously formed lung cavity or invades healthy lung tissue in immunocompromised individuals. Pulmonary aspergilloma and fungus ball are alternative names used to replace mycetoma.

People who inhale aspergillus particles when they come into contact with them do not normally develop mycetoma as the immune system destroys the fungus rapidly. However, patients who are immunocompromised or have an underlying lung disease, such as TB, COPD or cystic fibrosis, are more likely to develop the condition.

3 What treatment should be initiated for this gentleman?

The diagnosis of mycetoma uses a combination of CXR or CT, sputum samples, which are positive for *Aspergillus* spp. in 50% of patients, and a serum *Aspergillus* precipitin antibody test for the presence of IgG, IgM, and IgE.

Treatment is usually considered when the patient is symptomatic: haemoptysis is the most common symptom. Antifungal medication is first-line treatment, using various routes (IV, inhalation, and CT-guided percutaneous administration).

Embolisation of the pulmonary artery is beneficial in patients with life-threatening haemoptysis but is often a temporary measure as haemoptysis recurs due to collateral vessel formation.

Surgical resection of the cavity containing the mycetoma is beneficial in patients with recurrent haemoptysis providing their lung function is sufficient and often provides positive outcomes. However, it is not always without complications such as haemorrhage, haematogenous spread of fungal infection, and worsening shortness of breath.

Patients at risk of mycetoma must be educated to avoid environments that are likely to contain *Aspergillus* fungus, e.g. compost heaps, dead leaves, marshland, forests, and grain stores.

4 Discuss the spectrum of lung involvement that may be associated with this condition.

Aspergillus spp. causes a spectrum of clinical syndromes depending on the patient's immune system and the presence of pulmonary disease:

- Noninvasive.
    - Allergic bronchopulmonary aspergillosis (hypersensitivity reaction): background of asthma, atopy or cystic fibrosis.
    - Aspergilloma/mycetoma: background of cavitating lung disease (TB).
- Locally invasive.
    - Chronic necrotising aspergillosis: mildly immunocompromised or background of COPD.
- Severe disease.
    - Invasive pulmonary aspergillosis: immunocompromised.

LEARNING POINTS: MYCETOMA

- Mycetoma is a mass caused by a fungal infection, predominantly *Aspergillus* spp.
- More common in people who are immunocompromised or have an underlying lung disease such as asthma, COPD or cystic fibrosis.
- Treatment includes antifungal medications and surgical resection.
- Patients should be educated to avoid environments containing *Aspergillus*.
- *Aspergillus* causes a spectrum of syndromes, largely dependent on the immune status of the host.

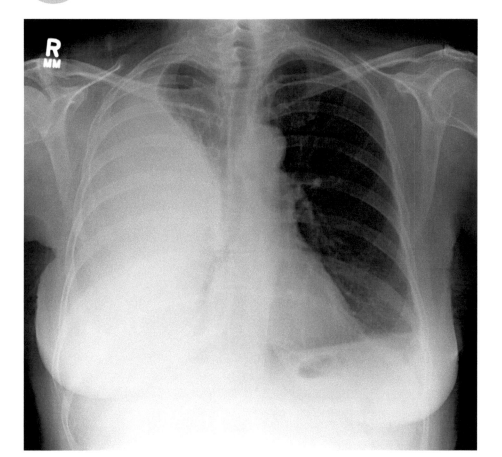

Fig. 5.13A PA CXR.

A 65-year-old female presents to the ED with a 2-month history of gradually worsening short-ness of breath associated with a dry cough and pleuritic chest pain. She had been diagnosed and treated for breast cancer 5 years previously.

On examination there is reduced expansion of the right hemithorax with stony dull percus-sion and absence of breath sounds on auscultation. She is mildly tachypnoeic at 24 bpm and her oxygen saturation on room air is low at 90%.

As part of her initial management, a CXR is arranged (**Figure 5.13A**).

CASE 5.13: QUESTIONS

1 What are CXR findings?
2 What is the diagnosis?
3 What further initial imaging investigation would be helpful?
4 How would you further manage this patient?

CASE 5.13: ANSWERS

1 What are the CXR findings?

The CXR shows near complete opacification of the right hemithorax with the presence of a meniscus at the superior margin (**Figure 5.13B**). The right hemidiaphragm and heart border are obscured. There is no significant mass effect or mediastinal shift. There are no bone lesions. Note the irregularity and reduction in size of the right breast shadow (consistent with previous breast surgery).

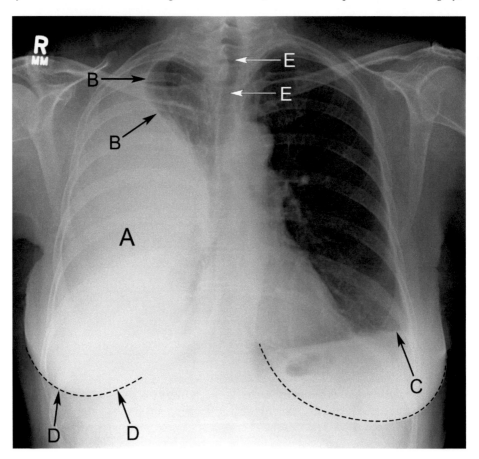

Fig. 5.13B CXR showing near complete opacification of the right hemithorax (A) with a meniscus at the superior margin (B). There is no mediastinal shift. Note blunting of the left costophrenic angle (C) and asymmetry of right breast outline (D). The trachea is central and undisplaced (E).

2 What is the diagnosis?

There are large right and small left pleural effusions – in the context of previous breast cancer, metastatic disease is to be excluded.

Types of pleural effusion:

- Hydrothorax (serous fluid).
- Haemothorax (blood).

- Chylothorax (chyle).
- Pyothorax (empyema).

3 What further initial imaging investigation would be helpful?

Further investigation of the pleural effusion is warranted and an US-guided diagnostic and/or therapeutic thoracocentesis is the next step. US guidance is recommended for all pleural procedures as it allows improved site identification and is safer. US can also identify pleural/lung solid lesions and whether an effusion is multiloculated, which will render drainage ineffectual. US is used to select a site for aspiration with sufficient volume, no intervening lung on maximal inspiration, and no adjacent structures (heart, liver, spleen) (**Figure 5.13C**).

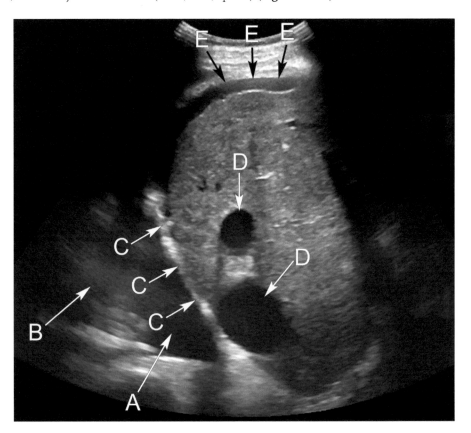

Fig. 5.13C Sagittal US image of the right lung base and liver showing a large pleural effusion (A), collapsed lung segment (B), diaphragm (C), liver with simple liver cysts (D), and ascites (E).

4 How would you further manage this patient?

Check carefully for other signs of breast metastatic disease – palpable nodes supraclavicular fossa or axilla, liver edge, and scar recurrence.

- ABCDE systematic approach with initial resuscitation of the patient and close monitoring.
- Early senior advice to be sought.
- Blood profile: FBC, U&Es, LFTs, bone profile, coagulation screen.

- ABG (identify type 1 respiratory failure, detect possible CO_2 retention).
- ECG and possibly echocardiogram (to assess LV function).
- Pleural US (to confirm the effusion, check for fibrous septations, and guide diagnostic/therapeutic thoracentesis or pleural drain insertion) (*Table 5.13A*).
- CT thorax (to identify lung pathology). If metastatic breast malignancy is suspected, a staging CT of the chest, abdomen, and pelvis, and a bone scan can be performed.

Pleural effusions can be transudates (protein <30 g/L) or exudates (protein >30 g/L). Light's criteria for exudates (causes *Table 5.13B*):

- Protein: effusion albumin/plasma albumin >0.5.
- LDH: effusion LDH/plasma LDH >0.6.
- LDH: effusion LDH >2/3 upper limit of the reference range for the serum LDH.

Table 5.13A Pleural fluid analysis

Macroscopic appearance	• Normal – light yellow and clear fluid (clear ultrafiltrate of plasma that originates from the parietal pleura) • Milky fluid – seen with chylothorax and is due to high triglyceride levels • Bloody fluid – seen after a traumatic thoracentesis and in traumatic haemopneumothorax, malignancy, pulmonary embolism, and TB • Purulent fluid – seen in empyema
Laboratory tests	• pH level • Gram stain and culture • Cell count and differential diagnosis • Glucose, protein, and LDH levels • Cytology • Amylase (if oesophageal perforation or pancreatitis is suspected) • Triglycerides (if chylothorax is suspected)

Table 5.13B Causes of pleural effusions

Transudative pleural effusion	Exudative pleural effusion
Liver cirrhosis	Malignant conditions
Cardiac	Metastatic pleural disease
Congestive cardiac failure	Carcinomatosis
Hypoalbuminaemia	Primary mesothelioma
Nephrotic syndrome	Meigs' syndrome
Protein-losing enteropathy	Infection
Miscellaneous	Empyema
Myxoedema	TB
Superior vena cava obstruction	Parapneumonic effusion
	Miscellaneous
	Connective tissue disease
	Vasculitis
	Sarcoidosis
	Pancreatitis
	Asbestos pleural effusion

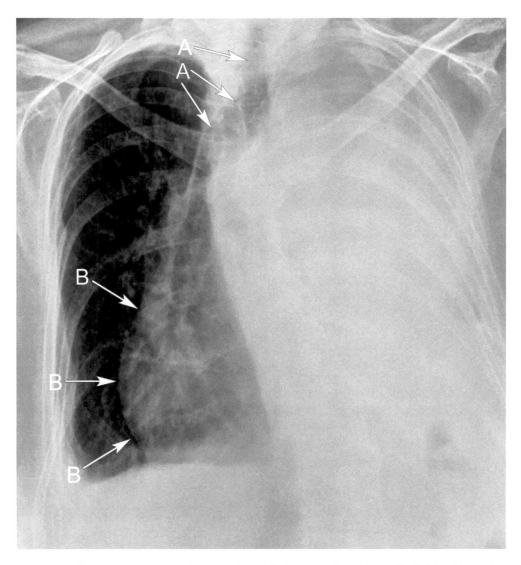

Fig. 5.13D Erect CXR in another patient with a large left pleural effusion with opacified left hemithorax. In this case the effusion has mass effect with mediastinal shift to the right – tracheal deviation (A) is present and the right heart border is also significantly displaced (B).

Another patient with a pleural effusion and mediastinal shift is demonstrated in **Figure 5.13D**. The causes of opacified hemithorax and its investigation are discussed elsewhere in this book, and it is important to be able to differentiate between lung collapse and pleural effusion on CXR. Assessment of the positioning of the mediastinum should allow this, with US being used in equivocal cases.

LEARNING POINTS: PLEURAL EFFUSION/OPACIFIED HEMITHORAX

Causes of an opacified hemithorax:

- Total lung collapse or pneumonectomy (trachea and heart displaced towards the opacified hemithorax, look for surgical clips).
- Consolidation (trachea remains central, look for air bronchograms).
- Pleural effusion (if large trachea plus heart pushed away from the opacified hemithorax).

Look for clues in the clinical assessment for either malignancy or infection.

US is useful to confirm the diagnosis and guide percutaneous drainage/aspiration.

Case 5.14

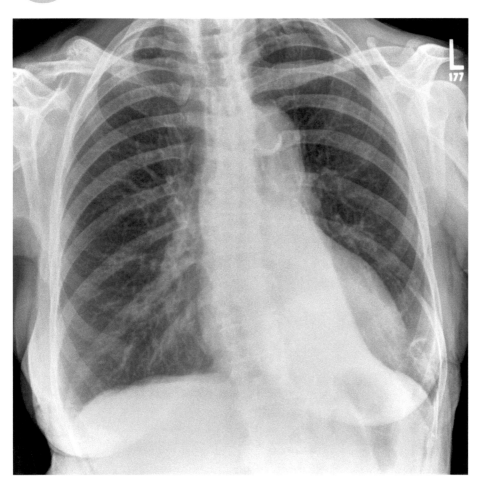

Fig. 5.14A CXR.

A 35-year-old female presents to the ED with acute breathlessness following a 1-week history of mild productive cough with thick green sputum. She has a history of asthma and currently uses a beclometasone dipropionate inhaler twice daily and salbutamol inhaler as needed.

On examination there is reduced expansion of the left hemithorax with reduced breath sounds on auscultation. She is tachypnoeic at 28 bpm, hypoxic with oxygen saturations on air of 85%, tachycardic at 110 bpm, and mildly hypertensive at 145/85 mmHg. As part of her initial investigations, a CXR is arranged (**Figure 5.14A**).

CASE 5.14: QUESTIONS

1 What are the CXR findings?
2 What is the diagnosis?
3 How would you manage this patient?

CASE 5.14: ANSWERS

1 What are the CXR findings?

There is reduced volume of the left hemithorax with a double contour of the LHB (*sail sign*, **Figure 5.14B**). There is loss of clarity of the medial left hemidiaphragm and the descending thoracic aorta (*silhouette sign*). The inferior mediastinum is also shifted towards the left. The right lung is clear.

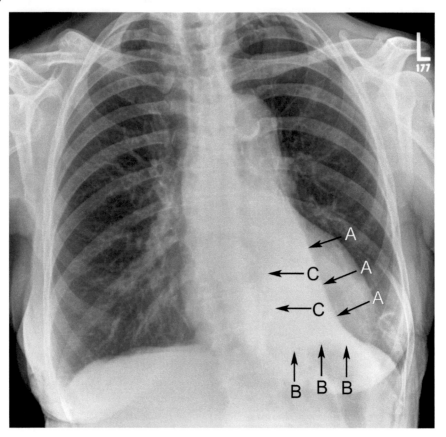

Fig. 5.14B CXR showing collapse of the left lower lobe causing a double LHB appearance (sail sign) (A), obscuration of the medial left hemidiaphragm (B), and descending thoracic aorta (C). The inferior mediastinum is deviated to the left, secondary to the collapse. Note reduced volume of left hemithorax and also increased translucency compared with the right owing to left upper lobe expansion.

2 What is the diagnosis?

Left lower lobe collapse. Given the history of recent infective exacerbation of asthma, the likely cause is a mucus plug obstructing the left lower lobe bronchus.

- Lobar collapse is recognised by an increase in density of an area of lung (in this case behind the heart) associated with loss of lung volume. General signs include:
  - Ipsilateral raised hemidiaphragm.
  - Displaced hilum (towards collapse).

- Tracheal (and mediastinal) shift towards the side of collapse.
  - Ipsilateral narrowing of the intercostal spaces.
- Left lower lobe collapse can be subtle as it is projected behind the heart. The key signs to look out for are the increased density with double heart border (sail sign) and obscuration of the medial aspect of the left hemidiaphragm (silhouette sign). *Silhouette sign* – on XR, borders of structures are often demarcated at the interface of tissues of different radiographic density. In this case, for example, the descending thoracic aorta and left hemidiaphragm are usually clearly seen as aerated/dark lung abuts soft tissue/white. When the lobe collapses this also becomes of soft tissue density and where it abuts the diaphragm/descending aorta the air/soft tissue interface is lost and is now soft tissue/soft tissue.
- Lobar collapse is usually related to endobronchial obstruction, which may be intrinsic or extrinsic. In adults the most common causes of intrinsic obstruction are tumours and mucus plugs. In the clinical context of a middle-aged or elderly smoker, lobar collapse should always be considered to be cause by bronchogenic carcinoma until proven otherwise (bronchoscopy needed). In children, inhaled foreign bodies or mucus plugs are most common. Extrinsic compression may be caused in any age by mediastinal lymphadenopathy or other mediastinal masses. Large pleural effusions can also cause external compression.

3 How would you manage this patient?

Initial management would follow an ABCDE approach with early senior advice. Investigations would include routine blood tests, ABG, CXR, continuous bedside monitoring, and peak expiratory flow rate (PEFR) every 15–30 minutes. Medical therapy for her asthma exacerbation will need to be commenced including:

- Supplementary oxygen, maintaining saturation pressure of oxygen (SPO_2) at 94–98%.
- Nebulised therapy: beta2-agonist bronchodilators (salbutamol), consider repeat doses every 15–30 minutes. Ipratropium bromide 0.5 mg every 4–6 hours.
- Steroid therapy (oral or IV).
- Antibiotics. Consider them only when evidence of bacterial infection is present: most asthma exacerbations are caused by viral infections.

The patient should be referred to the chest team and for urgent physiotherapy to dislodge the mucus plug. Early repeat CXR to confirm complete lung re-expansion – if collapse persists bronchoscopy will be needed.

Another left lung lobar collapse that can be difficult to recognise is left upper lobe collapse, where the upper lobe collapses anteriorly and medially. The result is that the main adjacent structures (AA and hilum) lose their clarity on CXR. This is demonstrated in **Figure 5.14C** and on CT in **Figure 5.14D** (both on page 118).

LEARNING POINTS: LEFT LOWER LOBE COLLAPSE

- In children, usually caused by inhaled foreign body.
- In young adults/asthmatics, mucus plug most common.
- In older patients/smokers, malignancy to be excluded.

Patients need respiratory team referral and early bronchoscopy if there is not prompt lung reinflation.

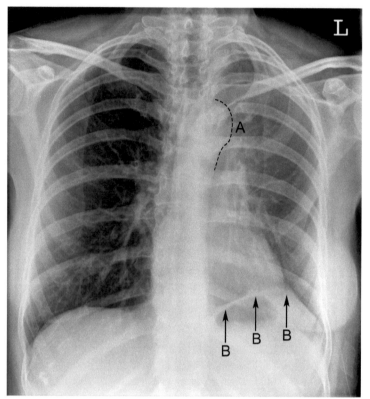

Fig. 5.14C CXR in a different patient showing left upper lobe collapse with a typical veil sign (the left lung field appears as though covered by a veil). The left upper lobe collapses anteriorly and medially, and as it encroaches upon the left hilum and aortic knuckle these structures will become obscured (silhouette sign again). The left hilum is also elevated towards collapse and is not well seen. Note obscuration of the aortic arch as collapsed lung lies against it (A) – as well as tenting/elevation of the left hemidiaphragm (B) with cardiac and minor tracheal shift to the left, and reduced volume of left lung. Left upper lobe collapse is usually caused by a central obstructing malignancy.

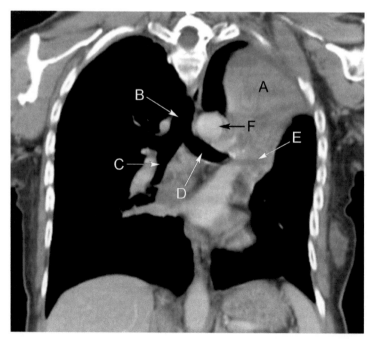

Fig. 5.14D Coronal CT image of the thorax showing left upper lobe collapse (A). Trachea (B), right main bronchus (C), and left main bronchus (D). Note collapsed lobe abutting upper pole left hilum (E) and aortic knuckle (F) with loss of aerated margin (silhouette sign).

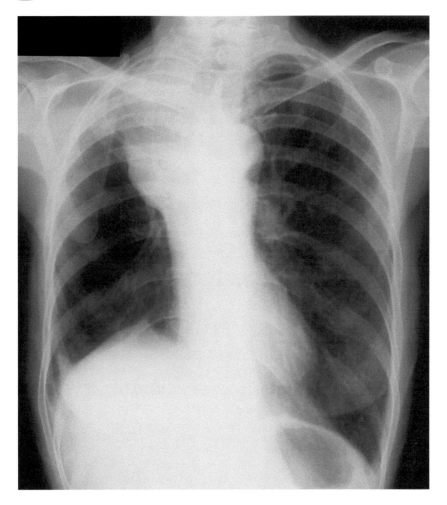

Fig. 5.15A CXR.

A 65-year-old male presents to the respiratory clinic referred by his GP with a 6-month history of gradually progressive shortness of breath, cough with haemoptysis, and weight loss. He is a smoker with a 45 pack-year history. He has no past medical history of note.

He is tachypnoeic at 35 bpm, tachycardic at 120 bpm, normotensive at 125/90 mmHg, hypoxic with SPO_2 of 88% on room air, and apyrexial.

As part of his initial investigations, a CXR is arranged (**Figure 5.15A**).

CASE 5.15: QUESTIONS

1 What are the CXR findings?
2 What is the diagnosis?
3 How would you investigate and manage this patient?

CASE 5.15: ANSWERS

1 What are the CXR findings?

The findings are (**Figure 5.15B**):

- Opacity of the right upper zone.
- Elevation and tenting of the right hemidiaphragm.
- Elevation of the right hilum. Note: the right hilum cannot be seen clearly but the curved S configuration of the hilum is suggestive of a mass (Golden's 'S' sign).
- Tracheal shift towards the collapsed side (right).
- Crowding of the ribs on the right side, reduced volume of the right hemithorax.

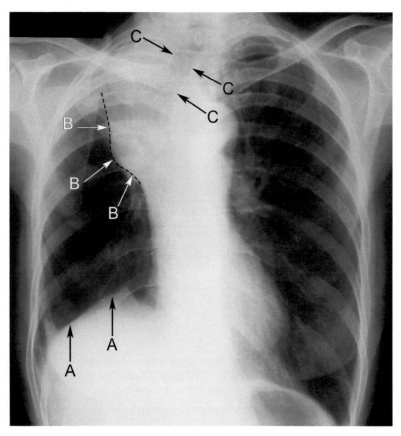

Fig. 5.15B
PA CXR. There is volume loss in the right hemithorax with elevation of the right hemidiaphragm (A). There is right upper zone opacity and the right hilum is elevated and blends with right upper zone opacity: an underlying mass is likely (Golden's "S" sign, B). The trachea is shifted to the right (C).

2 What is the diagnosis?

The CXR shows features of a collapsed right upper lobe likely caused by a central obstructing hilar mass: a diagnosis of lung malignancy is highly likely in this case.

Figures **5.15C** and **5.15D** are radiographs in another patient with middle lobe collapse (right lower lobe collapse is not dissimilar to left lower lobe collapse in terms of appearances in the collapsed lobe, **Figure 5.15E**).

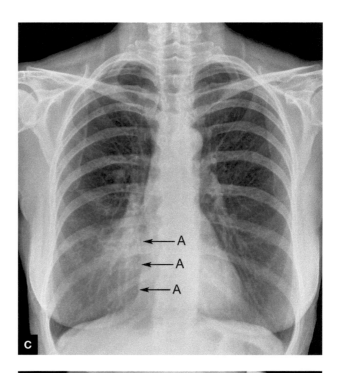

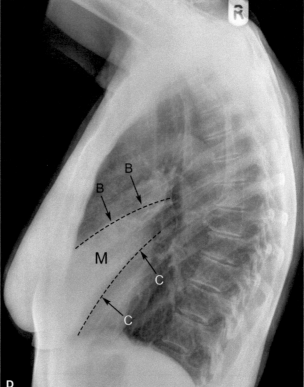

Figs. 5.15C, D PA and lateral CXRs, respectively. (Right) middle lobe collapse. Note the increased density adjacent to and obscuring the right heart border (A) with depression of the right hilum on the PA CXR. The collapsed dense middle lobe (M) is seen on the lateral view, outlined by the depressed horizontal fissure (B) and deviated oblique fissure (C).

121

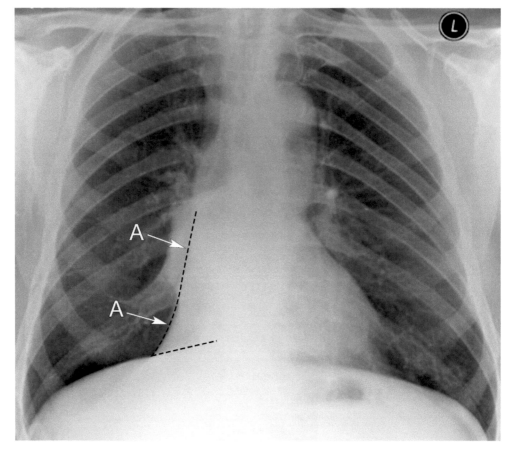

Fig. 5.15E CXR of right lower lobe collapse. Note the triangular shaped collapsed lower lobe (A), depressed hilum, and reduced volume in the right hemithorax.

Right middle lobe collapse radiological features:

- Difficult to identify on PA CXR owing to subtle changes.
- Ill-defined increased density of the right lower zone.
- Depressed right hilum.
- Silhouette sign, with loss of aerated middle lobe abutting the RHB; increased density in the right lower zone with loss of clarity of the RHB points to pathology in the middle lobe – consolidation or collapse.
- On the lateral CXR, a collapsed opacified middle lobe can be identified by outlining the depressed horizontal fissure and an elevated distorted right oblique fissure.

Right lower lobe collapse is also shown (**Figure 5.15E**).

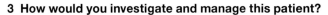

3 How would you investigate and manage this patient?

Use ABCDE as always initially, oxygen by mask, and monitoring. Routine bloods and discuss with seniors/respiratory team:

- Blood profile: FBC (anaemia), U&Es (SIADH), LFTs (metastatic liver disease, raised alkaline phosphatase (ALP) in metastatic bone disease), bone profile (high calcium levels secondary to metastatic bone disease or part of a paraneoplastic syndrome).
- Sputum cytology.
- Bronchoscopy.
- CT chest/abdomen.

LEARNING POINTS: RIGHT UPPER LOBE COLLAPSE

- The age of the patient and distribution of the lobar collapse is important in aetiology.
- Upper lobe collapse is more usually due to malignancy.
- Older patients/smokers need early bronchoscopy to exclude malignancy.

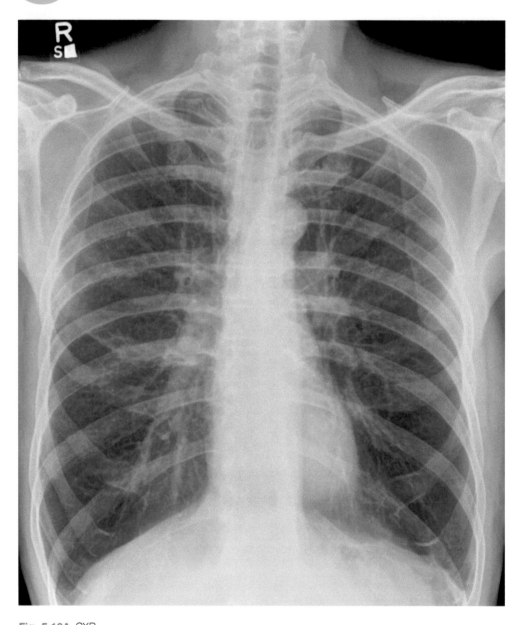

Fig. 5.16A CXR.

A 65-year-old male smoker presents to the medical assessment unit with a 6-month history of gradually worsening shortness of breath, dry cough, and decreased exercise tolerance. He describes no change in appetite and no recent weight loss. In the last 4 days he has noticed that his breathing has deteriorated acutely and his cough has become productive with small amounts of brown sputum.

He has been started on a bronchodilator inhaler by his GP with minimal improvement in symptoms. He has had recurrent chest infections over the past 6 months and has taken several courses of antibiotics.

On examination he is dyspnoeic, has a hyperexpanded chest, and on auscultation there is expiratory polyphonic wheeze and reduced breath sounds at the apices. He is afebrile, tachypnoeic at 35 bpm, tachycardic at 120 bpm, and normotensive at 130/70 mmHg. SPO_2 is 85% on room air.

As part of the initial assessment a CXR is arranged (**Figure 5.16A**).

CASE 5.16: QUESTIONS

1 What are the CXR findings?
2 What is the diagnosis?
3 How would you investigate and manage this patient?

CASE 5.16: ANSWERS

1 What are the CXR findings?

The CXR shows hyperexpansion of the lungs with flattening of diaphragms and reduced cardiac silhouette (**Figure 5.16B**). Lung vascular markings are significantly attenuated in the lower zones, which appear hyperlucent.

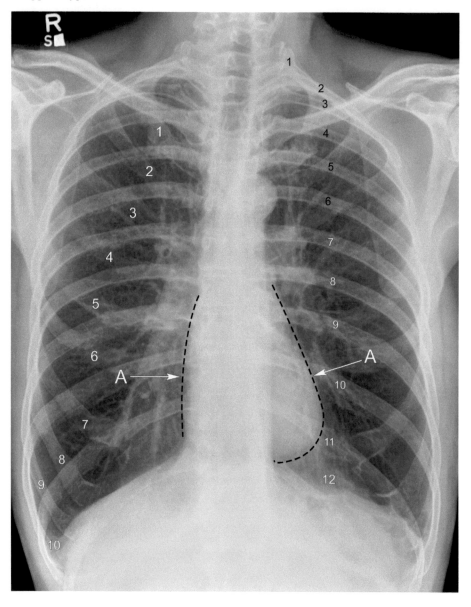

Fig. 5.16B CXR showing hyperexpanded lungs with flattened hemidiaphragms and small appearance of the heart (A). The lower zones are translucent. Note the increased visible anterior ribs (10 are visible, labelled on right, normal 5–7) and posterior ribs (12 are visible, labelled on left, normal 7–9).

2 What is the diagnosis?

These findings, associated with the clinical presentation, confirm a diagnosis of COPD with emphysematous changes. The current presentation can be attributed to a likely infective exacerbation of COPD.

- COPD is a progressive, poorly reversible condition of airflow limitation, caused by a persistent inflammatory response in the lungs. It is associated in most cases with smoking but can also be caused by atmospheric pollution or alpha-1-antitrypsin deficiency.
- In clinical practice, the radiographic assessment of hyperinflation is usually subjective but specific quantitative indices are sometimes applied. Thus, the diaphragm is considered low if the level of the right dome is at or below the anterior aspect of the 7th rib, and flat if the maximum curvature of the dome is less than 1.5 cm in height. Causes of hyperinflated lungs are shown in *Table 5.16*.

Table 5.16 Causes of hyperexpanded lungs

- Emphysema/chronic bronchitis/COPD
- Acute asthma attack
- Alpha-1-antitrypsin deficiency
- Cystic fibrosis

3 How would you investigate and manage this patient?

Investigations:

- Blood tests: FBC (raised WCC in associated infection, high Hb), consider serum albumin (severity), alpha-1-antitrypsin deficiency (younger patient with positive family history).
- ABG: type II respiratory failure (low P_aO_2 and high P_aCO_2).
- ECG and echocardiography: assess for features of cor pulmonale.
- CXR: hyperexpanded lungs, bullae, pneumothorax.
- Pulmonary function tests: obstructive ventilator defect with a low gas transfer coefficient.

Treatment of acute exacerbation:

- ABCDE resuscitation with early senior input.
- Controlled O_2 supplementation – aim for an O_2 saturation of 88–92%, to be administered through a Venturi mask, with monitoring for possible CO_2 retention and type II respiratory failure.
- Nebulised bronchodilators then oral steroids for 7 days.
- Antibiotics if evidence of an associated bacterial infection.
- Chest physiotherapy.
- Consideration of noninvasive ventilation in the presence of type II respiratory failure.
- High-resolution CT to look for features of lung disease, bullae, and fibrosis (**Figures 5.16C** and **5.16D**).
- Respiratory specialist review.
- Exclude an associated malignancy owing to the increased risk in smokers (cigarette smoking is linked to about 90% of lung cancers).

Long-term medical treatment:

- Smoking cessation.
- Long-term oxygen therapy if required.

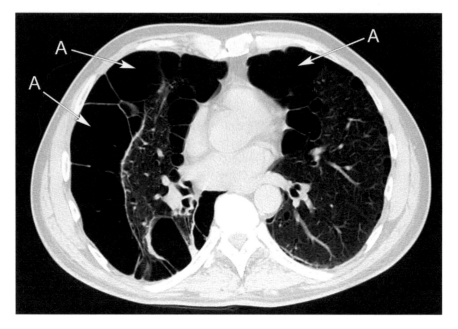

Fig. 5.16C Axial CT thorax using lung window setting, showing numerous large bullae (A) with thin septations in a different patient with severe COPD.

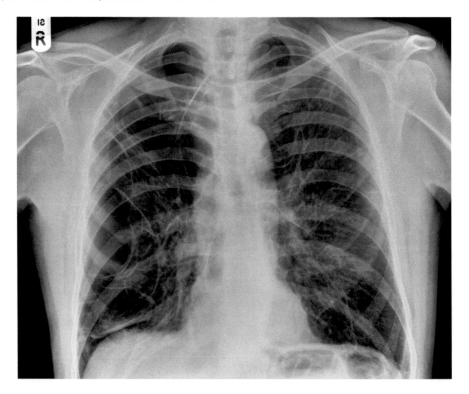

Fig. 5.16D CXR in a patient with more overt emphysematous changes, notably in the right lung.

- Pulmonary rehabilitation programmes should include multicomponent, multidisciplinary interventions, which are tailored to the individual patient's needs. The rehabilitation process should incorporate a programme of physical training, disease education, and nutritional, psychological, and behavioural intervention.
- Vaccinations – pneumococcal vaccination and an annual influenza vaccination should be offered to all patients with COPD.

Lung surgery (in selected, suitable patients):

- Bullectomy – patients who are breathless, have a single bulla on a CT scan, and an FEV1 less than 50% predicted should be referred for consideration of bullectomy.
- Lung reduction surgery – in patients with severe COPD who remain breathless with marked restrictions of their activities of daily living, despite maximal medical therapy and who are meeting specific criteria.
- Single lung transplant – patients with severe COPD who remain breathless with marked restrictions of their daily activities despite maximal medical therapy, bearing in mind comorbidities and local surgical protocols.

LEARNING POINTS: CHRONIC OBSTRUCTIVE PULMONARY DISEASE

- Emphysema/chronic bronchitis/COPD is the most common cause of hyperexpanded lungs.
- CXR findings include a flattened diaphragm, small appearance of the heart, and lucent bullae. Bullae and fibrosis, however, are better demonstrated on HRCT.
- Smoking is the most common cause, although alpha-1-antitrypsin deficiency should be considered in the young.
- Any discussion about long-term medical management should include mention of smoking cessation and long-term oxygen therapy.

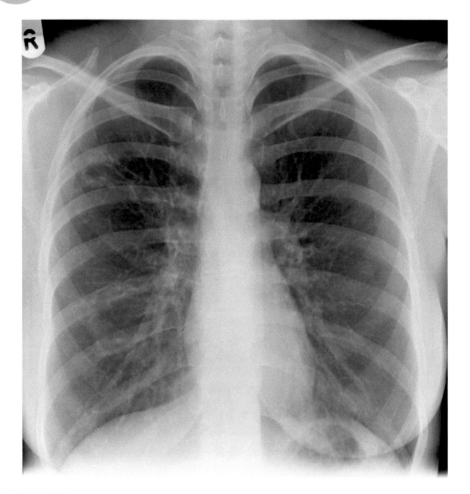

Fig. 5.17A CXR.

A 40-year-old female with a 15-year history of recurrent chest infections with a productive cough presents to the ED with an exacerbation of her cough, productive of purulent sputum, unwell, and febrile. She is a nonsmoker, keeps no pets, and with no history of recent foreign travel.

She is clubbed, pyrexial 37.5°C but otherwise well. On auscultation there are scattered inspiratory crackles and widespread inspiratory wheeze.

As part of her initial management a CXR is arranged (**Figures 5.17A** and **5.17B**).

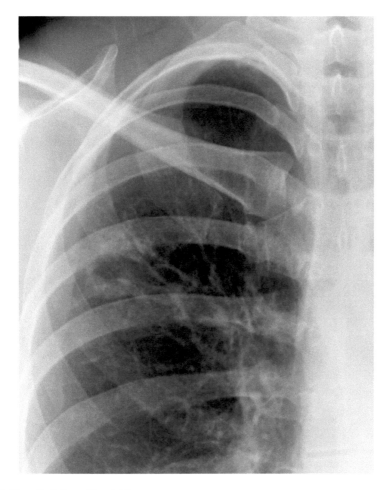

Fig. 5.17B Magnified view of the right upper zone.

CASE 5.17: QUESTIONS

1 What are the CXR findings?
2 What is the diagnosis?
3 How would you investigate and manage this patient?

CASE 5.17: ANSWERS

1 What are the CXR findings?

The CXR shows abnormal reticular 'tram-track' opacification in the right upper zone in keeping with grossly thickened and dilated bronchi. There is no associated volume loss or mediastinal lymphadenopathy (**Figure 5.17C**).

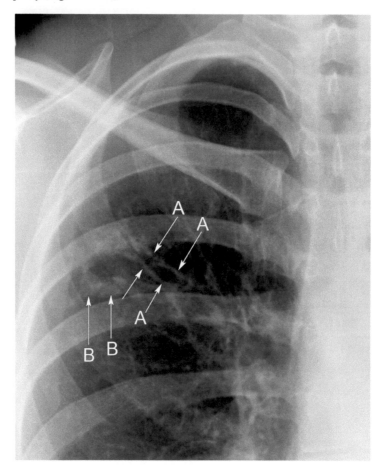

Fig. 5.17C CXR showing bronchiectasis in the right upper zone. 'Tram-track' lines represent a dilated, thick-walled bronchus (A). A tubular dilated opacified bronchus is present, likely containing mucus/pus (B).

2 What is the diagnosis?

The radiographic findings together with a history of recurrent chest infections and productive cough are consistent with a diagnosis of bronchiectasis:

- Bronchiectasis is a longstanding disease in which the bronchi become irreversibly thickened and dilated. It is caused by a combination of excess production of secretions with impaired clearance, often with impaired host defence mechanisms. It can be localised to a lobe or generalised. Bronchiectasis is a cause of clubbing.

- Types: cylindrical, varicose, cystic or traction. Recurrent infections cause recurrent bronchial wall damage, scarring, fibrosis, and dilatation.
- Causes:
  - Congenital: cystic fibrosis, Kartagener's syndrome, immunodeficiency, congenital kyphoscoliosis.
  - Acquired: infection (viral, bacterial, fungi), mechanical bronchial obstruction (mass, foreign body), recurrent aspiration or associated with autoimmune disorders (rheumatoid arthritis, inflammatory bowel disease).
  - Pathogens associated with bronchiectasis:
    - *Pseudomonas aeruginosa.*
    - *Haemophilus influenza.*
    - *Streptococcus.*
    - *Aspergillus* spp. (particularly in upper lobe bronchiectasis).
- Complications:
  - Pulmonary: recurrent infections, haemoptysis (can be life threatening), empyema, abscess, cor pulmonale, scarring and fibrosis of the lung.
  - Extrapulmonary: anaemia, cerebral abscess, secondary amyloidosis.
  - Cerebral abscess.

3 How would you investigate and manage this patient?

Investigations include CXR and HRCT (**Figure 5.17D**) to define the distribution of bronchiectasis and to look for a possible cause, as well as respiratory team referral. HRCT involves taking very thin CT slices through the chest but with small gaps between the slices.

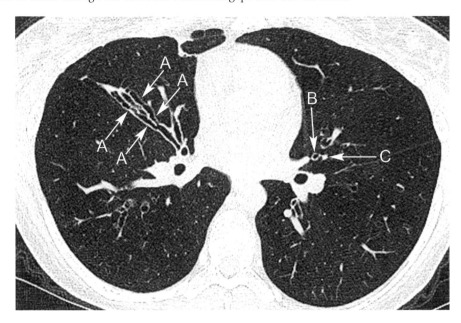

Fig. 5.17D Axial HRCT thorax using lung window setting showing cylindrical bronchiectasis and the signet ring sign. Note the dilated thick-walled bronchi in the middle lobe (A). In cross-section the bronchus and pulmonary artery branch should be the same size, whereas in bronchiectasis the bronchus is markedly dilated and thick walled appearing like a signet ring seen end-on. The dilated bronchus (B) is thick walled and can be seen to be larger than the adjacent pulmonary artery branch (C), the signet ring sign.

Additionally, blood tests (Hb and inflammatory markers), sputum cultures (including acid-fast bacilli and cytology), and pulmonary function tests (obstructive pattern with limited reversibility) should be performed.

To identify an underlying cause, cystic fibrosis sweat and genetic testing, TB elispot, serum immunoglobulins, serum electrophoresis and *Aspergillus* precipitins may be useful.

Bronchoscopy may be helpful in some cases.

Treatment (acutely):

- ABCDE initial approach with fluid/oxygen, resuscitation as needed, and early senior input.
- Routine bloods and blood cultures if pyrexial.
- Chest physiotherapy and postural drainage.
- Keep well hydrated – IV fluids if required.
- Bronchodilators (nebulised/inhaled).
- Mucolytics (carbocisteine).
- Antibiotics if evidence of bacterial infection.
- Treatment of underlying cause; might include surgery in carefully selected cases.

LEARNING POINTS: BRONCHIECTASIS

Radiographic features to look for on CXR:

- Dilated and thickened airways (tramlines, ring shadows).
- Mucus plugging with bronchoceles ('gloved finger sign').
- Volume loss secondary to consolidation.

HRCT is the diagnostic test of choice.

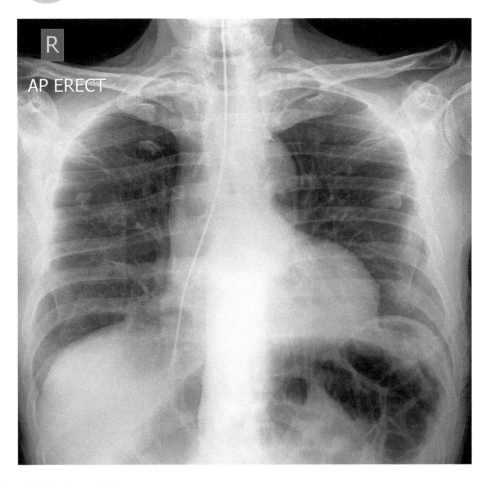

Fig. 5.18A AP erect CXR.

A 76-year-old male patient on the ward who has suffered a cerebrovascular accident coughs when drinking and recently choked on soft food. The nurses are worried about his ability to swallow and you have arranged for the speech and language therapists to assess him. The team decide that he should be fed for the time being via an NG tube. You have inserted this and want to check its position before it is used for feeding. Attempted aspiration did not yield enough fluid for the pH verification test and you therefore request a CXR (**Figure 5.18A**).

CASE 5.18: QUESTIONS

1 What does the CXR show and can feeding be commenced through the NG tube?
2 What are the possible complications of an incorrectly placed NG tube?
3 What other ways can correct NG tube placement be checked?
4 What other indications are there for NG tube insertion?

CASE 5.18: ANSWERS

1 What does the CXR show and can feeding be commenced through the NG tube?

The CXR shows incorrect placement of the NG tube. The tube has passed via the right main bronchus into the right lower lobe of the lung (**Figure 5.18B**). Feeding must not be commenced.

A correctly placed NG tube on CXR (**Figure 5.18C**) should:

- Follow the path of the oesophagus/avoid the contours of the bronchi.
- Clearly bisect the carina.
- Cross the diaphragm in the midline.
- Have a tip clearly visualised below the left hemidiaphragm.
- See **Figures 5.18D** and **5.18E** for another example.
- Owing to the close proximity of the oesophagus to the larynx, NG tube placement can be difficult as the tip can pass via the larynx into the trachea and into either the right or left main bronchus of the lung.

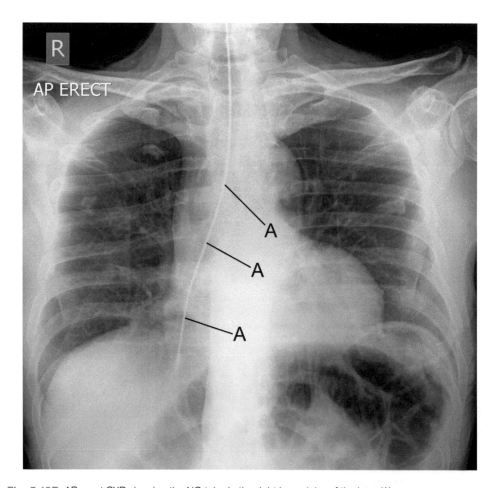

Fig. 5.18B AP erect CXR showing the NG tube in the right lower lobe of the lung (A).

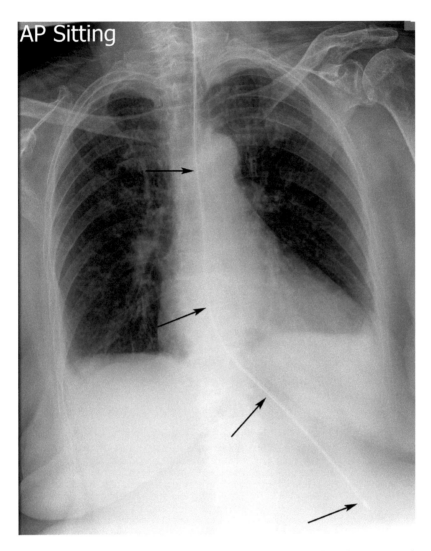

Fig. 5.18C CXR showing satisfactory NG tube placement. Note the arrows following the path of the tube, which bisects the carina and crosses the diaphragm in the midline. The tube tip lies well beneath the left hemidiaphragm.

KEY POINTS

If you are ever unsure of NG tube placement, always ask a senior doctor or radiologist to review the CXR before feeding. Document your findings and recommendations in the notes. Such decisions are best made in working hours when senior colleagues are freely available for advice.

Before confirming NG tube placement on CXR it is important to check the patient name, hospital number and date of birth. Additionally, check the time and date of the film you are reviewing. ITU patients may have several CXRs every day, so you must ensure that you are reviewing the correct one. Always document your findings in the patient notes.

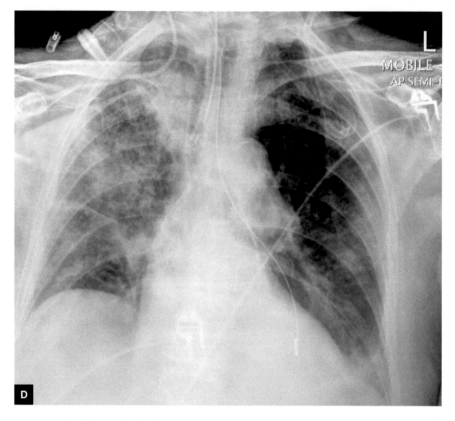

Figs. 5.18D, E (**5.18D**) Mobile AP CXR in a different patient showing consolidation in the right lung, likely caused by aspiration pneumonia. Although the radiopaque NG tube tip is projected below the left hemidiaphragm, the tube clearly does not bisect the carina and has passed into the left main bronchus. The dashed line (A) shows the expected path of a normally positioned NG tube. The solid black line (B) shows the actual passage of the NG tube down the left main bronchus. (**5.18E**) The outline of the trachea and the carina (C) are shown in a solid black line. Note that although the tip of the NG tube is below the left hemidiaphragm, there is failure of the tube to bisect the carina (C) and the actual path of the tube overlaps the left main bronchus due to incorrect positioning. This patient also has an incorrectly placed right subclavian central venous line, which passes cranially up the right internal jugular vein (D).

2 What are the possible complications of an incorrectly placed NG tube?

Complications of NG tube placement include:

- Immediate.
  - Epistaxis.
  - Oesophageal perforation.
  - Intracranial placement of the tube.
- Early.
  - Incorrect placement of tube in the lung.
  - Pneumonitis.
  - Lung collapse.

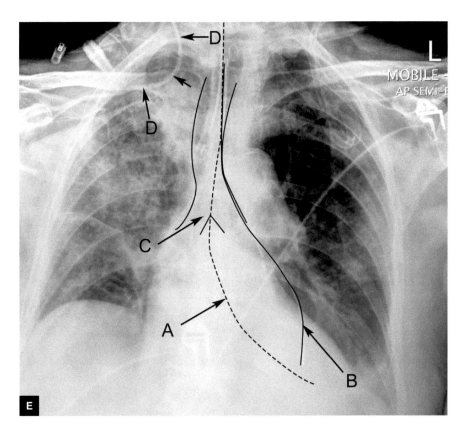

Fig. 5.18E

- Late.
  - Aspiration pneumonia.
  - Tube obstruction.
  - Feed related complications: diarrhoea, abdominal cramps, nausea.

Note: In an exam situation when asked for complications of a procedure, split this into immediate, early, and late complications. This is a good way to classify the information you give and ensures that you do not forget anything.

3 What other ways can correct NG tube placement be checked?

The National Patient Safety Agency (NPSA) issued guidance in 2005 for safe placement and position checking of nasogastric tubes. There are two methods that can be used to check NG tube placement:

- First-line check is by aspiration of gastric fluid and measurement of pH of the aspirate using pH indicator paper. If the aspirate pH is below 5.5 then feeding can commence.
- CXR is indicated as second line test (not routine) and can only be checked by those trained to do so. If there is any uncertainty, the CXR should be checked by a radiologist.
- Other methods have been highlighted as insufficient, such as the 'whoosh' test (listening for bubbling sounds after air entry) or use of litmus paper in testing acidity.

TOP TIPS

- Know what a correctly placed NG tube should look like on CXR (**Figures 5.18C** and **5.18D, E**).
- Follow the NG tube down from the most superior aspect where it is first seen on the CXR.
- The NG tube should bisect the carina centrally.
- Ensure it follows the central line of the oesophagus and not down a main bronchus.
- The tip should be within the stomach/duodenum, which is on the left side below the diaphragm.
- Take senior advice if you are unsure and document your findings. Arrange NG tube changes/CXR if possible in working hours, when senior advice is readily available. Delay any feeding until correct position confirmed.

---

4 What other indications are there for NG tube insertion?

The indications are:

- Evaluation of an upper GI bleed.
- Aspiration of gastric contents.
- Administration of radiographic contrast to the GI tract.
- Gastric or small bowel decompression.
- Feeding* or administration of medication.

LEARNING POINTS: NASOGASTRIC TUBE PLACEMENT AND ASSESSMENT

- NG tube position can be checked using pH assessment of gastric aspirate. If pH is below 5.5, it confirms correct NG tube position.
- CXR is a second line investigation. If correctly placed, the NG tube should follow the line of the oesophagus, bisect the carina and cross the diaphragm in the midline, tip lying beneath the left hemidiaphragm.
- If there are any concerns over the positioning, review the CXR with a senior colleague, make a record in the medical notes, and do not commence feeding.

---

* NG tubes are used for short-term feeding for up to 6 weeks in patients with dysphagia or for those on ventilators. Longer-term feeding is better delivered via a gastrostomy or jejunostomy tube.

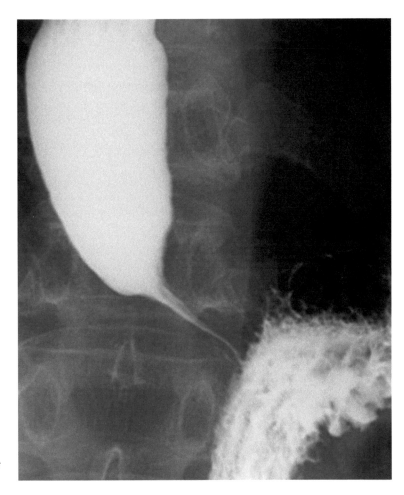

Fig. 5.19A Spot image from an upper GI contrast study.

A 53-year-old male presents to his GP with difficulty in swallowing solids and liquids over the past 6 months, often with regurgitating of his food. This is associated with retrosternal chest pain. Otherwise he feels well and has not lost any weight recently. He has no relevant past medical or family history.

His observations are normal. Abdominal examination reveals a soft and nontender abdomen with no organomegaly or palpable masses. His GP performs a set of routine bloods that reveals a Hb of 129 g/L (130–180 g/L) and refers to the gastroenterology team. The patient could not tolerate an upper GI endoscopy and therefore the following imaging test is arranged (**Figure 5.19A**).

CASE 5.19: QUESTIONS

1 What is the imaging modality shown?
2 What is the abnormality demonstrated?
3 How would you further investigate this condition?
4 How would you manage this patient?

CASE 5.19: ANSWERS

1 What is the imaging modality shown?

The imaging (**Figure 5.19A**) shows an upper GI contrast study called a barium swallow. Barium solution is swallowed and coats the lining of the oesophagus, stomach, and duodenum.

- Barium studies of the upper GI tract have largely been replaced by upper GI endoscopy, which allows more accurate mucosal assessment, avoids irradiation, and also provides a biopsy facility. Barium studies still have a role, however, in the investigation of motility disorders and in patients who cannot tolerate endoscopy.

2 What is the abnormality demonstrated?

There is a tight, smooth, narrowing of the lower oesophagus and gastro-oesophageal junction, characteristic of achalasia. Prestenotic dilatation of the lower oesophagus is also noted. Contrast has passed through the constriction into the stomach (**Figure 5.19B**).

- The constriction has a smooth tapered margin ('bird's beak' sign). This is important in differentiating it from a malignant stricture. The imaging shows no features of malignancy, with no shouldering or visible mucosal erosion.

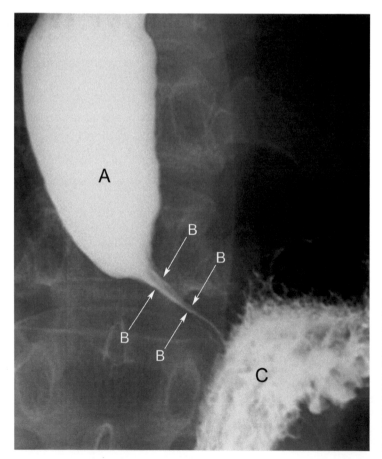

Fig. 5.19B Spot image from a barium swallow showing dilation of the lower oesophagus with pooling of contrast (A) above a tight smooth narrowing ('bird's beak' sign) of the lower oesophageal sphincter (B). Some contrast has passed through into the fundus of the stomach, with visible rugae (C).

Features of achalasia:

- Primary achalasia is failure of organised oesophageal peristalsis.
- There is impaired relaxation of the lower oesophageal sphincter.
- This is due to denervation of the muscles in the lower oesophagus, with unknown cause.
- This results in dilatation of the oesophagus and food stasis (**Figure 5.19C**).
- Both solids and liquids are equally affected, dysphagia is nonprogressive.
- Little or no weight loss.
- Involves a short segment (<3.5 cm) of the distal oesophagus.

Complications of achalasia:

- Oesophageal carcinoma, 5% of cases caused by chronic irritation of the mucosa by stasis of food and secretions.
- Aspiration pneumonia.
- Candida oesophagitis.
- Acute airway obstruction (emergency) requiring NG tube decompression.

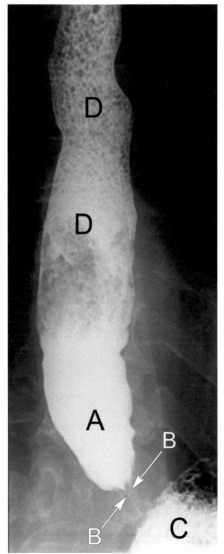

Fig. 5.19C Barium swallow image from a different patient with achalasia. This also shows prestenotic dilatation of the lower oesophagus with pooling of contrast (A). There is smooth tapering of the oesophageal stricture with a 'bird's beak' abnormality (B). Air and contrast (C) are seen within the fundus of the stomach. Note the food residue in the dilated upper oesophagus (D).

> ### DIFFERENTIAL DIAGNOSIS OF ACHALASIA OF THE OESOPHAGUS
>
> When presented with an image you will usually be asked for a differential diagnosis. In this case the following need to be considered:
>
> - Benign stricture.
>   - Achalasia (bird's beak).
>   - Chagas disease (caused by protozoan *Trypanosoma cruzi*, endemic to Latin America with multiple-organ involvement including myocarditis).
> - Malignant stricture.
>   - Oesophageal malignancy or gastric carcinoma (irregular margin or shouldering of the stricture. Clinical signs are also important).

3 How would you further investigate this condition?

Upper GI endoscopy, to exclude malignancy, is usually the first investigation for dysphagia. Early signs of achalasia, however, can be subtle endoscopically and findings may appear normal. Following endoscopy, patients with suspected achalasia will usually undergo a barium swallow. Visualisation of barium passage in real time is most accurate in demonstrating dysmotility. In the early stages, barium swallow may show loss of normal peristalsis and delayed emptying before formation of a typical beak-like narrowing.

CT is only used if malignancy is suspected but may show a dilated thin-walled oesophagus filled with fluid or food debris. It may also show evidence of aspiration pneumonia.

4 How would you manage this patient?

Treatment is aimed at allowing adequate drainage of the oesophagus into the stomach. A gastro-enterologist usually manages this condition. Management options include:

- Calcium channel blockers (used as a bridge to definitive management).
- Endoscopic dilatation (85% effective).
- Local botulinum toxin injection at the level of the gastro-oesophageal sphincter (risk of scarring to submucosa).
- Surgical myotomy (usually alongside Nissen fundoplication owing to risk of later reflux).

> ### LEARNING POINTS: ACHALASIA OF THE OESOPHAGUS
>
> - Achalasia classically produces a smooth, beak-like narrowing of the distal oesophagus, best demonstrated on barium swallow.
> - It is important to differentiate achalasia from a malignant stricture that presents with progressive dysphagia and weight loss and produces an irregular stricture on barium swallow.
> - 5% of patients with achalasia progress to develop oesophageal carcinoma.
> - Endoscopic dilatation of achalasia is the mainstay of management; this also allows biopsies to be taken in cases where malignancy is suspected.

Case 5.20

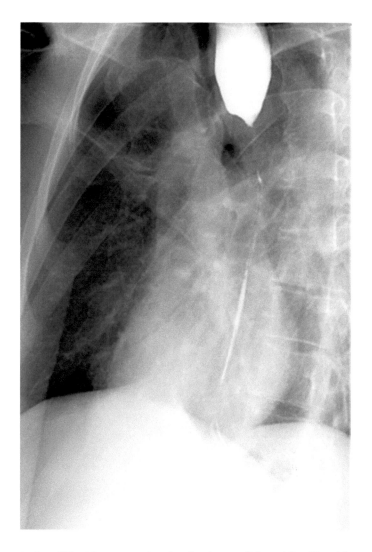

Fig. 5.20A Lateral oblique image from a barium swallow series.

A 67-year-old female presents to her GP with progressive dysphagia to solids and liquids with absolute dysphagia over the past 24 hours. She regurgitates anything swallowed. Six months ago she weighed 75 kg but today weighs 64 kg. She has been feeling more lethargic recently. She is a heavy smoker with a 40 pack-year history and drinks 2–3 glasses of wine per night.

An upper GI endoscopy was attempted but could not pass the midoesophagus. A barium swallow is performed to further delineate the oesophageal anatomy (**Figure 5.20A**).

CASE 5.20: QUESTIONS

1 What does the barium study show?
2 How would you manage this patient initially?

3 What therapeutic options are available for symptomatic treatment of this condition and what are the complications?

CASE 5.20: ANSWERS

1 What does the barium study show?

The image shows an abrupt irregular stricture of the midthoracic oesophagus with mucosal irregularity and shouldering (**Figure 5.20B**). There is prestenotic oesophageal dilatation and minimal passage of contrast through the stricture into the stomach.

- Features that favour a malignant cause for the stricture include a history of a progressive then absolute dysphagia, recent weight loss, and smoking. Long-term reflux or Barrett's oesophagus are also significant risk factors (not present in this case).
- Examination findings might include cachexia and palpable cervical lymph nodes, particularly Virchow's node in the left supraclavicular fossa (Troisier's sign), which is associated with upper GI malignancy. Examine also for metastatic liver enlargement and features of lung aspiration pneumonia.
- The tightness of the stricture and the asymmetric shouldering of the stricture margin also suggest malignancy.

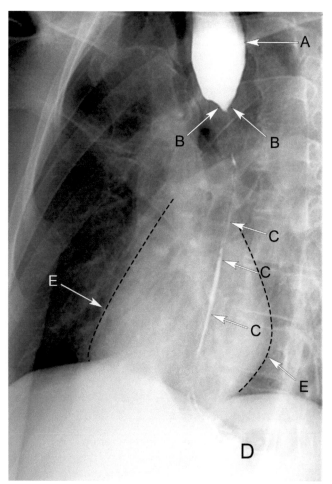

Fig. 5.20B Lateral oblique image from a barium swallow series showing a tight midoesophageal stricture. There is prestenotic dilatation and pooling of contrast (A) and irregular shouldering of the oesophagus at the level of the stricture (B). Minimal contrast bypasses the stricture (C) to enter the stomach (D). The normal cardiac outline is also labelled (E).

2 How would you manage this patient initially?

Management of the patient depends on the likelihood of malignancy. She requires urgent assessment and admission to hospital under gastroenterology because of the absolute dysphagia. This patient has a number of the *red flag symptoms* for malignancy:

- Dysphagia.
- Vomiting.
- Anorexia.
- Weight loss.
- Upper GI bleeding (haematemesis or melena).
- Rapidly progressing symptoms.
- Iron deficiency anaemia.
- Abdominal mass.

These symptoms should point you towards the diagnosis and the need for further investigation. Be aware, however, that symptoms can overlap with benign conditions and formal investigation and diagnosis is necessary in all cases.

A sensitive discussion with the patient should be had with support from a specialist nurse or relatives to explain that malignancy is a diagnosis that is being considered.

Following review from a senior gastroenterologist the following investigations may be performed:

- Repeat endoscopy with biopsy for histological diagnosis.
- Endoscopic US to look for enlarged paraoesophageal nodes.
- A CT chest and abdomen for tumour staging (**Figure 5.20C**).
- PET-CT is often used as a supplementary staging technique.

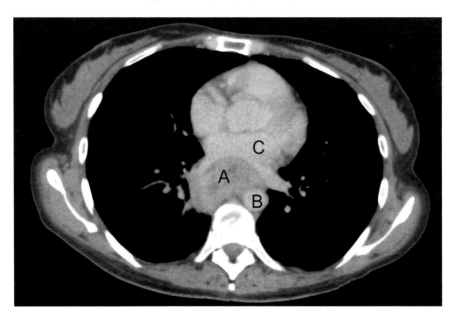

Fig. 5.20C Axial CT of the same patient with an obstructing oesophageal malignancy. This large tumour (A) compresses the oesophageal lumen, which is no longer visible. The normal descending aorta (B) and left atrium (C) are also labelled. CT will demonstrate mediastinal lymph node involvement (endoscopic US more sensitive and allows biopsy), also lung/liver/bone/abdominal lymph node metastases.

The differential diagnoses of an oesophageal stricture are:

- Benign oesophageal stricture – results from scarring from long-term reflux disease and Barrett's oesophagus (lower oesophagus).
- Postoperative stricture.
- Malignant oesophageal stricture.
- Oesophageal webs.
- Eosinophilic oesophagitis.
- Extrinsic compression of the oesophagus (from a lung mass, nodal mass or vascular anomaly).

3 What therapeutic options are available for symptomatic treatment of this condition and what are the complications?

Oesophageal malignancy carries a poor prognosis and management is often palliative. In operable patients with early stage tumours, oesophagectomy is the treatment of choice. Chemo-radiation may be used in some patients preoperatively, and is the main form of treatment for more advanced tumours.

Stents may be inserted using radiological or endoscopic techniques to relieve the stricture for palliative symptomatic control. The stent is measured so that it crosses the full length of the stricture and is self-expanding; a degree of 'waisting' in the middle is expected initially where the stent traverses the tumour (**Figure 5.20D**).

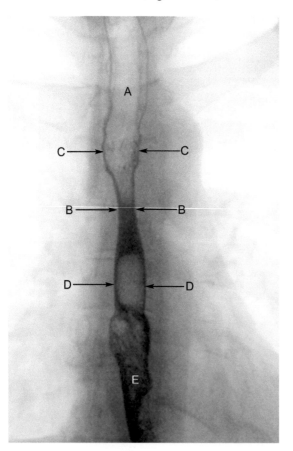

Fig. 5.20D An oesophageal malignancy after stenting. The proximal oesophagus is visualised above the upper part of the stent (A). There is compression/waisting from the tumour on either side of the stent (B) between the upper (C) and lower part of the stent (D). Contrast is seen passing through the stent into the distal oesophagus (E).

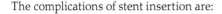

The complications of stent insertion are:

- Immediate.
  - Oesophageal perforation.
- Early.
  - Failure of the stent to relieve the obstruction owing to tumour overgrowth or incomplete coverage of the stricture by the stent (sometimes additional stents are needed).
- Late.
  - Proximal or distal stent migration.
  - Aspiration pneumonia.

The types of oesophageal malignancy are:

- Adenocarcinoma (arises from glandular cells, lower one-third of oesophagus).
  - Associated with reflux and obesity.
  - Follows Barrett's oesophagus owing to longstanding inflammation causing metaplasia and then dysplasia of the squamous cells to columnar cells and adenocarcinoma.
- Squamous cell carcinoma (arises from epithelial cells lining oesophagus).
  - Associated with alcohol, smoking, and achalasia.

LEARNING POINTS: OESOPHAGEAL CARCINOMA

- If there are any red flag symptoms for malignancy refer to gastroenterology urgently using the 2-week-wait rule.
- A malignant oesophageal stricture may have an irregular contour with asymmetric shouldering on barium swallow.
- Management is often palliative and based on symptom control.
- Endoscopic or radiological stent placement can palliatively relieve the obstruction.

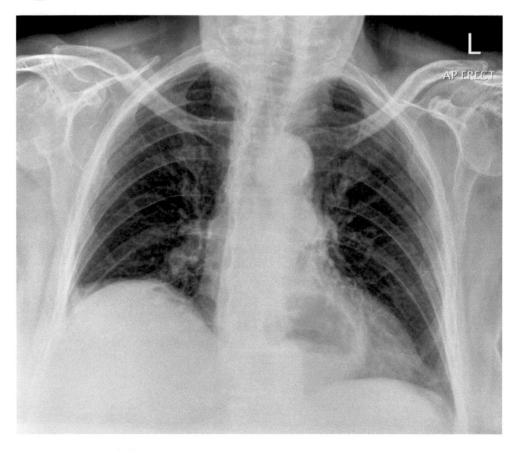

Fig. 5.21A AP erect CXR.

A 65-year-old male presents to his GP with heartburn, a chronic dry cough, and excess burping that has been present for the past year. He denies any weight loss, anorexia or shortness of breath and is otherwise fit and well. He has tried a 4-week course of omeprazole, which has not improved his symptoms, and he has had an *Helicobacter pylori* stool antigen test, which is negative.

On examination he has a body mass index (BMI) of 33. His heart sounds are normal and chest is clear. His abdomen is soft and he has minimal tenderness on palpation of the epigastrium.

A CXR is performed (**Figure 5.21A**).

CASE 5.21: QUESTIONS

1 What does the CXR show?
2 What are the long-term complications of this condition?
3 How would you manage this condition?

CASE 5.21: ANSWERS

1 What does the CXR show?

The CXR shows a large hiatus hernia, with the gastric fundus projected behind the heart, and a clear air–fluid level (**Figure 5.21B**).

- The gastric fundus has protruded through the oesophageal hiatus of the diaphragm into the thoracic cavity.
- These are usually sliding hiatus hernias (90%) where the gastro-oesophageal junction has displaced through the oesophageal hiatus. Rolling paraoesophageal hernias (10%) occur when the gastro-oesophageal junction remains in its normal position while a portion of the stomach herniates above the diaphragm.
- Most hiatus herniae are asymptomatic, some may present with reflux symptoms, postprandial fullness, chest pain or nausea and vomiting.
- Risk factors for hiatus hernia are those that raise intra-abdominal pressure, such as obesity, heavy lifting, chronic cough, and pregnancy.
- The main differential for this appearance on a CXR is a cavitating lung mass. It is often possible, however, to differentiate between the two on CXR but ask for senior advice if unsure. CT is helpful in equivocal cases or to aid with hernia repair surgical planning (**Figure 5.21C**).

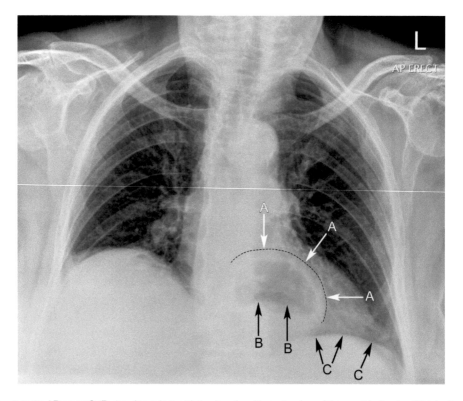

Fig. 5.21B AP erect CXR showing a large hiatus hernia with protrusion of the gastric fundus (A) into the thorax with an air–fluid level (B) above the left hemidiaphragm (C).

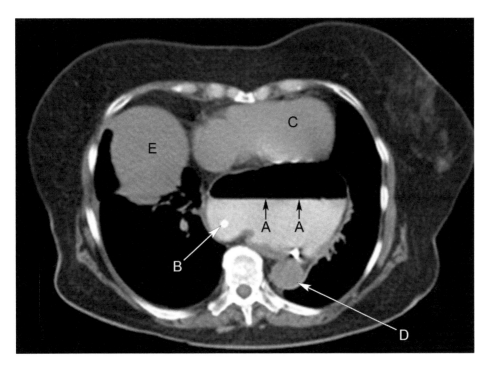

Fig. 5.21C Axial CT of the thorax confirming a large sliding hiatus hernia. The gastric fundus with air–fluid level (A) and NG tube (B) is seen above the diaphragm, behind the heart (C). The normal descending thoracic aorta (D) and liver (E) are also labelled.

2 What are the long-term complications of this condition?

The long-term complications include the risks of developing incarceration of the herniated bowel or development of a gastric volvulus. Associated gastro-oesophageal reflux disease (GORD) over many years can lead to the development of strictures, ulcers, and subsequent bleeding. Additionally, with long-term reflux the risk of oesophageal adenocarcinoma secondary to Barrett's oesophagus is increased and this condition will require endoscopic surveillance.

> **EXAM TIP**
>
> When asked about complications of a condition in an exam, make sure to structure your answer. The easiest way to do this is to break it down into immediate, early, and late complications. This is especially helpful in surgical conditions where, for example, bleeding may be an immediate complication, sepsis an early complication, and failure of the procedure a late complication.

3 How would you manage this condition?

Management options depend on whether the hernia is symptomatic or not. Most are incidental findings on CXR or endoscopy that require no specific management. Some, as in this case, are found through investigation for chronic acid reflux. Another CXR case is shown in **Figure 5.21D**.

Upper GI endoscopy may be used to determine any complications associated with GORD such as strictures, bleeding or ulceration, which can happen over time in severe cases.

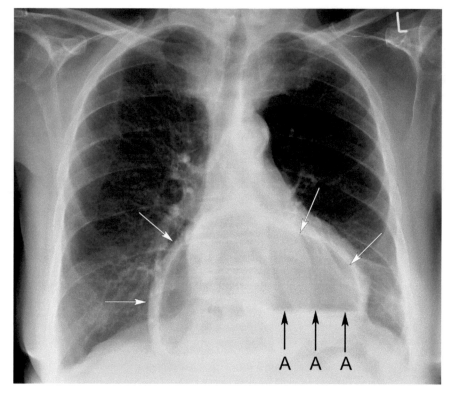

Fig. 5.21D A large hiatus hernia (white arrows) projected overlying the cardiac silhouette. Note the air–fluid level (A).

Management of hiatus hernias can be divided into conservative, medical, and surgical options:

- Conservative: if asymptomatic then there is no indication for treatment.
- Medical: if reflux symptoms are troubling then a trial of proton pump inhibitors (such as omeprazole or lansoprazole) may be helpful alongside lifestyle modification (e.g. smoking cessation and weight loss).
- Surgical: if medical management of GORD has failed and there are complications of the hiatus hernia (e.g. strictures, ulcers, bleeding). Those patients with large, symptomatic paraoesophageal hernias are at risk of incarceration and surgical repair is usually advised prior to this happening. Nissen fundoplication is the procedure most often performed for both types of hernia.

LEARNING POINTS: HIATUS HERNIA

- Hiatus herniae are usually asymptomatic and picked up incidentally on CXR.
- There are two main types of hiatus hernia: sliding (90%) and paraoesophageal (10%).
- Complications can be related to the hernia itself, such as incarceration in paraoesophageal hernias, or to long-term reflux symptoms such as ulceration.
- Surgical repair is indicated in most paraoesophageal hernias or for sliding hernias that are particularly large or associated with resistant symptoms.

Case 5.22

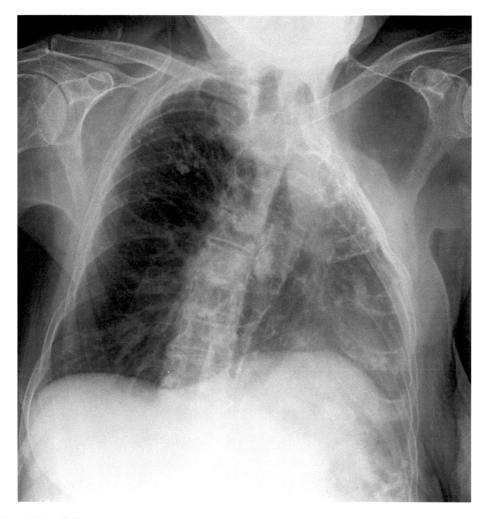

Fig. 5.22A CXR.

A 87-year-old male patient presents to his GP with recent discomfort over his left chest. On examination there is obvious deformity over his left thorax and there is minor tenderness of the left upper ribs, which he noticed after gardening. He appears otherwise well. A CXR is arranged for further assessment (**Figure 5.22A**).

CASE 5.22: QUESTIONS

1 What are the CXR findings?
2 What is the diagnosis?
3 What surgical treatments were used for this condition in the past?

CASE 5.22: ANSWERS

1 What are the CXR findings?

The CXR shows a severe thoracic deformity with crowding of abnormally modelled ribs and absent ribs in the left upper zone (**Figure 5.22B**). There is left hemithoracic volume loss with tracheal deviation to the left and a raised left hemidiaphragm. The left costophrenic angle is blunted, likely related to pleural thickening. Calcified granulomas are noted in the right upper zone and left lung.

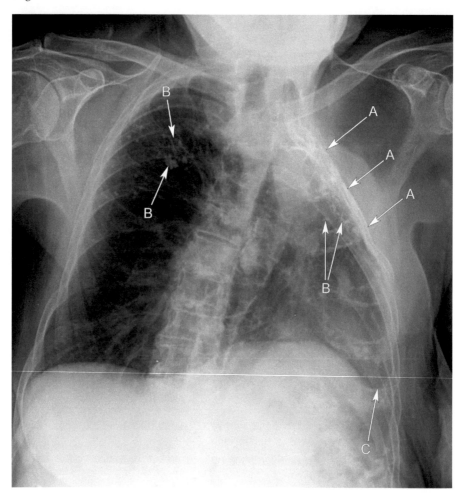

Fig. 5.22B A CXR showing loss of volume in the left hemithorax. The left upper ribs are deformed and crowded (A) and calcified granulomata can be seen in both lungs (B). The costophrenic angle on the left is blunted, likely longstanding (C).

2 What is the diagnosis?

The patient has had a previous left thoracoplasty with rib resection for TB, as evidenced by the CXR findings. Old calcified lung granulomata are indicative of previous TB infection.

3 What surgical treatments were used for this condition in the past?

Thoracoplasty was used from the early 1900s through to the late 1950s as one form of collapse therapy for TB prior to anti-TB medical therapy (**Figure 5.22C**). These historical techniques are re-emerging as a treatment option owing to the increasing incidence of multidrug resistant TB strains.

Collapse therapy was based on the observation that healed TB cavities were closed and that closing the cavities helped to inactivate the disease. In thoracoplasty this was achieved through resection of multiple ribs.

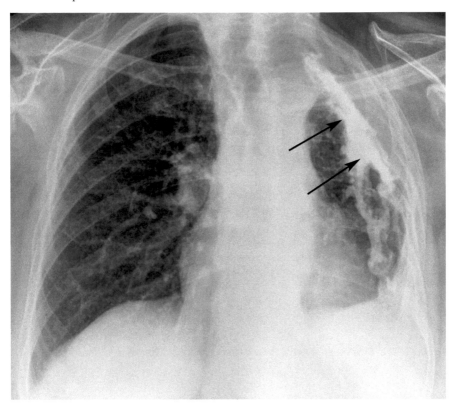

Fig. 5.22C Another patient (female) with evidence of previous left thoracoplasty. Note the extensive left pleural calcifications (arrows) – this is likely to be the result of a healed TB empyema, although oleothorax may also cause a pleural calcified lesion (oleothorax tends to be more circumscribed).

Procedure types are:

- Intrapleural thoracoplasty: involves multiple rib excisions as well as resection of the parietal pleura, periosteum, intercostal muscles, and intercostal neurovascular bundles.
- Extrapleural thoracoplasty: the rib periosteum, intercostal muscle, and parietal pleura are preserved.
- Plombage thoracoplasty: Plombe or filler (well-circumscribed radiopaque or radiolucent densities) are inserted in the space created between the rib cage, endothoracic fascia, and periosteum (**Figure 5.22D**).
- Phrenic nerve crush: diaphragm paralysis (look for scar in the supraclavicular fossa), often used in combination with an artificial pneumothorax.

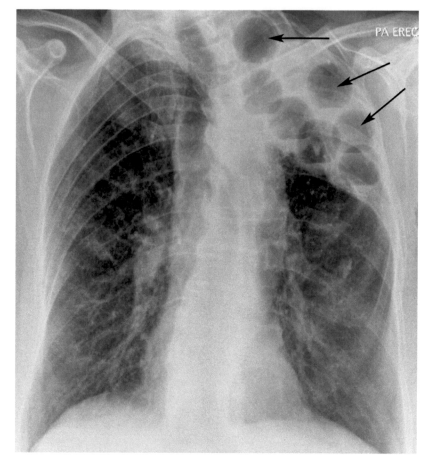

Fig. 5.22D CXR showing previous left plombage treatment. Note the multiple lucent spheres in the left upper zone (arrows) and also calcified lung granulomata.

- Apical lobectomy.
- Recurrent medical pneumothoraces.
- Oleothorax: involved insertion of an oil filled capsule between ribs and pleura to collapse adjacent lung. These lesions may be seen as calcified pleural masses.

4 How would you manage this patient?

This patient has no clinical evidence to suggest TB recurrence and has reassuring chest radiograph findings. His rib discomfort is likely to be musculoskeletal in origin after gardening. He can be discharged with an invitation to return if the thoracic discomfort persists/worsens.

> **LEARNING POINTS: THORACOPLASTY**
>
> - Thoracoplasty was used to treat TB prior to the introduction of medical therapy and is recognisable on CXR as upper zone volume loss with chest wall deformity.
> - Other forms of surgical collapse treatment included plombage and oleothorax.
> - The radiological findings are characteristic and once seen are readily recognisable.

Case 5.23

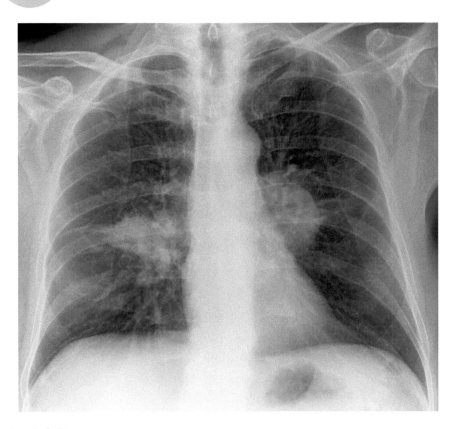

Fig. 5.23A CXR.

A 55-year-old Caucasian male presents to his GP with a persistent dry cough that has been present for 2 months. He has been feeling more lethargic than usual and has noticed about 6 kg of recent weight loss.

On examination, there is palpable, firm, nontender cervical lymphadenopathy. The chest is clear, heart sounds are normal, and the abdomen is soft with no palpable masses. A set of bloods is performed and a CXR is arranged (**Figure 5.23A**). His blood results are:

Hb	116 g/L (130–180 g/L)	Potassium	4.2 mmol/L (3.2–5.1 mmol/L)
MCV	92 fL (80–100 fL)	Urea	4.2 mmol/L (1.7–8.3 mmol/L)
WBC	4.6 × 10⁹/L (4.0–11.0 × 10⁹/L)	Creatinine	86 micromol/L (62–106 micromol/L)
CRP	9 mg/L (<5 mg/L)	Corrected calcium	2.65 mmol/L (2.15–2.55 mmol/L)
Sodium	140 mmol/L (135–146 mmol/L)		

CASE 5.23: QUESTIONS

1 What is the key radiological finding?
2 What are the differential diagnoses?
3 What further imaging is necessary?

4 How would you further investigate this patient?

CASE 5.23: ANSWERS

1 What is the key radiological finding?

The CXR shows bilateral symmetrical lobulated enlargement of the hila secondary to lymph-adenopathy (**Figure 5.23B**).

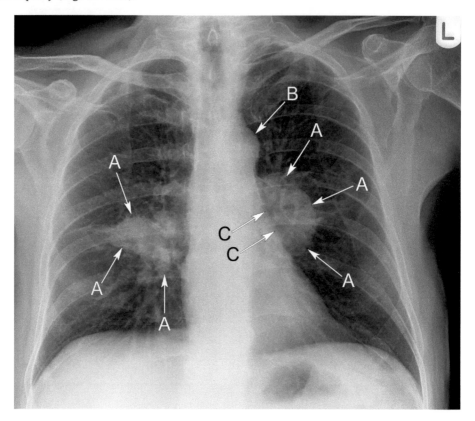

Fig. 5.23B CXR showing bilateral hilar lymphadenopathy (A). The pulmonary arteries cannot be separated from the hilar masses, confirming the origin of the masses to the hila. Also note the normal aortic arch (B) and left heart border (C) seen clearly separate to the mass, confirming the mass is not anterior and abutting the heart (border would be lost).

2 What are the differential diagnoses?

The differential diagnoses for bilateral hilar lymphadenopathy are:

- Symmetrical.
  - Sarcoidosis.
  - Lymphoma.
  - Chronic lymphoid leukaemia (CLL).
- Asymmetrical (or unilateral) – note symmetrical causes may also cause asymmetric changes.
  - Tuberculosis.
  - Lung malignancy.

In this patient, the clinical information and CXR suggest sarcoidosis; however, it is usually not possible to distinguish the cause of bihilar lymphadenopathy without further investigations.

> **EXAM POINT**
>
> Know a little about each of the causes of bilateral hilar lymphadenopathy as they are common and should not be missed:
>
> - Bilateral.
>   - Malignancy (CLL, lymphoma).
>   - Sarcoidosis.
> - Asymmetrical.
>   - Tuberculosis.
>   - Malignancy (lung, metastases).

3 What further imaging is necessary?

CT of the thorax and abdomen is necessary to confirm the findings and allow differentiation of the masses within the hilum. It also allows visualisation of the lungs and a review for abnormalities and lymph nodes elsewhere.

A CT thorax of the same patient is shown (**Figure 5.23C**). Try to identify the normal and abnormal structures yourself.

> **EXAM POINT**
>
> When asked in an exam what investigations you would perform, remember to structure your answer. Always remember to mention you would take senior advice prior to arranging more advanced investigations, after bedside baseline tests.
>
> - Bedside tests – bloods, urine dip/MSU, ECG, cardiac monitoring, blood cultures, ABG/VBG (as applicable, be able to say why you would perform each test).
> - Imaging – be specific about which part of the body you wish to image, which investigation, and why.
> - More invasive investigations – e.g. endoscopy, biopsy, interventional radiology.

- Sarcoidosis is a disease of unknown aetiology involving abnormal collections of inflammatory noncaseating chronic granulomas. Initially it tends to affect the lungs, skin or lymph nodes; however, it can affect multiple other organs such as the heart, liver, brain, and eyes. Often there are few or no symptoms but it may cause shortness of breath and cough. An early sign is a high blood serum calcium level (with normal parathyroid hormone). Later clinical findings in progressive respiratory disease are due to lung fibrosis, which can cause severe right-sided heart failure.
- Thoracic sarcoidosis is staged according to the imaging findings:
  - Stage 0 - normal CXR findings.
  - Stage I - bilateral hilar lympadenopathy.
  - Stage II - bilateral hilar lymphadenopathy and pulmonary infiltrates.
  - Stage III - pulmonary infiltrates alone.
  - Stage IV - end-stage lung disease with pulmonary fibrosis and honeycombing.

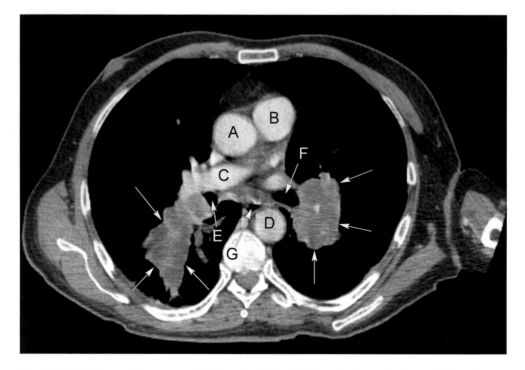

Fig. 5.23C CT thorax of the same patient showing bilateral hilar lymphadenopathy (arrows). Normal mediastinal structures including the ascending aorta (A), pulmonary trunk (B), right pulmonary artery (C), descending aorta (D), and air-filled oesophagus (G) are demonstrated. Note the normal black and air-filled right (E) and left main bronchi (F).

4 How would you further investigate this patient?

Further investigations are necessary to confirm the diagnosis and to assess the extent of lung disease. These may be started by the GP but would also require a referral to a specialist respiratory consultant.

- Bloods: FBC and CRP to look for infection and a blood film to look for leukaemic cells. Check serum calcium as this can be high in sarcoidosis and malignancy. Serum ACE is also increased; however, this is a nonspecific marker and rarely used.
- CT scan, for the reasons discussed above. HRCT reformats are used to look at the lungs in more detail.
- Image-guided core biopsy of an accessible lymph node, (this patient had an US-guided core biopsy of a cervical lymph node that confirmed sarcoid granuloma infiltration).
- Bronchoscopy with washout if sarcoidosis or TB suspected, with biopsy of any lesions for histology and confirmation of diagnosis.
- Pulmonary function tests and a diffusion capacity of the lung for carbon monoxide (DLCO) test are used routinely in evaluation and follow-up of patients with sarcoidosis and chronic lung disease.

Treatment with corticosteroids is only required if the patient is symptomatic. NSAIDs are used for any associated arthralgia (which is common). In patients who do not respond to steroid therapy or where it is not tolerated, immune modulating therapy is used (e.g. methotrexate, aza-thioprine, infliximab).

Sarcoid eye disease with neuro-ophthalmic involvement can present with diplopia owing to cranial nerve palsies or decreased vision caused by optic nerve infiltration/oedema. Ocular sarcoidosis presents with symptoms of uveitis (blurred vision, photophobia, floaters, redness, and pain). Mass lesions can also develop. These need urgent review by an ophthalmologist owing to the risk of blindness. Systemic disease is more likely to be progressive in these patients.

> **TOP TIP**
>
> You will be expected to recognise bihilar lymphadenopathy on CXR and suggest a differential diagnosis as well as further investigations such as bloods, imaging (CT), and referral to a respiratory consultant. Be able to discuss differential diagnoses such as sarcoidosis, tuberculosis, and lung malignancy.

> **LEARNING POINTS: SARCOIDOSIS, BILATERAL HILAR LYMPHADENOPATHY**
>
> ■ Bilateral hilar lymphadenopathy is a common exam scenario and you should be able to recognise the CXR findings.
> ■ Common causes of bilateral hilar lymphadenopathy include sarcoidosis, lymphoma, and tuberculosis.
> ■ Thoracic sarcoidosis is the most common form and is staged according to the imaging findings, which range from normal to significant fibrosis.
> ■ Diagnosis is best confirmed with lymph node or lung nodule biopsy or via bronchoscopy.

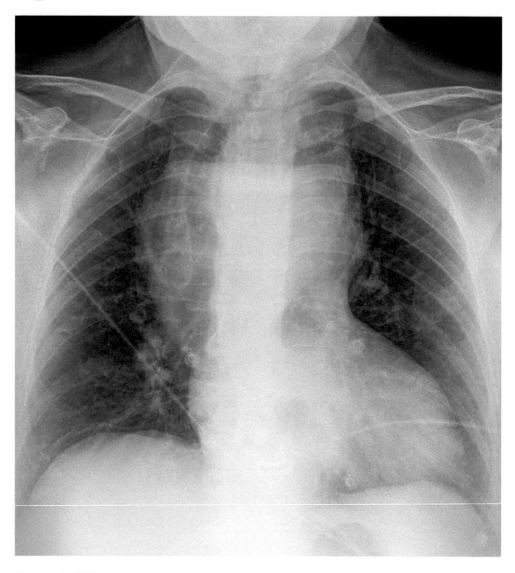

Fig. 5.24A CXR.

A 75-year-old female presents to her GP with a sensation of fullness in her neck, worse when she lies flat and also mildly increasing shortness of breath on exercise. On clinical examination there is a firm, nontender swelling in her neck, palpable above the manubrium. A CXR is arranged initially (**Figure 5.24A**).

CASE 5.24: QUESTIONS

1 What are the CXR findings?
2 What is the diagnosis? Is there a differential diagnosis?
3 How would you investigate and manage this patient?

CASE 5.24: ANSWERS

1 What are the CXR findings?

The CXR shows a large mediastinal mass with a lobulated contour that involves the superior, anterior, and middle mediastinum. The trachea is deviated to the right (**Figure 5.24B**).

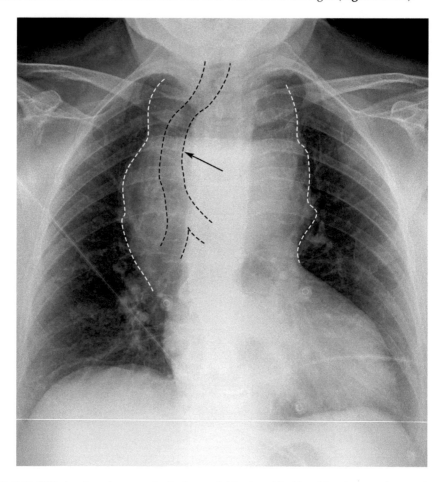

Fig. 5.24B CXR showing a large mediastinal mass (white dotted line) involving the superior, anterior, and middle mediastinum. Note the silhouette of the pulmonary vessels is obliterated by the mass, indicating contact with the hila in the middle mediastinum (hilum overlay sign). The trachea is deviated to the right (arrow). Note also the mediastinal mass extends up to and above the clavicles but the supraclavicular portion is not well defined.

2 What is the diagnosis? Is there a differential diagnosis?

The likely diagnosis is that of a multinodular goitre of the thyroid with retrosternal, intrathoracic extension. As can be seen from the CXR, the intrathoracic component is significant and the patient describes symptoms of mass effect with pressure effects in the neck and shortness of breath, which may relate to tracheal compression/deviation. Dysphagia may also occur in large thyroid lesions.

Clinically patients with goitre are often hypothyroid, although a toxic nodule within the goitre may cause hyperthyroidism.

As described this is a large mediastinal lesion involving several compartments. Typically an intrathoracic goitre tends to involve the anterior mediastinum and is one of the causes of an anterior mediastinal mass.

Causes of an anterior mediastinal mass – think of the 4 'Ts':

- **T**hyroid.
- **T**eratoma.
- **T**hymus (thymic tumour, e.g. thymoma).
- 'Terrible' lymph nodes, usually lymphoma.

Radiologically on CXR, the anterior mediastinum does not extend above the clavicles, therefore any mass that clearly extends above this level towards the root of the neck is likely to be extending from the neck itself (cervicothoracic sign).

3 How would you investigate and manage this patient?

This patient requires full history and examination. Look particularly for evidence of hypo/hyperthyroidism in the history/examination. A thyroid lump is a common OSCE scenario; familiarise yourself with thyroid examination.

Baseline bloods, i.e. FBC/TFTs, clearly are important.

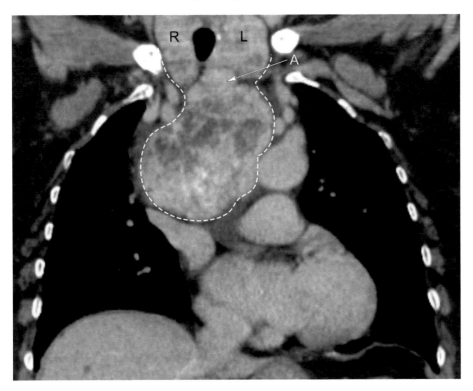

Fig. 5.24C Coronal postcontrast thoracic CT confirming a large lobulated multinodular goitre with retrosternal extension into the mediastinum (white dotted line). Note the right (R) and left (L) lobes of the thyroid and communication of the mediastinal thyroid mass with the left lobe (arrow A).

In view of the significant intrathoracic extension of the goitre and evidence of mass effect plus possible airway compromise, this patient requires urgent referral to an ear, nose, and throat (ENT) department.

Once in hospital, imaging investigations will include:

- US neck/thyroid to confirm multinodular nature of the goitre and demonstrate any suspicious intrathyroid lesions requiring fine-needle aspiration cytology. US will also assess the neck for suspicious nodes, but will not be able to access the intrathoracic component.
- CT neck/chest – to accurately delineate the size and extent of the thyroid enlargement (**Figure 5.24C**). This will precisely gauge the degree of tracheal deviation/compression and also the relationship of the goitre to intrathoracic vessels. The need for surgical intervention will depend on the operative fitness of the patient and whether airway compression is of concern (surgery will require ENT/cardiothoracic approach).

LEARNING POINTS: MULTINODULAR THYROID/SUPERIOR MEDIASTINAL MASS

- Multinodular goitres are seen more commonly in women aged 35–50 years. The gland may be hyperfunctioning or hypofunctioning.
- Nodules may harbour malignancy and US is performed to look for any suspicious features or dominant nodules, (large, hypervascular, with microcalcifications) that may require fine-needle aspiration and cytology.
- Thyroid goitre is on the differential list for an anterior/superior mediastinal mass on CXR, and is associated with the cervicothoracic sign and also deviation of the trachea.
- CT can be useful to fully characterise the extent of a retrosternal goitre.
- Treatment may be indicated if the goitre is symptomatic (hyperfunctioning or hypofunctioning thyroid) or if it is causing significant mass effect.

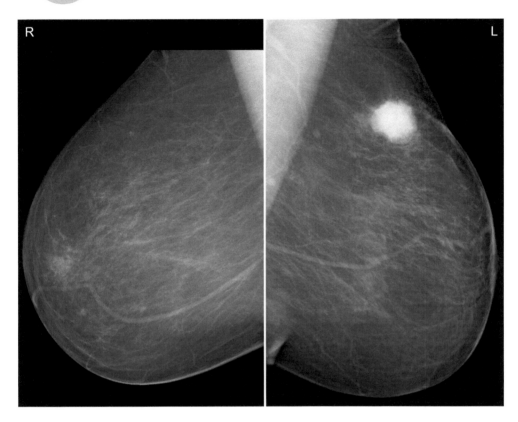

Fig. 5.25A Lateral oblique mammographic views of both breasts (R/L).

A 57-year-old female presents to her GP having felt a lump in her left breast. On examination there is a fixed, nonmobile nodule in the upper outer quadrant of her left breast. The GP refers the patient urgently to the local breast unit. A mammogram is arranged following clinical assessment (**Figure 5.25A**).

CASE 5.25: QUESTIONS

1 What are the imaging findings?
2 What are the indications for mammography?
3 What do you know about mammography?
4 How would you further investigate and manage this patient?

CASE 5.25: ANSWERS

1 What are the imaging findings?

The mammogram shows a lobulated dense, ill-defined mass in the superior aspect of the left breast with overlying skin retraction, in keeping with malignancy (**Figure 5.25B**). Benign lesions tend to be circumscribed and smooth with no associated parenchymal or skin changes – all cases will need US for further characterisation.

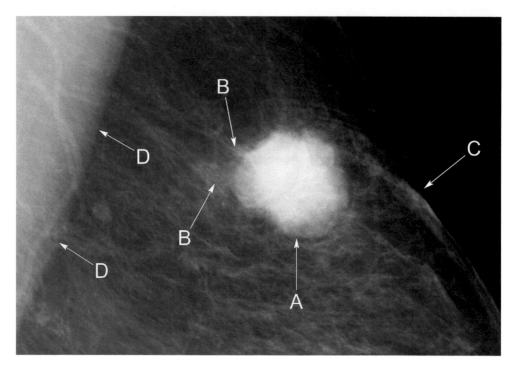

Fig. 5.25B Magnified lateral oblique mammographic view of the left breast showing a mass in the upper breast (A). This is lobulated and poorly defined in part, and there is distortion of the adjacent breast parenchyma (B). Note the overlying skin retraction (C – clinically this will appear as a dimple) and normal pectoralis major muscle shadow (D).

2 What are the indications for mammography?

Indications for mammography:

- Screening programme (in the UK ages vary, currently screening is being offered to women aged 47–73 years).
- Assessment of symptomatic breast patients (usually >35 years old).
- Follow-up of previously treated breast cancer patients.

3 What do you know about mammography?

Mammography is a dedicated radiographic technique for imaging the breast. It is used for both screening and diagnostic symptomatic imaging. Two standard views are obtained, craniocaudal (CC) and mediolateral oblique (MLO).

Digital mammography (full field digital mammography: FFDM) is a newer technique that provides higher resolution imaging and is more sensitive in younger women with denser breast tissue. Mammography does involve a radiation dose to the breast, although this is not large and is reduced in newer digital units.

4 How would you further investigate and manage this patient?

The assessment of the symptomatic breast involves the concept of triple assessment: *this is the key phrase to mention in the exam.* Triple assessment of the symptomatic breast includes:

- Clinical assessment (examination of both breasts and axillae and supraclavicular fossae/neck if there is a lump). In the exam you will usually encounter a mannequin or actor with a prosthetic breast. Remember the axillae and always check you are not hurting the patient. Warn the patient if you have cold hands before you examine her!
- Imaging with either mammography and/or US.
- US only for women <35 years old.
- Mammography for women >35 years old (due to the less dense breasts) and US of breast and ipsilateral axilla if palpable or mammographic abnormality (**Figures 5.25C** and **5.25D**).
- US-guided core biopsy and histology if needed.

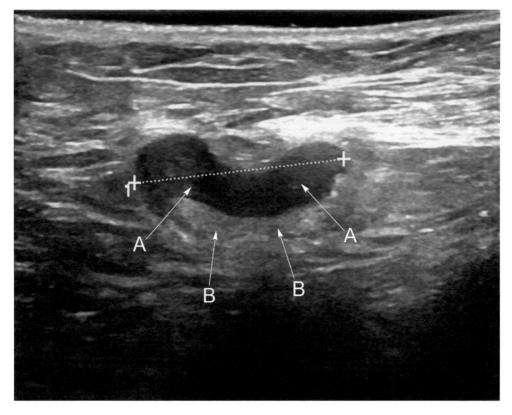

Fig. 5.25C US of a left axillary lymph node (callipers) showing features of malignant infiltration including enlarged size, eccentric thickened cortex (A), and a displaced node hilum (B).

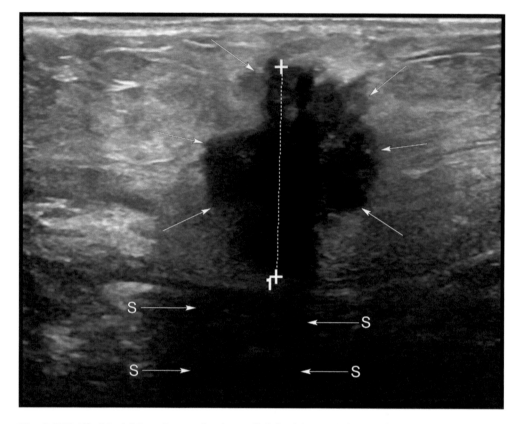

Fig. 5.25D US of the left breast mass showing an ill-defined, hypoechoic mass (arrows) with posterior acoustic shadowing (arrows S) consistent with a carcinoma.

MRI of the breasts is not used in initial assessment but has a valuable role as a problem-solving tool – MRI is also excellent in the evaluation of the treated breast and breast implants.

Further investigation and management includes completion of the triple assessment with US-guided core biopsy of the breast mass and core biopsy or fine-needle aspiration of any suspicious axillary lymph nodes.

A score is given for each aspect of the triple assessment (Examination, Imaging, and Cytology) between 1 and 5. The higher the score, the greater the suspicion of malignancy. The above patient received a score of E4 (suspicious lump on examination), M5/U5 (malignant on mammogram and US), and B5 (malignant on histology).

These results are discussed at a multidisciplinary team meeting involving surgeons, oncologists, radiologists, histopathology, and nurse specialists.

The results are then carefully explained to the patient with counselling offered and discussion of management options. Management is likely to involve surgery to the breast (wide local excision or mastectomy) and also axillary surgery. Postoperatively, the patient may require chemotherapy or radiotherapy depending on tumour type and node status.

PATHOLOGY OF BREAST CANCER

Virtually all breast cancers are adenocarcinomas (tumour derived from epithelial cells of glands or ducts):

- Preinvasive carcinomas are tumours confined to the ducts or the acini of the lobules without infiltration of the basement membrane. These are called either ductal or lobular carcinomas in situ (DCIS/LCIS).
- Invasive carcinomas are malignant tumours that have penetrated the basement membrane of the tissue of origin and spread to other tissues. Of these, 80% are invasive ductal carcinoma and 10–15% are invasive lobular carcinomas.

Tumours may spread either locally (directly into the surrounding tissue), via lymph nodes (to the axillary and periclavicular nodes) or via the blood (to the lungs, bones, liver, brain, and adrenal glands).

TREATMENT OPTIONS FOR BREAST CANCER

- Surgery gives the best outcomes with either wide local excision or mastectomy. Surgery is combined with sentinel axillary node sampling or axillary clearance depending on tumour type and patient.
- Adjuvant radiotherapy is given to the chest wall after mastectomy for tumours with a high risk of local recurrence.
- Adjuvant chemotherapy improves survival, particularly in younger patients with node-positive disease. Anthracyclines are usually combined with other agents. Hormone therapy (tamoxifen blocks oestrogen receptors, aromatase inhibitor blocking oestrogen production) is used longer term postsurgery in oestrogen-positive tumours. Some breast cancers are stimulated by human epidermal growth factor receptor 2 (HER-2), while biological therapy, e.g. trastuzamab, blocks the effects of HER-2.

LEARNING POINTS: BREAST LUMPS/BREAST CARCINOMA

- Examination of a breast lump is a common OSCE scenario.
- Triple assessment, involving clinical examination, imaging, and biopsy with discussion at a MDT meeting, is key to initial management.
- Mammography is less effective at detecting the early changes of breast cancer in women <35 years, as their breast tissue is often dense. US usually initially preferred in patients below this age with a palpable abnormality.
- Always review both CC and MLO images for any mammogram and be able to orientate yourself. Comment on any asymmetry, masses, calcification, skin changes, and enlarged axillary nodes.

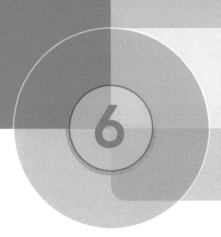

Cardiovascular cases

6

HANNAH ADAMS, SARAH HANCOX,
CRISTINA RUSCANU, AND
DAVID C HOWLETT

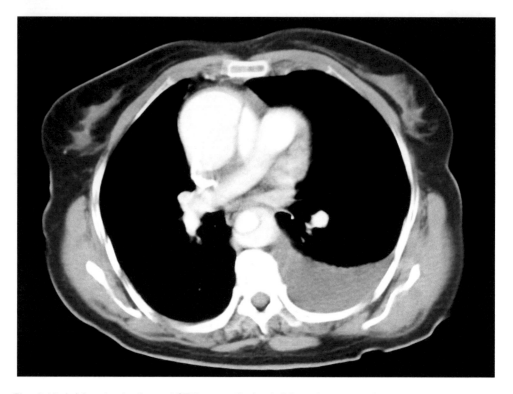

Fig. 6.1A Axial contrast-enhanced CT thorax at the level of the pulmonary trunk.

A 63-year-old male presents to the ED with a severe, constant, sharp, central chest pain radiating to his back, which started 1 hour ago. He is on medication for hypertension and has a 40 pack-year smoking history.

On examination he looks pale. Heart sounds are normal and his chest is clear. He is tachycardic at 110 bpm and has a BP in the right arm of 140/96 mmHg and in the left arm of 104/74 mmHg. Radial pulses are present but weaker in the left than the right and femoral pulses also are weak.

The ECG shows a sinus tachycardia and the CXR reports a small left pleural effusion only. After discussion with a senior colleague, you organise a CT thorax (**Figure 6.1A**).

CASE 6.1: QUESTIONS

1 What does the CT thorax show?
2 What is the likely diagnosis?
3 How would you manage this patient?
4 What are the complications of this condition?

CASE 6.1: ANSWERS

1 What does the CT thorax show?

This CT demonstrates an aortic dissection with an intimal dissection flap involving both the descending and ascending aorta. The following structures are identifiable (**Figure 6.1B**):

- Ascending aorta true lumen with visible intimal flap and false lumen.
- Descending aorta with intimal flap and false lumen.

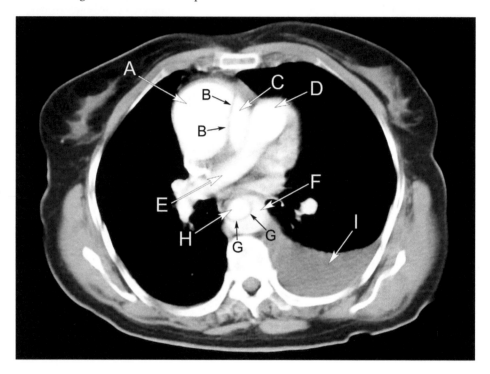

Fig. 6.1B Postcontrast CT thorax at the level of the pulmonary trunk. The ascending aorta true lumen is seen (A) with visible intimal flap (B) and false lumen (C). Descending aorta true lumen (F), intimal flap (G) and false lumen (H). Note: left basal pleural effusion (I), normal main pulmonary artery (D), and right main pulmonary artery (E).

2 What is the likely diagnosis?

The history and imaging findings are consistent with a diagnosis of aortic dissection. This is where there is a tear in the tunica intima of the aorta causing blood to flow between the layers of the wall of the aorta and forcing the layers apart. This classically presents with severe, tearing chest pain, radiating to between the scapulae. This is often in a patient with cardiac risk factors such as smoking, high blood pressure or high cholesterol.

If suspected, then an urgent CT aortogram with contrast is necessary alongside an echocardiogram to look at the aortic root (as this is more accurate for diagnosis of this type of dissection where the dissection extends to involve the aortic root and there may be acute aortic regurgitation, pericardial effusion, and also coronary artery involvement). You will need support from senior colleagues and both ITU and cardiothoracic involvement.

There is a system of classification dependent on the extent of the dissection diagnosed on imaging and this informs the management (*Table 6.1* and **Figure 6.1C**).

Table 6.1 Stanford system of classification of aortic dissection

Type A	Involves the ascending aorta and the aortic arch (AA) (proximal to the origin of left subclavian artery) +/– descending aorta. The tear can originate in the ascending aorta, the AA or in the descending aorta
Type B	Involves the descending aorta or AA (distal to the origin of left subclavian artery), without involvement of the ascending aorta/arch proximal to the left subclavian artery

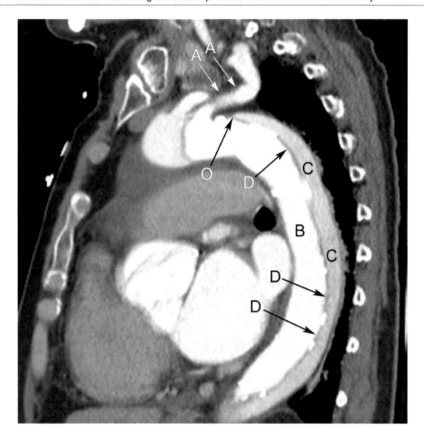

Fig. 6.1C A sagittal reconstruction of a CT aortogram postcontrast in another patient. It shows a type B aortic dissection with origin (O) distal to the left subclavian artery (A) involving the descending thoracic aorta (B) with a false lumen on the outside (C) and visible intimal flap (D). It does not involve the ascending aorta or arch thereby classifying it as a type B dissection.

3 How would you manage this patient?

Management is via an ABCDE approach. These patients can become unstable very quickly; therefore, it is necessary for continuous cardiac monitoring with initial management in a specialist cardiology/cardiothoracic unit:

- Bloods – FBC to check Hb levels, U&Es as patient can be in shock, clotting factors as any derangement will need to be corrected, serum troponin to ensure that there is no concurrent myocardial infarction (MI), and cross match as patient could need a transfusion.

- It is important to perform an ECG and check cardiac enzymes as cardiac blood supply can be affected in type A dissections.
- Early imaging is vital for prompt diagnosis and decision on management.

Acute aortic dissection can be treated surgically or medically. This is dependent on the patient's current clinical condition, comorbidities, and type of dissection (extent):

- Type A: emergency surgical repair.
- Type B: if a complicated type B dissection, then surgery is indicated. Otherwise, medical management is the mainstay of treatment.

4 What are the complications of this condition?

Complicated type B dissections involve the following:

- Propagation of aorta (increasing diameter).
- Increasing size of haematoma.
- Compromise of major branches of the aorta.
- Impending rupture.
- Persistent pain despite adequate pain management.
- Bleeding into the pleural cavity.
- Development of saccular aneurysm.

Medical management remains the treatment of choice for type B dissections unless they are leaking, ruptured or complicated (see above). The principles also relate to patients awaiting surgery in order to decrease the intimal tear and propagation of the dissection, and also postoperatively. Antihypertensive treatment in the form of beta-blockers (IV labetolol) is usually used with continuous cardiac monitoring.

Surgical management aims to alleviate the symptoms and decrease the frequency of complications. Ultimately the surgeon aims to prevent aortic rupture and death. The affected layers of the aorta are sutured together and the aorta is reinforced with a Dacron graft. Advances in stenting technology have also allowed this technique to be used by interventional radiologists in more stable type B dissections.

TOP TIPS

A history of severe, sudden-onset, tearing chest pain with unequal four limb blood pressures in a susceptible patient should raise your suspicion of aortic dissection. ABCDE management and early involvement of a senior doctor is important. Prompt imaging will help with your diagnosis.

LEARNING POINTS: AORTIC DISSECTION

- Aortic dissection presents with severe, sudden-onset, tearing chest pain radiating between the scapulae.
- CT imaging will show a false lumen within the aorta but an echocardiogram is more accurate for evaluation of aortic root involvement.
- Dependent on the level of the dissection, it can be classified as type A (involving ascending aorta) or type B (descending aorta only below the level of the left subclavian artery).
- Emergency management of type A dissection is surgical while type B is often managed medically.

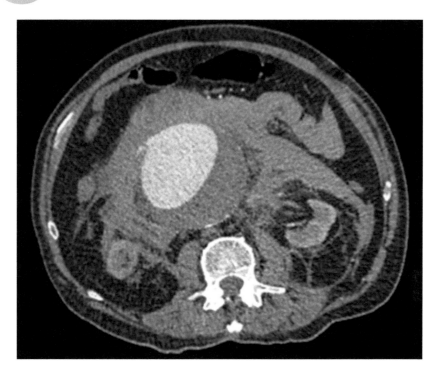

Fig. 6.2A Axial arterial enhanced CT ('aortogram') at the level of the umbilicus.

A 68-year-old male presents to the ED with generalised abdominal pain that has been worsening over the last 24 hours and now radiates to his back. He does not report any change in bowel habit or recent weight loss. He is on antihypertensive medication and reports that he has a high cholesterol level. He smoked a pipe for 40 years but has now given this up.

On examination, he appears pale and is in some discomfort. He has a BMI of 32. He is hypotensive at 110/72 mmHg and tachycardic at 90 bpm. He has an SPO$_2$ of 98% on air. Heart sounds are normal and his chest is clear. His abdomen is generally tender, most marked at the umbilicus, but not distended and there is no palpable tenderness in the loins or down the spine. His blood results are as follows:

Hb	109 g/L (130–180 g/L)	LFTs	normal
WBC	9 × 10⁹/L (4.0–11.0 × 10⁹/L)	Serum amylase	normal
CRP	8 mg/L (<5 mg/L)		

The initial FAST scan (focused assessment with sonography for trauma) performed in the ED is nondiagnostic owing to bowel gas, and a CT scan is arranged (**Figure 6.2A**).

CASE 6.2: QUESTIONS

1 What does the CT scan show?
2 What other imaging might show this abnormality in an emergency situation?
3 How would you manage this patient?
4 How might this condition be prevented in the older population?

CASE 6.2: ANSWERS

1 What does the CT scan show?

The CT 'aortogram' shows a ruptured AAA, which is a surgical emergency (**Figures 6.2B** and **6.2C**). There is a contained leak from the AAA, which will lead to further bleeding and ultimately death. Urgent surgical (or radiological) intervention is necessary.

Leaking AAA can present with very nonspecific symptoms ranging from abdominal pain to back pain, and can often be misdiagnosed as renal colic or pyelonephritis. A retroperitoneal haematoma may compress the ureter and cause dipstick-positive haematuria causing further potential confusion with renal colic.

AAA may be associated with:

- Atherosclerosis (most common).
- Chronic aortic dissection.
- Vasculitis, e.g. Takayasu arteritis.
- Connective tissue disorders, e.g. Marfan's or Ehlers–Danlos syndrome.

Complications of AAA are:

- Bleeding due to leak or rupture.
- Fistula (aortoenteric would cause life-threatening bleeding into the bowel).

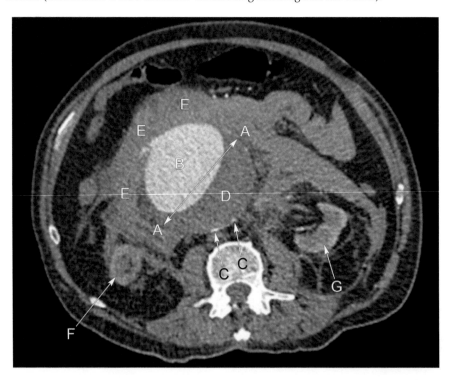

Fig. 6.2B CT 'aortogram' showing a ruptured AAA. Note the large 9 cm aortic aneurysm (A), aortic lumen with contrast (B), mural calcification (C), mural thrombus (D), and retroperitoneal haemorrhage (E). Also demonstrated are the chronically scarred and atrophic right (F) and left (G) kidneys. Note the anterior and right margins of the aneurysm are not well seen owing to adjacent retroperitoneal haematoma.

2 What other imaging might show this abnormality in an emergency situation?

CT angiography is ideal for confirming the diagnosis and for preoperative planning as it accurately determines the size and shape of the AAA and its relationship to branch arteries and the aortic bifurcation. It is also superior to US in detecting and sizing common iliac artery aneurysms. Patients must be haemodynamically stable and monitored closely when they are referred to CT.

There are, however, a number of other imaging modalities that may detect a AAA:

- AXR: this is an insensitive test but may outline the curvilinear arterial calcification of an aneurysm.
- US: this is simple, quick, inexpensive, and commonly used technique in the ED in patients with nonspecific symptoms or where a AAA is suspected. It is not sensitive for detecting leaks or rupture and may be limited by overlying bowel gas (as in this case) or abdominal tenderness. US is, however, used for routine AAA screening of men over 65 years old in the UK.

3 How would you manage this patient?

Management of this patient is via an ABCDE approach. This is a surgical emergency and, therefore, urgent discussion with the surgical team and anaesthetist is required.

Do not forget:

- IV access with two large bore cannulae in the antecubital fossae.
- Bloods. Check Hb, U&Es, and clotting, and cross match 8–10 units.
- ECG and portable CXR, VBG, and cardiac monitoring.
- Imaging. US in the ED if sufficient expertise is available may show the aneurysm. CT aortogram is the technique of choice following urgent senior surgical and radiological discussion.

If there is a suspicion of a ruptured AAA, careful BP control with hypotensive resuscitation is advised, under the guidance of an acute medicine physician. Raising the BP too high may cause clot migration and rebleeding. The ideal replacement fluid is blood but local resuscitation protocols will apply. If the AAA is confirmed to be leaking then either open or endovascular aneurysm repair (EVAR) will be required, depending on available expertise and the clinical condition of the patient.

AAA repair options:

- EVAR (radiology and surgical collaboration). A stent-graft is inserted via the femoral artery in the groin up to the aorta, and deployed over the aneurysmal section. This supports the aneurysm and restores normal blood flow.
- Open aneurysm repair (surgical). The abdomen is opened and the aorta exposed and repaired with a graft. This is still the standard procedure in many institutions.

EVAR is less invasive than open surgery, has a lower morbidity and mortality rate, and reduces postoperative recovery time. It is performed in elective aneurysm repairs as well as in patients undergoing emergency repair for rupture. Not all aneurysms, however, are suitable for EVAR and a CT aortogram is always required for preprocedural planning.

TOP TIPS

Elective management of AAA can be classified as conservative, medical, or surgical:

- Conservative: screening programme, monitoring of aneurysms >3 cm.
- Medical: risk factor management (BP, cholesterol, weight, smoking).
- Surgical: aneurysms >5.5 cm or growing >1 cm/year or after leak/rupture.

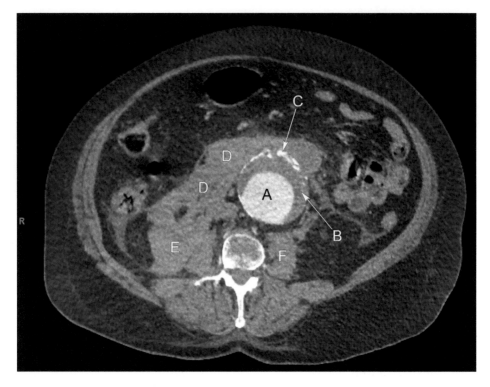

Fig. 6.2C CT aortogram of a different patient with aneurysmal dilation of the infrarenal aorta, measuring 6 cm diameter, with contrast in the aortic lumen (A), mural thrombus (B), and mural calcification (C). There is also a large para-aortic haematoma (D), which has tracked into the retroperitoneum along the right iliopsoas (E), which is enlarged (this finding may be visible on AXR). This contrasts with the normal looking left iliopsoas (F).

4 How might this condition be prevented in the older population?

Owing to the mortality associated with a large AAA, the UK has a screening programme for at-risk patients (males over 65 years old). Men are offered an US examination at the age of 65 years and small aneurysms (>3 cm diameter) are followed up. If >5.5 cm or growing >1 cm in 1 year then intervention is recommended.

LEARNING POINTS: LEAKING ABDOMINAL AORTIC ANEURYSM

- Rupture of a AAA is a surgical emergency with a high mortality rate and can present with collapse in a patient who is cardiovascularly unstable.
- AAAs >5.5 cm are at risk of rupture and should be considered for either elective open or endovascular repair.
- A leaking AAA can present with nonspecific symptoms, such as abdominal or back pain, and may be misdiagnosed as renal colic.
- US is accurate for AAA screening; however, CT angiography (in stable patients) is the reference standard test for diagnosis and preoperative planning.

Case 6.3

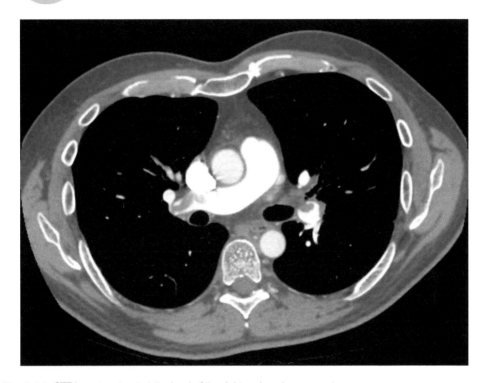

Fig. 6.3A CTPA postcontrast at the level of the right main pulmonary artery.

A 63-year-old female presents to the ED at night having woken with sudden onset shortness of breath and sharp, right-sided, chest pain, which is worse on inspiration. She is undergoing chemotherapy for breast cancer and had a left mastectomy 2 months ago. She is a previous smoker with a 20 pack-year history.

On examination, she is normotensive at 128/74 mmHg, tachycardic at 110 bpm, tachypnoeic at 30 bpm, and has an SPO_2 of 88% on air. Chest and cardiovascular examinations are normal. Her ECG shows a sinus tachycardia.

A CTPA is arranged (**Figure 6.3A**). ABG results (on air) are as follows:

P_aO_2	7.2 kPa (11.1–14.4 kPa)	Bicarbonate	24.2 (22–28)
P_aCO_2	4 kPa (4.7–6.4 kPa)	Base excess	+1 (−2–+2)
pH	7.48 (7.35–7.45)	Lactate	1.2 mmol/L (0.5–2.2 mmol/L)

CASE 6.3: QUESTIONS

1 From the history alone, what are your differential diagnoses?
2 What does the blood gas show?
3 What does the CTPA scan show?
4 What are the important factors in deciding when to perform a CTPA?
5 How would you manage this patient?

CASE 6.3: ANSWERS

1 From the history alone, what are your differential diagnoses?

Sudden onset shortness of breath with a background of malignancy suggests:

- Pulmonary embolus.
- Myocardial infarction with acute heart failure.
- Malignant pleural effusion.
- Pneumonia secondary to chemotherapy (immunosuppression).
- Pneumothorax.
- Rib fracture.
- Metastases (lung or bone).

The sudden onset with severe hypoxia and pleuritic chest pain, however, makes pulmonary embolism (PE) most likely.

2 What does the blood gas show?

The ABG results show a mild respiratory alkalosis with significant hypoxia. This is indicative of type 1 respiratory failure. There does not seem to be any metabolic compensation (as shown by the normal bicarbonate and base excess), which suggests an acute insult.

3 What does the CTPA scan show?

The CTPA shows large filling defects within the main pulmonary arteries bilaterally (**Figures 6.3B–6.3D**). These are pulmonary emboli, outlined by the contrast within the vessels. The lungs are clear without evidence of infarction.

> **TOP TIPS**
>
> Risk factors for pulmonary embolism:
> - Non-modifiable.
>   - Malignancy.
>   - Pregnancy.
>   - Inherited clotting disorder.
>   - Immobility.
>   - Previous PE/deep vein thrombosis (DVT).
> - Modifiable.
>   - Smoking, obesity, age, combined oral contraceptive pill.

4 What are the important factors in deciding when to perform a CTPA?

Having taken a history and assessed modifiable and nonmodifiable risk factors for thromboembolism, a Wells score should be calculated. This scoring system is used to decide whether or not a PE is likely and, therefore, requires further investigation with a CTPA (**Table 6.3**).

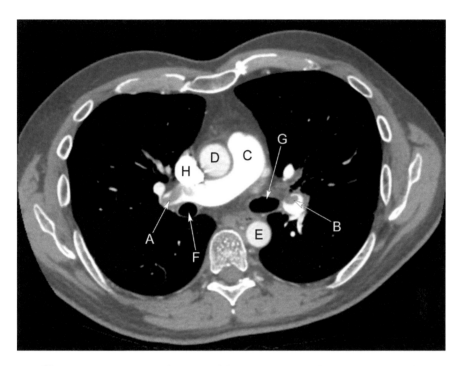

Fig. 6.3B CTPA with large emboli within the right (A) and descending left (B) pulmonary arteries. Note: normal pulmonary trunk (C), aortic root (D), and descending aorta (E). The normal air-filled right (F) and left (G) main bronchi are also demonstrated. Superior vena cava (H).

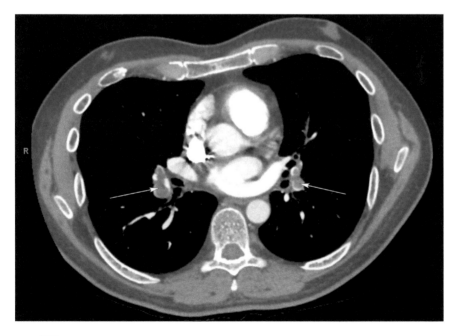

Fig. 6.3C CTPA of the same patient (more inferior slice) showing further emboli (arrows) outlined by contrast within the lower lobe pulmonary arteries.

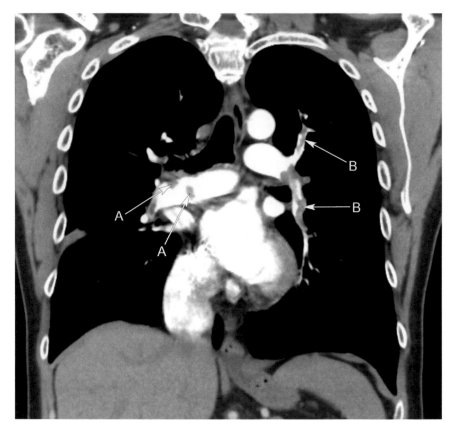

Fig. 6.3D Coronal CTPA with thrombus in the right main pulmonary artery (A) and left upper and lower lobe pulmonary arteries (B).

Table 6.3 PE Wells score

Clinical feature	Points
Clinically suspected DVT	3
Alternative diagnosis is less likely than PE	3
Tachycardia (HR >100)	1.5
Immobilisation (≥3 days)/surgery in previous 4 weeks	1.5
History of previous DVT or PE	1.5
Haemoptysis	1
Malignancy (with treatment within 6 months) or palliative	1
Clinical probability scores	
PE *likely* (consider diagnostic testing)	More than 4 points
PE *unlikely* (consider D-dimer to rule out PE)	4 points or less

- D-dimer is a useful test but only when used correctly. It is a fibrin degradation product, a small protein fragment present in the blood after a blood clot is degraded by fibrinolysis. The absence of a raised concentration implies no recent thromboembolic event. A positive concentration, however, is fairly nonspecific and is found in malignancy, infection, and pregnancy as well as thrombosis.
- It is, therefore, useful to rule out thromboembolic disease when the Wells score probability is low.

5 How would you manage this patient?

The patient should be resuscitated with an ABCDE approach. A large PE is a potential cause for cardiac arrest and close monitoring is therefore required. An ABG should be performed and CTPA will confirm the diagnosis. *Remember:* O_2 by mask, analgesia, IV access, and bloods.

Other important investigations include:

- ECG. The most common finding is sinus tachycardia. Less commonly the ECG may show a $S_1Q_3T_3$ pattern (a large S wave in lead I, a Q wave in lead III, and an inverted T wave in lead III indicates acute right heart strain).
- CXR to rule out pneumothorax as a cause of the pain. The CXR is usually normal in PE but may show atelectasis.
- Echocardiogram. This is usually performed in patients presenting with suspected PE to look for right-sided heart strain.

Once PE is confirmed, IV thrombolysis may be considered if the patient is haemodynamically unstable. Direct pulmonary angiography with embolectomy may also be considered (in patients with a massive embolus and where interventional radiology facilities are available).

Initially in the majority of cases, patients will be treated with a treatment dose of low molecular weight heparin (LMWH). This can then be converted to oral medication such as warfarin, or the more recently introduced rivaroxaban, on discharge.

LEARNING POINTS: PULMONARY EMBOLISM

- CTPA is the diagnostic test of choice for PE and has largely replaced ventilation/perfusion (V/Q) scanning. (Nuclear medicine perfusion scanning alone is sometimes used in pregnant patients to reduce maternal radiation dose).
- The Wells score allows assessment of patients on an individual basis to determine whether further tests are necessary to rule out thromboembolism.
- PE can be fatal and, therefore, it is important to get early senior help in managing patients to ensure prompt diagnosis and treatment.
- Long-term management is with anticoagulation and the length of treatment is dependent on precipitating factors.

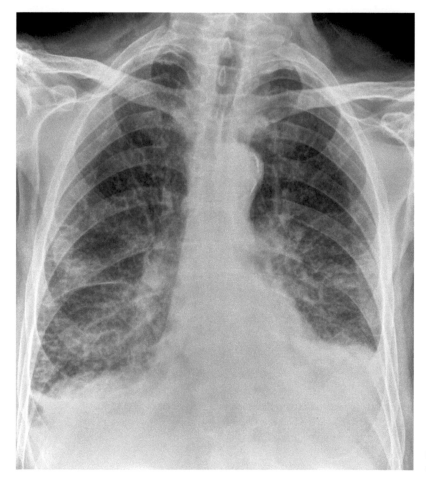

Fig. 6.4A Erect AP CXR.

A 78-year-old male presents to the ED having woken up in the night severely short of breath. He does not report any chest pain. He had an MI 1 year ago and since then has been increasingly short of breath on exertion (SOBOE), only being able to walk about 50 metres at a time. His regular medications include amlodipine, ramipril, furosemide, simvastatin, and aspirin. He is a past smoker with a 30 pack-year history.

On examination he is visibly breathless while sitting upright. There are fine crepitations with reduced air entry in both lung bases. Heart sounds are normal and his abdomen is soft and non-tender. There is no peripheral or sacral oedema. His SPO_2 is 88% on air, BP 135/84 mmHg, HR 96 bpm, respiration rate 26 bpm, and temperature 36.4°C. You arrange an urgent CXR (**Figure 6.4A**).

CASE 6.4: QUESTIONS

1 What does the CXR show?
2 What other investigations would you perform?
3 How would you manage this patient?

CASE 6.4: ANSWERS

1 What does the CXR show?

The CXR shows widespread interstitial oedema with septal lines in the lower zones. There are bilateral pleural effusions with fluid tracking along the horizontal fissure. The heart is not enlarged. These changes are consistent with acute pulmonary oedema (**Figure 6.4B**). There is upper lobe blood diversion (indicting pulmonary venous hypertension with upper lobe venous blood redistribution).

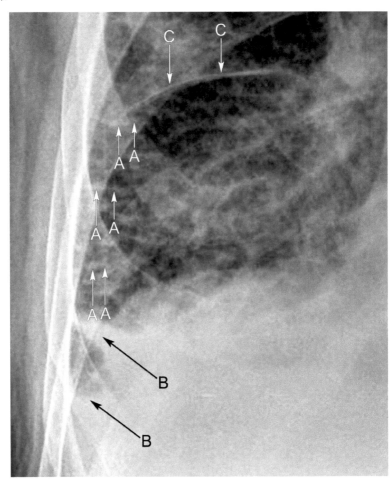

Fig. 6.4B
Magnified view of the right lower zone, better demonstrating the small, subpleural, peripheral horizontal septal lines of interstitial oedema (A). There is also a small pleural effusion (B) with fluid tracking into the horizontal fissure (C).

TOP TIPS

A way to remember the CXR features of heart failure (ABCDE):

Alveolar oedema (bat wing appearance).

Kerley **B** lines (septal lines of interstitial oedema).

Cardiomegaly.

Dilated prominent upper lobe vessels.

Effusion (pleural).

Heart failure is when the heart is unable to pump blood sufficiently to maintain the body's needs. The cause may be acute or chronic, or acute on chronic, and is usually multifactorial:

- Acute: MI, fluid overload or arrhythmia.
- Chronic: coronary heart disease, hypertension, cardiomyopathy, anaemia, hyperthyroidism.

Kerley B lines (also known as septal lines) represent interstitial oedema in the interlobular lymphatics. Causes include pulmonary oedema, lymphangitis carcinomatosa, and sarcoidosis. A good history and examination will help differentiate these. It is also helpful if you can compare with any previous CXRs. Remember that in acute, 'flash' pulmonary oedema the heart size may be normal, with enlargement occurring later in the disease process. Initially, interstitial oedema may be seen and fluid may extend into the airspace/alveolus also, and then has the appearance of consolidation, radiopaque and often perihilar (**Figure 6.4C**).

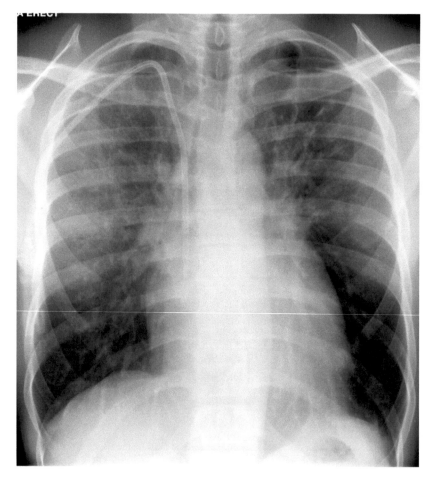

Fig. 6.4C CXR showing the typical perihilar (bat wing) appearance of pulmonary oedema (in a patient on dialysis). There is a central venous catheter placed within the superior vena cava. The heart is slightly enlarged and there are no pleural effusions. This appearance is nonspecific, and infection (particularly atypical, e.g. *Pneumocystis jiroveci* [formerly known as *P. carinii*] pneumonia) could also explain these XR appearances.

It is important to distinguish pulmonary oedema from other causes of consolidation on CXR, such as pneumonia. Always ask for help if unsure. As well as the clinical differences (SOBOE, crackles, hypertension versus cough and fever), there are a few helpful radiological differences (*Table 6.4A*).

Table 6.4A Differentiation of causes of consolidation on CXR

Pulmonary oedema	Pneumonia
Usually bilateral	Usually unilateral
Typically perihilar	Typically lobar, segmental or focal
Associated interstitial densities (septal lines) and cardiomegaly	Usually a single and denser area of opacity. No interstitial markings
Usually bilateral pleural effusions	Possible associated unilateral pleural effusion

2 What other investigations would you perform?

Other investigations are:

- ECG to exclude an acute MI.
- Blood tests.
  - FBC and CRP for concurrent infection and to rule out anaemia.
  - Troponin/cardiac enzymes to rule out acute MI.
  - TFTs to check for hyperthyroidism as a cause.
  - U&Es as diuretics are a mainstay of management.
  - Brain natriuretic peptide (BNP) for diagnosis and management of chronic heart failure.
  - Echocardiogram, to evaluate cardiac function.

3 How would you manage this patient?

Initial management is via an ABCDE approach. This includes sitting the patient up, administering high-flow oxygen, taking a more detailed history, getting IV access, taking bloods (see above), and arranging an ECG and CXR with early senior review.

Medical management then aims to reduce preload and afterload pressures on the heart:

- Preload: sublingual GTN and diuretics (oral or IV furosemide).
- Afterload: long-term BP management with ACE inhibitors and angiotensin receptor blocker (ARB) agents.
- In the acute and unstable setting, inotropic agents may be necessary with ICU support.

The New York Heart Association (NYHA) classification of chronic heart failure is shown in *Table 6.4B*.

TOP TIPS

When asked how to manage a patient with acute cardiogenic pulmonary oedema start with the ABCDE approach, a full history, and investigations including bloods, ECG, and CXR. Mention senior clinical review before talking about the use of GTN and diuretics to offload fluid from the lungs. The examiners want to know that you can comfortably manage a patient like this in an acute setting.

Table 6.4B NYHA classification of heart failure

This is a simple way of classifying the functional extent of heart failure and is widely used in the management of patients. It often comes up in exams, both written and practical, so is handy to remember:

I	Cardiac disease but no symptoms or limitation in ordinary physical activity
II	Mild symptoms (mild shortness of breath and/or angina) and slight limitation during ordinary activity
III	Marked limitation in activity due to symptoms, even during less-than-ordinary activity, e.g. walking short distances (20–100 m), comfortable only at rest
IV	Severe limitations with symptoms at rest (mostly bed-bound patients)

LEARNING POINTS: CARDIAC FAILURE

- CXR changes in a patient with heart failure do vary but include alveolar oedema, 'Kerley B' septal lines of interstitial oedema, cardiomegaly, dilated prominent upper lobe vessels, and pleural effusions.
- Try to differentiate the consolidation seen in pulmonary oedema from that seen in pneumonia, although this can be difficult (bilateral symmetrical versus unilateral asymmetrical).
- Management is via an ABCDE approach with high-flow oxygen, GTN, and IV diuretics to offload the heart. Always exclude an acute MI.
- NYHA classification is used to determine functional status in chronic heart failure.

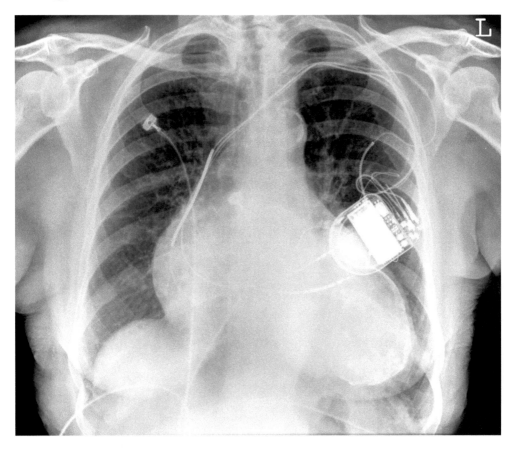

Fig. 6.5A CXR.

A 78-year-old female is admitted to hospital with sudden-onset, left-sided weakness and dysarthria. She has a CT of her brain, which shows early signs of an acute right middle cerebral artery stroke. She had an anterior MI 4 years previously and has been under the care of cardiology, and in the last few months she has been complaining of lethargy, nonspecific chest pains, and palpitations.

As part of her initial investigations she has a CXR performed (**Figure 6.5A**).

CASE 6.5: QUESTIONS

1 What are the CXR findings?
2 What is the CXR diagnosis?
3 How would you investigate and manage this patient?

CASE 6.5: ANSWERS

1 What are the CXR findings?

The CXR shows cardiomegaly (**Figure 6.5B**). The left atrium and ventricle are particularly enlarged with splaying of the carina secondary to left atrial enlargement. There is calcification of the left ventricle (LV) wall at the apex. A dual lead pacemaker with implantable cardiac defibrillator (ICD) is *in situ*. The lungs are clear.

Cardiomegaly in adults is defined as a cardiothoracic ratio (CTR) that exceeds 50% on a PA projection CXR. In this case the left side in particular of the heart is enlarged:

- Left atrial enlargement: double RHB (caused by the enlarged left atrium), enlarged left atrial appendage, and splaying of the carina (>70°).
- Left ventricular enlargement, with globular chamber enlargement.

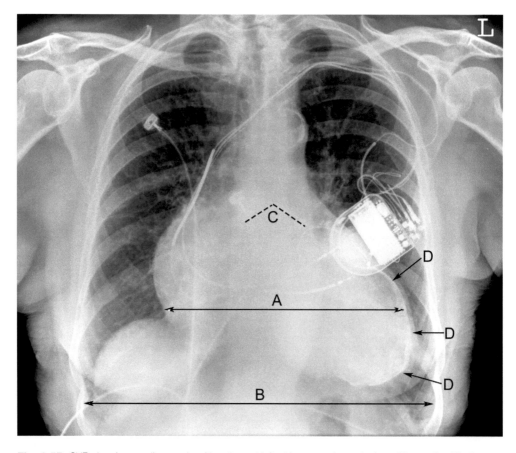

Fig. 6.5B CXR showing cardiomegaly with enlarged left atrium, causing splaying of the carina (C): the normal carina angle is <60–70°, splaying occurs with left atrial or subcarinal nodal enlargement. The cardiothoracic ratio (A/B) is >50% – this widest point of transverse cardiac diameter/widest intrathoracic diameter from inner rib margins in adults should be <50%. There is curvilinear left ventricular myocardial calcification (D). Note: implantable defibrillator/pacing device.

2 What is the diagnosis?

The diagnosis is a calcified left ventricular aneurysm (LVA), likely secondary to her previous MI:

- Myocardial calcification is a sign of prior infarction, while pericardial calcification is strongly associated with constrictive pericarditis. Therefore, detecting and recognising calcification related to the heart on chest radiography and other imaging modalities, such as fluoroscopy, CT, and echocardiography, may have important clinical implications.
- Aneurysmal myocardial calcification is identified as thin and curvilinear shaped and usually appears toward the apex of the LV. There is often an associated bulge in the ventricular contour and myocardial calcification is deeper than pericardial, which tends to outline the periphery of the cardiac silhouette. Myocardial calcification follows the ventricular contour and will not cross the midline following the pericardium.
- LVA is a rare complication of a MI that can cause serious morbidity or death (4% of cases). Acute MI damages the muscle wall and this can then bulge and develop into a true aneurysm, where there is a full-thickness breach in the myocardial lining with a broad neck. Acutely this may rupture, or there may be fibrosis, scarring, and healing with a chronic aneurysm and this may calcify (*Table 6.5*). Rarely the rupture is contained by the pericardium, creating a false aneurysm.

Table 6.5 Complications of LVA

Acute	• Sudden death/cardiac rupture
Chronic	• Thromboembolism (embolic events from thrombus within the aneurysmal sac)
	• Ventricular arrhythmia (note the presence of pacemaker) often refractory to drug treatment
	• Congestive heart failure
	• Refractory angina

3 How would you investigate and manage this patient?

Investigations:

- ECG: it is important for identifying evidence of acute or prior myocardial ischaemia, as well as associated arrhythmias. A LVA acutely can cause persistent ST elevation.
- Blood profile: troponin (to exclude acute MI), FBC (anaemia or infection can exacerbate pre-existing heart failure), U&Es (renal impairment, hyponatraemia, establish baseline electrolytes prior to starting diuretics or ACE inhibitors), LFTs, blood glucose (to detect underlying diabetes mellitus).
- Echocardiography: assess atrial and ventricular sizes, global left and right ventricular systolic function, diastolic function of the LV, regional wall abnormalities, and mural thrombus and valve abnormalities.

Refer for cardiology specialist review (further management depends on whether the presentation is acute or chronic).

Treatment (in chronic cases):

- Lifestyle advice: stopping smoking, control BP/diabetes, weight loss.
- Anticoagulation.
- Heart failure medication for symptom control (ACE inhibitors also help to prevent ventricular remodelling and the formation of aneurysms).

- Arrhythmia management.
- Definitive surgery with left ventricular reconstruction is often not needed in chronic cases, particularly with smaller aneurysms.

LEARNING POINTS: LEFT VENTRICULAR ANEURYSM

- A chronic left ventricular (true) aneurysm is an area of well-delineated, thinned, and fibrotic myocardial wall, devoid of muscle, that is a result of a healed transmural MI. Lesions may calcify when healed and are associated with arrhythmias and thromboembolic events.
- A ventricular pseudoaneurysm (false aneurysm) develops after an acute MI that has been complicated by cardiac wall rupture that is contained by localised pericardial adhesions. These lesions are at high risk of cardiac rupture with sudden death, and urgent surgical intervention is needed.

Case 6.6

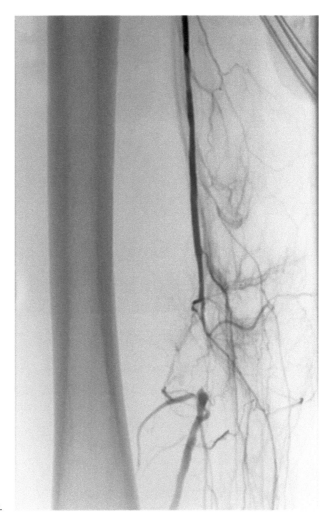

Fig. 6.6A Digital subtraction angiogram of the right upper leg/thigh.

A 58-year-old male presents to his GP complaining of pain at rest in his right leg for the previous week and numbness in the foot and calf. This was preceded by several months of pain in the calf and foot on minimal exertion. He is taking medication for hypertension and is a smoker of 10 cigarettes a day.

On examination the right foot is pale and cold to touch. There is reduced sensation, pedal pulses are absent, and the popliteal pulse is weak. There are no abdominal masses. Femoral pulses are present. He is referred to the hospital for an urgent vascular assessment.

As part of his management he undergoes femoral angiography (**Figure 6.6A**).

CASE 6.6: QUESTIONS

1 What are the angiographic findings?
2 What is the diagnosis?

3 How would you investigate and manage this patient?

CASE 6.6: ANSWERS

1 What are the angiographic findings?

The angiogram of the right upper leg shows an occlusion of the superficial femoral artery just above the adductor canal with collateral circulation and reconstitution of the artery more distally (**Figure 6.6B**). The adductor canal is a common site of occlusion/stenosis as it is an area of potential narrowing/vascular compression as the artery passes through the fascia at this level.

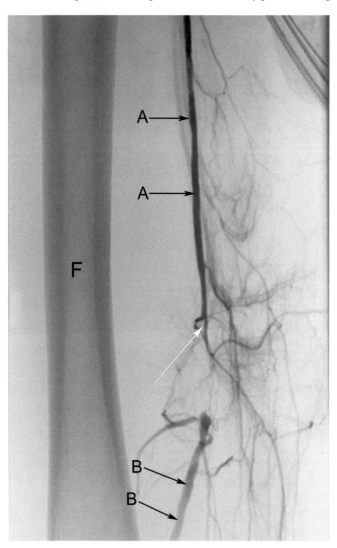

Fig. 6.6B Digital subtraction angiogram of the right upper leg showing occlusion (white arrow) of the right superficial femoral artery (A) with reconstitution of the distal femoral artery (B) via collateral circulation. Femur (F).

2 What is the diagnosis?

This patient has occlusion of the right superficial femoral artery that will need urgent treatment. The likely aetiology is acute thrombosis on a background of pre-existing chronic stenosis of the distal superficial femoral artery.

Possible aetiologies of acute vascular occlusion include:

- Thrombosis: acute on chronic (embolus from rupture of proximal atherosclerotic plaque) or chronic (gradual extension of thrombus with development of collateral circulation). This is peripheral artery occlusive disease (PAOD), which has presented with claudication/pain.
- Embolism: secondary to atrial fibrillation, post-MI, prosthetic heart valves, aortic aneurysm, proximal atheromatous stenosis or malignancy.
- Trauma: penetrating injury with laceration of the vessel.
- Raynaud's syndrome: peripheral arterial spasm when exposed to cold temperatures, smoking, or emotional stress.
- Compartment syndrome: occurs when perfusion pressure falls below tissue pressure in a closed anatomical space. This may follow orthopaedic (fracture), vascular (haemorrhage) or soft tissue (crush, burn) injury.

There are several limb ischaemia classification systems. *Fontaine's four stages* are the easiest to remember:

- Stage I: asymptomatic.
- Stage IIa: intermittent claudication >200 m walk.
- Stage IIb: intermittent claudication <200 m walk.
- Stage III: rest pain.
- Stage IV: ischaemic ulcers or gangrene.

The clinical features of an acutely ischaemic limb ('the 6 Ps') are:

- Pale.
- Pulseless.
- Painful.
- Paralysed.
- Paraesthetic.
- 'Perishing with cold'.

3 How would you investigate and manage this patient?

Investigations would include:

- Doppler US of both feet to identify any distal arterial flow.
- Blood tests including FBC (anaemia can worsen the ischaemia), ESR (giant cell arteritis or other connective tissue disorders), glucose (diabetes mellitus), lipids, thrombophilia screen, and coagulation screen.
- Investigations to identify an embolic source including ECG and echocardiogram.
- CT or MR angiography to assess the abdominal aorta and limb vasculature, and the stenosis and collateral circulation.
- Digital subtraction angiography (DSA), as performed above. This is an invasive technique that involves femoral catheter insertion. It is the reference standard technique for assessing stenoses, occlusions, and collateral circulations, and is performed in interventional radiology and usually as a precursor to radiological treatment of the stenosis.

Management (remember ABCDE) includes:

- Urgent admission (this is a surgical emergency).
- IV heparin (may double the limb salvage rate).
- Analgesia.

Short-term management has a number of options depending on patient condition and find-ings. Radiological intervention is most common in the first instance (remember in the exam to mention that you would seek urgent senior advice).

- If thrombotic: intra-arterial thrombolysis, angioplasty or bypass surgery.
- If embolism: radiological or surgical embolectomy or local intra-arterial thrombolysis; bypass graft if the embolectomy fails.
- If the limb is irreversibly ischaemic: amputation will be required.
- If significant arterial stenosis: radiological angioplasty with or without a stent (**Figure 6.6C**).

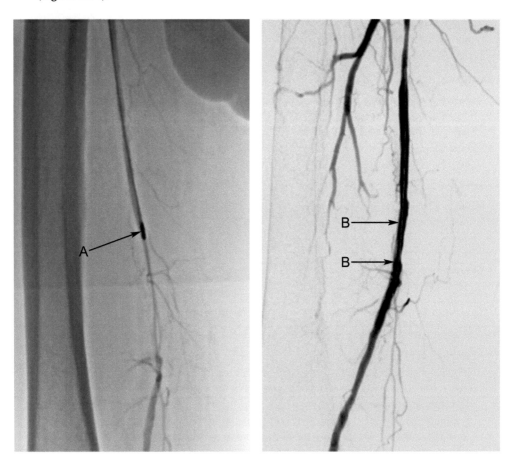

Fig. 6.6C Digital subtraction angiogram before (left) and after (right) catheter thrombectomy and angioplasty in the same patient. Note: contrast opacified superficial femoral artery with central catheter tip (A) just proximal to the stenosis on the left image. The postprocedural image on the right shows contrast flowing normally through the previously stenotic portion of femoral artery after balloon dilatation angioplasty (B). In this procedure the catheter is deployed near the stenosis and a guidewire navigated over the stenosis. The catheter is then advanced and a balloon inflated to reduce the stenosis. This process can be repeated and if unsuccessful a metallic stent can be deployed.

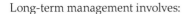

Long-term management involves:

- General management for underlying cardiovascular disease: exercise, smoking cessation, treatment of hypertension and hyperlipidaemia, and achieving optimal diabetes control.
- Low-dose aspirin or clopidogrel.
- ACE inhibitor therapy: reduces the morbidity and mortality of cardiovascular disease in patients with peripheral arterial disease by up to 25%.

LEARNING POINTS: ISCHAEMIC LEG

- Thrombolysis usually takes between 6 and 72 hours to achieve clot lysis, hence patients with limb-threatening ischaemia are not usually candidates for local thrombolysis and require urgent radiological/surgical intervention.
- Without revascularisation, complete acute ischaemia can lead to extensive tissue necrosis within 6 hours.
- Ischaemia is considered acute if the symptoms and signs have developed over less than 2 weeks.
- Management involves close collaboration between vascular surgery and interventional radiology.

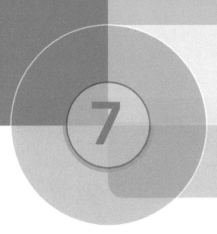

Abdomen and pelvis cases

7

FAYE CUTHBERT, AMANDA JEWISON, AND OLWEN WESTERLAND

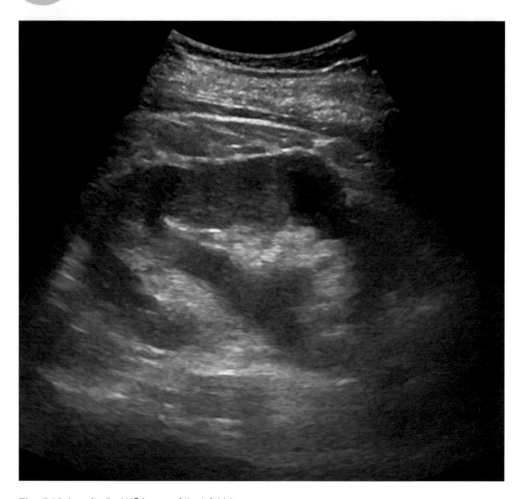

Fig. 7.1A Longitudinal US image of the left kidney.

A 74-year-old male presents to urology with a 4-week history of painless haematuria. He describes 'rosé' coloured urine but no clots. He denies pain, weight loss or dysuria.

On examination he is well. He has tar stains on his fingers and is a heavy smoker of 20 cigarettes per day for over 40 years. There is no abdominal tenderness or any palpable masses. Observations are stable. Urinalysis shows blood +++ but no leucocytes, nitrites or glucose. Blood tests reveal mild normochromic, normocytic anaemia, and slightly elevated urea and creatinine.

A renal US is requested (**Figure 7.1A**).

CASE 7.1: QUESTIONS

1 What does the US show?
2 What are the possible causes?
3 What investigation should be carried out next?
4 How should this patient be managed?

CASE 7.1: ANSWERS

1 What does the US show?

The US shows mild hydronephrosis of the left kidney (**Figure 7.1B**). Hydronephrosis is dilatation of the renal pelvis and calyceal system, usually caused by obstruction of urine outflow. It can be physiological, for example in pregnant women where the gravid uterus compresses the ureters, or pathological. It can be unilateral or bilateral, acute or chronic.

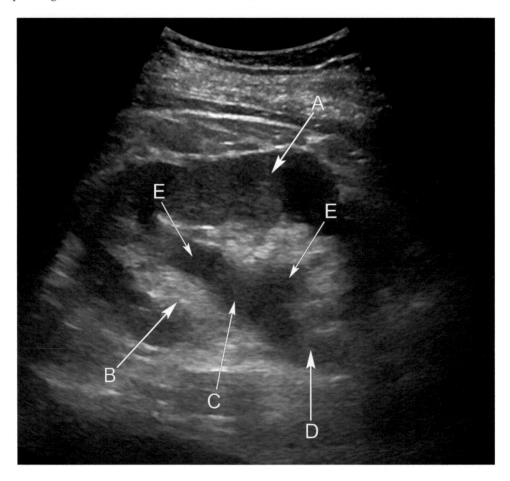

Fig. 7.1B Longitudinal ultrasound image of a left kidney showing mild hydronephrosis. Renal cortex (A). Renal sinus fat, which is bright (B). Dilated renal pelvis (C). Dilated proximal ureter (D) and dilated upper and lower pole calyces (E). The upper pole of the kidney lies to the left of the image. Note the preservation of thickness of renal cortex, which may suggest an acute/subacute cause (longer standing obstruction will usually cause cortical loss/damage and thinning).

2 What are the possible causes?

Common causes of urinary tract obstruction are shown in *Table 7.1*. Obstruction can occur at any level from the pelvicalyceal system to the urethra. In this case, the obstruction is unilateral and painless, therefore malignancy is the cause to be excluded.

Table 7.1 Common causes of urinary tract obstruction

Intrinsic (within the lumen or wall)	Extrinsic (external compression or infiltration)
Calculi	Malignancy (retroperitoneal mass, lymph nodes, pelvic malignancy)
Blood clot	Prostatic enlargement
Malignancy (transitional cell carcinoma)	Congenital (pelviureteric junction obstruction)
Ureteric or urethral stricture	Retroperitoneal fibrosis

3 What investigation should be carried out next?

The patient should be referred urgently to urology for a cystoscopy to look for a bladder tumour. The patient will also require a CT IVU or CT urogram: this involves a precontrast study through the renal tract to look for stones and then a postcontrast examination to look for other lesions, and in particular transitional cell carcinoma of the urinary tract, which may occur from renal pelvis to bladder and may be multifocal.

4 How should this patient be managed?

Management of the patient depends on the underlying cause and whether the renal function is compromised. If the renal function is compromised or there is suspicion of infection, the patient may require ureteric stenting. This involves passing a thin tube up the ureter to relieve the obstruction (usually cystoscopically) or inserting a percutaneous nephrostomy tube into the renal pelvicalyceal system to decompress the kidney. If malignancy is found, it will need to be staged and discussed at the urology MDT meeting in order to plan appropriate treatment. Transitional cell carcinoma can involve the urothelium anywhere in the renal tract. Smoking is an important risk factor.

This patient had a cystoscopy and CT, which revealed a large mass in the bladder causing obstruction of the left ureter at the vesicoureteric junction (**Figure 7.1C**). Biopsy confirmed transitional cell carcinoma. The ureters and upper tracts were, however, normal on CT.

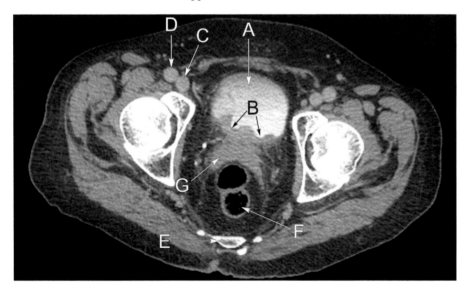

Fig. 7.1C Axial CT image at the level of the bladder. Contrast in the bladder (A) helps to demonstrate that the posterior wall of the bladder is irregular and thickened, in keeping with a bladder tumour (B). Femoral vessels: vein medial (C), artery lateral (D). Coccyx (E), rectum (F), seminal vesicles (G).

> ### LEARNING POINTS: HAEMATURIA/HYDRONEPHROSIS
>
> - Painless haematuria is caused by malignancy until proven otherwise and warrants an urgent referral to urology.
> - CT urogram and cystoscopy are first-line investigations.
> - It is important to exclude infection clinically because an infected obstructed system can lead to rapid loss of function unless urgently decompressed.
> - Hydronephrosis can be caused by intrinsic blockage or external compression at any level of the urinary tract.
> - Common causes of hydronephrosis include urinary tract calculi, ureteric or bladder tumours, pelvic masses, and congenital pelviureteric junction obstruction.

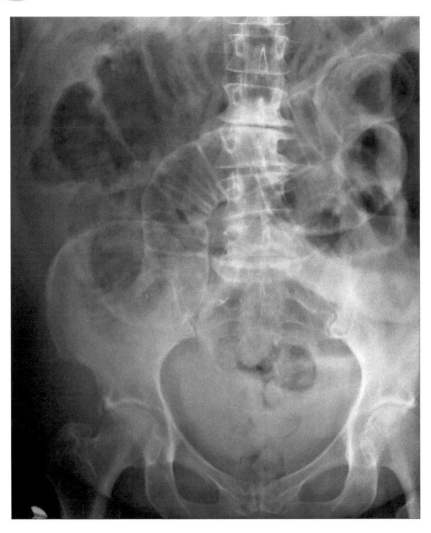

Fig. 7.2A AXR.

A 65-year-old male presents to the ED with sudden-onset severe abdominal pain. On examination he is pale and sweaty. He has generalised abdominal tenderness with reduced bowel sounds and guarding in the upper abdomen. Observations reveal tachycardia 120 bpm, BP 80/60 mmHg, and temperature 37.5°C. A supine AXR is performed amongst other initial investigations (**Figure 7.2A**).

CASE 7.2: QUESTIONS

1 What radiological sign is shown and what does it indicate?
2 What is the most likely cause?
3 How should the patient be managed?

CASE 7.2: ANSWERS

1 What radiological sign is shown and what does it indicate?

The AXR shows Rigler's sign. This is when air is seen on both sides of the bowel wall (**Figure 7.2B**). It indicates pneumoperitoneum, so air outlines the bowel wall clearly, with air within the bowel lumen and also outside of the bowel. Rigler's sign was first described by L.G. Rigler in 1941; a positive Rigler's sign does require relatively large amounts of free intraperitoneal air.

Other abdominal radiographic features of free intraperitoneal air include:

- 'Football' sign, oval-shaped free air in the upper abdomen, which may outline the falciform ligament.
- Triangular free air collection in Morrison's pouch beneath right lobe of liver.
- Perihepatic free air.
- 'Cupola' sign, free air trapped beneath the central tendon of the diaphragm.

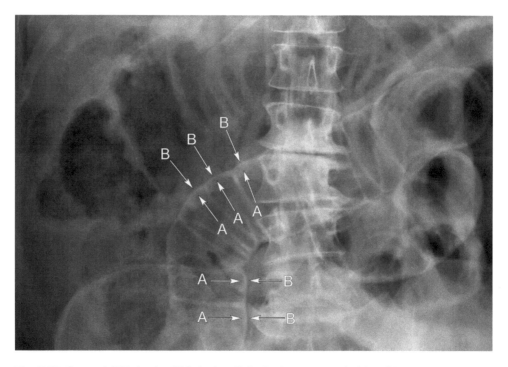

Fig. 7.2B Cropped AXR showing Rigler's sign. Air is clearly seen on both sides of the bowel wall (within lumen A, outside bowel B).

2 What is the most likely cause?

Pneumoperitoneum is free intra-abdominal gas, either as a result of recent surgery or visceral perforation. The most common sites of a perforated viscus are the duodenum and sigmoid colon, although a perforation can occur at any part of the GI tract. Common causes include a peptic ulcer, bowel obstruction, and inflammatory processes such as diverticulitis or appendicitis.

Another example of Rigler's sign is shown in **Figure 7.2C**.

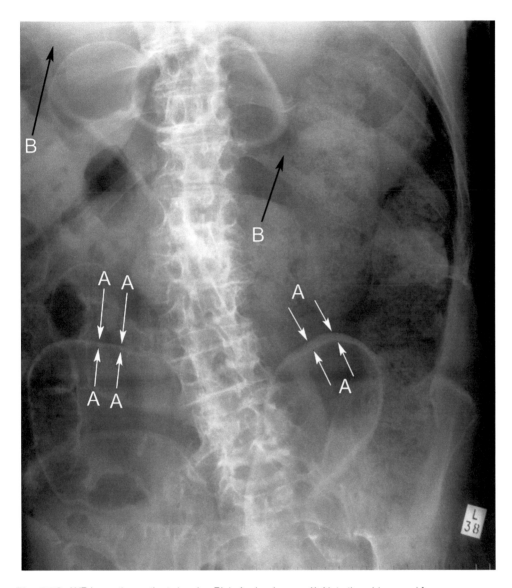

Fig. 7.2C AXR in another patient showing Rigler's sign (arrows A). Note the widespread free intraperitoneal air throughout abdomen (arrows B).

3 How should the patient be managed?

The patient is unwell and needs a structured ABCDE approach initially, including IV access and fluid resuscitation. It is important to state in an OSCE situation that you would seek senior input early. Bowel perforation carries high mortality if untreated because the leaked bowel contents cause inflammation and infection in the peritoneum (peritonitis) and can rapidly lead to severe sepsis and death. Therefore, urgent surgery is usually the most appropriate next management step in order to repair or resect the area of bowel that has perforated and to thoroughly wash out the abdomen.

Often, a CT scan of the abdomen and pelvis (**Figure 7.2D**) is requested, if patient condition allows, prior to surgery in order to confirm the presence of pneumoperitoneum and help guide the surgeon to the site and cause of perforation.

Do also remember that an erect CXR is far more sensitive than an AXR in the detection of free intraperitoneal air. CT is the technique of choice for difficult or equivocal cases and can detect tiny amounts of free gas. A good quality erect CXR can detect amounts of free intraperitoneal air down to 1 mL.

In this patient the majority of free gas was located in the upper abdomen, and there was no evidence of diverticular disease or colonic tumour on CT, therefore it was thought that the likely source of perforation was the upper GI tract. A perforated duodenal ulcer was confirmed at laparotomy.

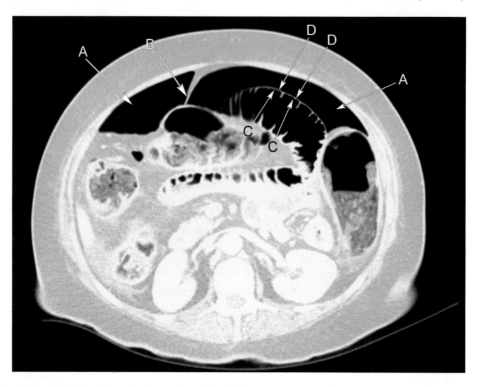

Fig. 7.2D Axial CT on lung window setting to help further evaluate the patient from this case. Free gas is present in the peritoneal cavity (A). Note the falciform ligament (B) surrounded by air. One can appreciate how Rigler's sign appears on AXR; air within small bowel lumen (C) and free air outside the bowel (D) outline the small bowel wall.

LEARNING POINTS: PNEUMOPERITONEUM

- Rigler's sign is where air is seen on both sides of the bowel wall. It indicates pneumoperitoneum.
- An erect CXR is more sensitive and more useful than an AXR at detecting pneumoperitoneum.
- Always ask about recent surgery.
- Free gas on AXR indicates a large volume of free gas. Smaller volumes can be present without being visible on CXR or AXR, therefore high clinical suspicion of perforation should prompt further investigation with CT.

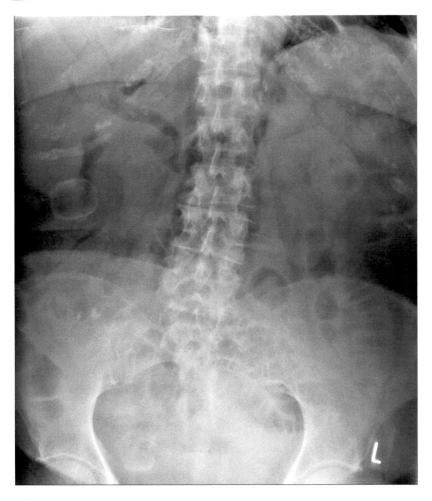

Fig. 7.3A Supine AXR.

A 75-year-old male presents to the ED with a 3-day history of abdominal pain and distension. He reports no bowel movements for 4 days and is not passing flatus. He complains of nausea and has vomited once. He has no past medical history of note.

On examination, observations are temperature 36.5°C, BP 100/70 mmHg, HR 100 bpm, and respiratory rate 18 bpm. He has a distended abdomen and is tender in the epigastrium. Tinkling bowel sounds are present.

An AXR is requested (**Figure 7.3A**).

CASE 7.3: QUESTIONS

1 What three key radiological signs are present?
2 What is the likely diagnosis?
3 How should the patient be managed?

CASE 7.3: ANSWERS

1 What three key radiological signs are present?

The AXR (**Figure 7.3B**) shows small bowel dilatation, biliary air (aerobilia), and a calcified gall-stone lying outside of the expected position of the gallbladder. Note the dilated small bowel is subtle, not the classic dilated air-filled loop. The dilated small bowel in this patient in the left iliac fossa is largely fluid filled with only bubbles of air seen lying on top of the fluid.

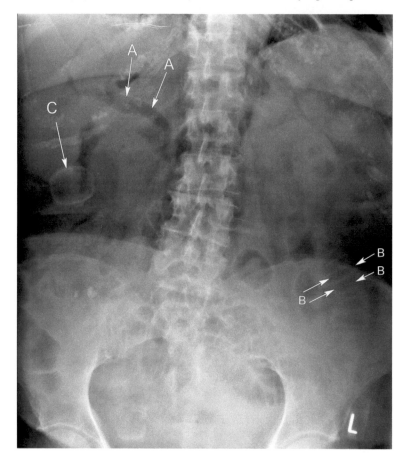

Fig. 7.3B AXR showing gas in the biliary tree (A), dilated small bowel (B), and a calcified gallstone (C).

2 What is the likely diagnosis?

The likely diagnosis is gallstone ileus. This term is actually a misnomer as it describes small bowel obstruction due to a gallstone that has passed through the gallbladder wall into the small bowel. Gallstone ileus comprises about 1% of cases of bowel obstruction.

- The gallstone often becomes lodged at the ileocaecal valve, a site of physiological bowel narrowing, and causes mechanical small bowel obstruction. It is a rare complication of chronic cholecystitis where the long-standing inflammation allows a fistula to form between the gallbladder and adjacent bowel wall and air passes from bowel into the biliary tree. Small stones will pass into the colon and then exit the bowel in stool.

Rarely a stone may pass in a fistula to the duodenum and obstruct at the duodeno-jejunal flexure: Bouveret's syndrome.

- Classic gallstone ileus on an AXR consists of three radiological features: small bowel dilatation, biliary air, and a gallstone. However, beware that not all gallstones are calcified therefore all three features may not be present. It is also usually very hard to detect gallstones when they lie in fluid-filled bowel. Air within the bile ducts is often not seen as the cystic duct may be inflamed and occluded so air cannot enter the bile ducts, although air may still be seen in the gallbladder itself.

3 How should the patient be managed?

The patient has small bowel obstruction and should be managed as such. He will need IV fluids, insertion of a NG tube to decompress the stomach and close monitoring of input and output. Urgent senior and surgical review are required. A CT may be helpful if the diagnosis is in doubt, or to look for complications such as bowel ischaemia or pneumoperitoneum (**Figures 7.3C** and **7.3D**). Treatment of gallstone ileus is surgery in most cases. This may involve just a minilaparotomy in the first instance with removal of the obstructing stone from the bowel lumen. CT can help significantly in planning minimally invasive surgery. The gallbladder region is often avoided at initial surgery owing to chronic inflammation and adhesions, although it can be targeted at a later date.

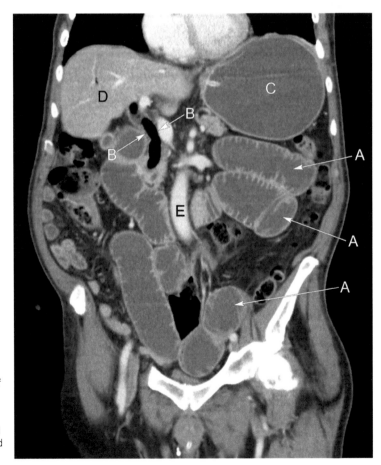

Fig. 7.3C Coronal contrast-enhanced CT of the abdomen and pelvis showing dilated small bowel (A) and gas in the biliary tree (B). Distended stomach (C), liver (D), and aorta (E).

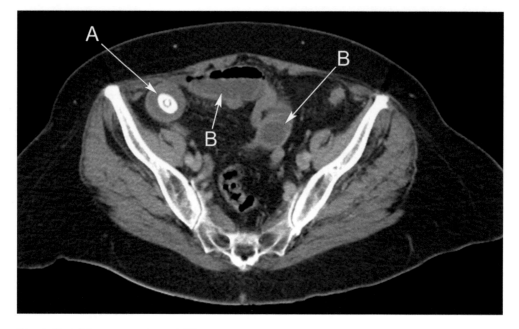

Fig. 7.3D Axial contrast-enhanced CT at the level of the right iliac fossa showing an obstructing gallstone in the small bowel lumen in the right iliac fossa (A) and dilated loops of small bowel (B).

LEARNING POINTS: GALLSTONE ILEUS

- A rare complication of chronic cholecystitis.
- A gallstone passes through a fistula from the gallbladder into the small bowel and causes small bowel obstruction.
- The impacted gallstone often becomes lodged at the ileocaecal valve.
- Key radiological features are:
  - Small bowel dilatation.
  - Air in the biliary tree.
  - Gallstone in the right lower quadrant.

Case 7.4

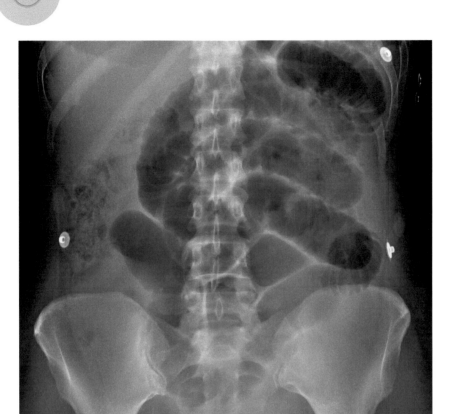

Fig. 7.4A Supine AXR.

A 46-year-old female presents to the ED with abdominal pain and vomiting, she cannot keep any fluids down, and is only passing small amounts of flatus. Her past medical history includes two caesarean sections and a laparascopic sterilisation.

Examination reveals she is afebrile, with HR 100 bpm, and BP 120/80 mmHg. There is abdominal distension and general tenderness, and bowel sounds are tinkling and loud. She has evidence of abdominal surgical scars consistent with a previous caesarean section and laparoscopic surgery.

An AXR is requested (**Figure 7.4A**).

CASE 7.4: QUESTIONS

1 What does the AXR show?
2 What are the most common causes?
3 How should the patient be managed?

CASE 7.4: ANSWERS

1 What does the AXR show?

The AXR shows dilated loops of small bowel in the central abdomen (**Figure 7.4B**). There is minimal bowel gas distally in the large bowel or rectum. No free gas. There are metal sterilisation clips in the pelvis. The dilated loops of bowel, together with the clinical history and findings, indicate small bowel obstruction (SBO). Remember that both obstruction and ileus will cause bowel dilatation and the two are not distinguishable on XR alone: the clinical findings should help differentiate.

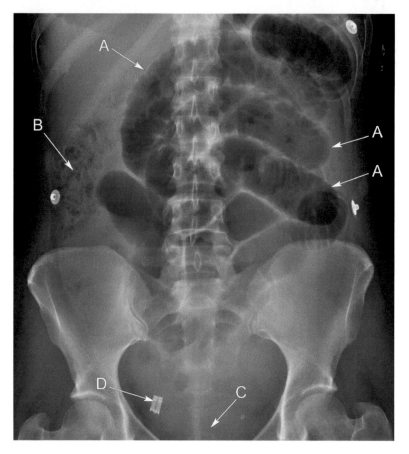

Fig. 7.4B AXR showing central dilated small bowel loops (A), faeces in the nondistended right colon (B), absence of bowel gas in the expected position of the rectum (C), and sterilisation clips in the pelvis (D). These dilated small bowel loops are arranged in what is sometimes called a 'stepladder' configuration.

Why is this small bowel?

- It is centrally located.
- It does not contain faeces.
- It contains valvulae conniventes (**Figures 7.4C** and **7.4D**).
- It is dilated >3 cm but not markedly so (e.g. 7–10 cm), which would be more consistent with large bowel.

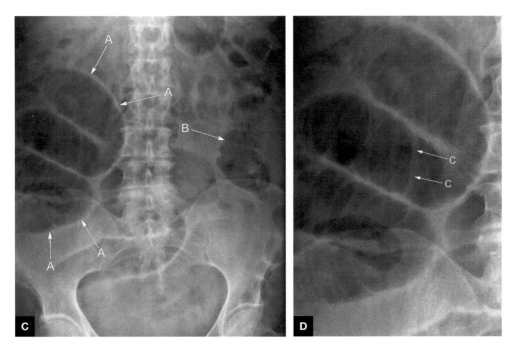

Figs. 7.4C, D Another example of SBO on AXR (magnified view of upper right quadrant shown in **Figure 7.4D**). There are dilated small bowel loops (A) and absence of gas within the rectum, normal calibre large bowel (B). Note the presence of valvulae conniventes, and mucosal folds that traverse the small bowel lumen (C), unlike mucosal mural indentations – haustra – seen in the large bowel.

TOP TIPS

When faced with small bowel dilatation on an AXR in an obstructed patient, look for clues with regards to the cause of obstruction, for example:

- Surgical clips (previous surgery increases the likelihood of adhesions).
- Bowel gas below the inguinal ligament (this indicates the presence of a hernia, which can become strangulated).
- Biliary gas and a gallstone in the right iliac fossa suggestive of gallstone ileus.

---

2 What are the most common causes?

The most common causes of SBO in adults are shown in *Table 7.4*. Taking a careful history from the patient will give important information to help determine the cause.

Table 7.4 Common causes of SBO

- Adhesions (>90% of cases) from previous surgery
- Malignancy (carcinoma, lymphoma)
- Inflammatory bowel disease (Crohn's disease with strictures)
- Hernia (obstructed inguinal or femoral)
- Small bowel volvulus
- Gallstone ileus

3 How should the patient be managed?

The patient needs close monitoring and a senior review. Initial management should consist of insertion of a NG tube and administration of IV fluids, known as 'drip and suck'. She will also need an erect CXR to exclude a perforation. The patient must be kept nil by mouth, will need routine blood tests to look for evidence of infection or dehydration, and may require a CT scan in order to determine the location and cause of obstruction. Subsequent management depends on the cause. If the patient has had no previous abdominal surgery (a 'virgin abdomen'), the obstruction is less likely to resolve with conservative management and to require surgical exploration. CT will often help make this decision.

- In this case, a CT was requested (**Figure 7.4E**), which showed dilated small bowel with a point of calibre change in the pelvis. No obstructing mass was demonstrated: therefore, the cause was thought likely to be adhesions. After a day of conservative management, the symptoms did not settle therefore a laparotomy was performed to relieve the obstruction and treat the adhesions.

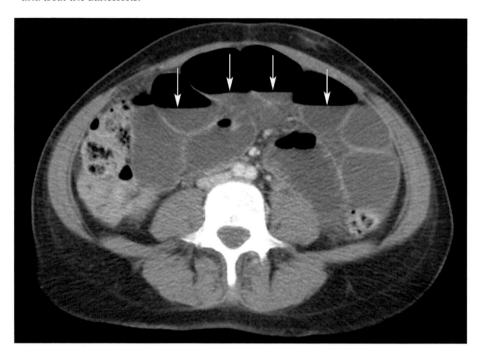

Fig. 7.4E Axial contrast-enhanced CT of the abdomen showing loops of dilated small bowel containing air/fluid levels (arrows).

LEARNING POINTS: SMALL BOWEL OBSTRUCTION

- \>3 cm can be used as an approximate cut-off for small bowel dilatation.
- Always take a careful history including past surgical history.
- When small bowel dilatation is seen on an abdominal radiograph, check for clues as to the cause (e.g. surgical clips/anastomoses, gas below the inguinal ligament, aerobilia, and calcified gallstone outside the gallbladder).

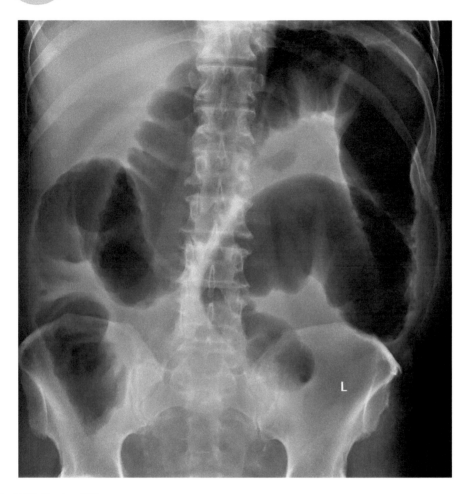

Fig. 7.5A Supine AXR.

A 60-year-old male presents to the ED with 2 days of abdominal pain and absolute constipation. He has not vomited. He describes alternating diarrhoea and constipation for several months and feeling generally tired and lethargic.

On examination, he is pale but afebrile with normal BP and mild tachycardia. His abdomen is distended and tympanic. Digital rectal examination reveals an empty rectum. Initial blood tests show microcytic anaemia but normal renal function, electrolytes, and inflammatory markers.

An AXR is requested (**Figure 7.5A**).

CASE 7.5: QUESTIONS

1   What does the AXR show?
2   What is the likely diagnosis?
3   What is the next most appropriate imaging investigation?
4   How should the patient be managed?

CASE 7.5: ANSWERS

1 What does the AXR show?

The AXR shows gas-filled dilated large bowel down to the level of the sigmoid colon. The small bowel is not dilated. *Table 7.5A* and **Figures 7.5B** and **7.5C** show a key difference between small and large bowel on AXR.

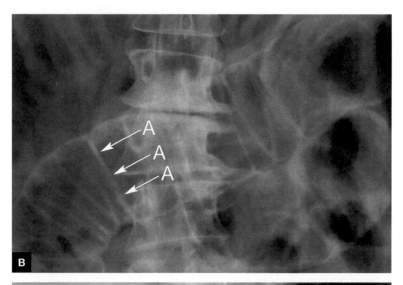

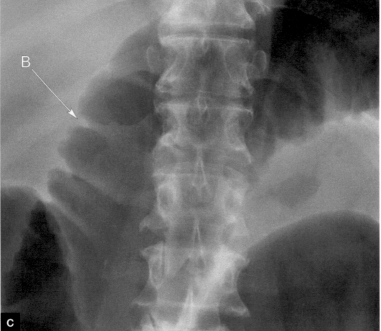

Figs. 7.5B, C
Valvulae conniventes in small bowel (A) and haustra in large bowel (B). Valvulae conniventes traverse the lumen and haustra indent, although sometimes haustral folds can also traverse.

Table 7.5A Radiological differentiation of dilated small and large bowel on AXR

Small bowel	Large bowel
Smaller calibre (>3 cm)	Larger calibre (>6 cm)
Central location	Peripheral location
Valvulae conniventes	Haustrations
No faecal matter	May contain faeces

2 What is the likely diagnosis?

The most likely diagnosis at this stage is large bowel obstruction (LBO). Common causes of LBO in adults are listed in *Table 7.5B*.

Table 7.5B Common causes of LBO in adults

- Malignancy (colorectal carcinoma)
- Inflammatory strictures, most commonly complicating diverticulitis
- Volvulus (sigmoid)
- Intussusception, less common

3 What is the next most appropriate imaging investigation?

Assuming the patient's condition does not require urgent laparotomy, the patient will require an erect CXR (as in most cases of acute abdomen) to exclude a perforation; it will also demonstrate lung metastases. A CT scan of the abdomen and pelvis is often requested to determine the cause of the obstruction and to look for evidence of complications such as perforation or bowel ischaemia. CT will also allow staging of tumours.

In this case, the CT scan showed a tumour in the sigmoid colon causing luminal obstruction, without perforation.

4 How should the patient be managed?

Initial management will depend on the clinical status of the patient. Dehydration and electrolyte disturbances should be corrected and a nasogastric tube should be inserted if the patient is vomiting. Subsequent management is guided by the cause of the obstruction and whether there is evidence of perforation. If there is a perforation or bowel ischaemia, the patient will likely require emergency surgery without delay for further imaging. Sometimes conservative management may be appropriate.

In cases of an obstructing tumour, if time allows the patient will need to be discussed at the colorectal MDT meeting in order to stage the cancer and decide what treatment should be offered. A colonic stent might be appropriate to relieve the obstruction, which can be palliative or a temporary measure prior to surgical resection. Colonic stents are inserted radiologically (**Figure 7.5D**). Colonic stents are being increasingly used to relieve acute LBO; they are used for more distal lesions and allow patient resuscitation to facilitate safer surgery if indicated.

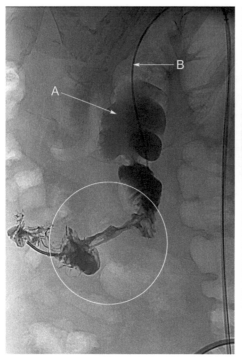
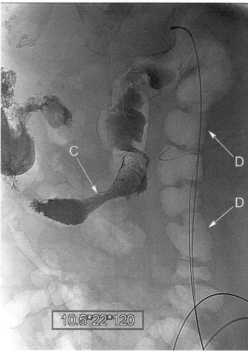

Fig. 7.5D Fluoroscopy images during colonic stent insertion. First, contrast (A) introduced by a rectal catheter is used to demonstrate the location of the tumour (circled) and the degree of stenosis. A wire (B) is guided per rectum through the narrowing caused by the tumour then a self-expanding metallic stent (C) is fed per rectum over the guidewire and the wire removed. The stent expands and relieves the obstruction. This is a classical 'applecore' stricture of carcinoma, in this case in the distal transverse colon. The wire (B) lies in the splenic flexure. Note the air-filled descending colon (D) and also 'waisting' of the stent (C) where the stent traverses the stricture.

LEARNING POINTS: LARGE BOWEL OBSTRUCTION

- It is important to distinguish between small and large bowel on AXR.
- Small bowel dilatation often coexists secondary to LBO.
- Common causes are malignancy and inflammatory strictures.
- A CT scan can help determine the cause of the obstruction, which will in turn guide management.
- When discussing management of a patient, always use an ABCDE approach initially and be able to discuss several different options of further treatment.

Case 7.6

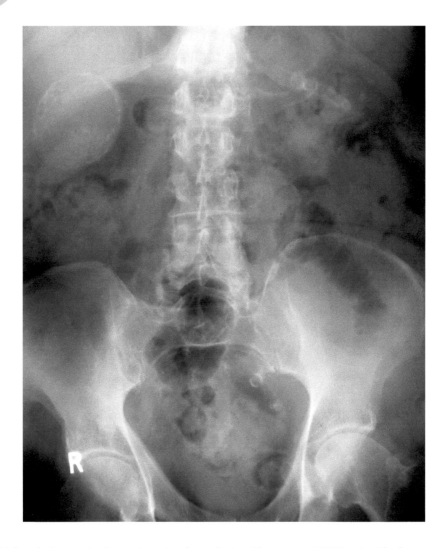

Fig. 7.6A
Supine AXR.

A 48-year-old female is seen in the gastroenterology clinic with recurrent RUQ pain. She has a history of diet-controlled type 2 diabetes, gastro-oesophageal reflux disease, and fibroids. Clinical examination reveals mild tenderness in the RUQ but is otherwise unremarkable. Observations are normal. Blood tests including a full blood count, urea and electrolytes, inflammatory markers, and LFTs are within the normal range. She has had an US, arranged in the community by her GP, of the RUQ, which showed 'shadowing' in the gallbladder fossa of uncertain significance.

An AXR is requested (**Figure 7.6A**).

CASE 7.6: QUESTIONS

1 What does the AXR show?
2 What could the abnormality represent?

3 What should the next management step involve?

CASE 7.6: ANSWERS

1 What does the AXR show?

It shows a peripherally calcified lesion in the RUQ (**Figure 7.6B**). There is no biliary gas. The bowel gas pattern is normal.

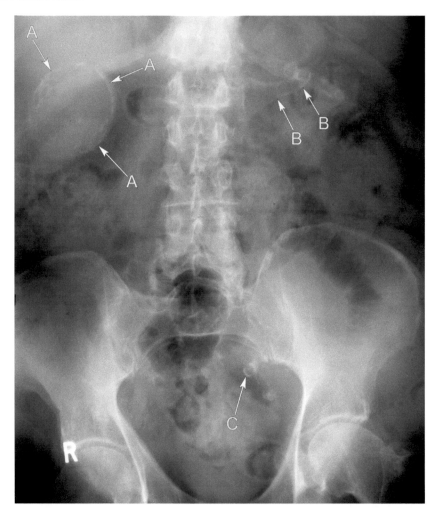

Fig. 7.6B Porcelain gallbladder (dense calcification in the RUQ [A]). Note the curvilinear splenic artery (B) and left iliac artery (C) calcification.

2 What could the abnormality represent?

The RUQ density is peripherally calcified, a pattern known as 'eggshell calcification'. This lesion could be within liver, gallbladder fossa or at the upper pole of the right kidney. The rim-like nature of the calcification suggests it is likely to be within the gallbladder wall. This is called a 'porcelain gallbladder'. This condition is associated with gallstones and chronic cholecystitis, and also an increased risk of gallbladder carcinoma.

3 What should the next management step involve?

The diagnosis and recognition of porcelain gallbladder is important as this condition carries an increased risk of malignancy (up to 7–10% incidence); therefore, once porcelain gallbladder is diagnosed the treatment is normally cholecystectomy. An appropriate next investigation would be CT to confirm that the calcification is within the gallbladder (**Figure 7.6C**) and also to exclude an invasive gallbladder mass, nodes or liver metastases, following which there can be a discussion with the patient regarding an elective cholecystectomy. US is less useful in this condition as calcific shadowing obscures the gallbladder (as in this case).

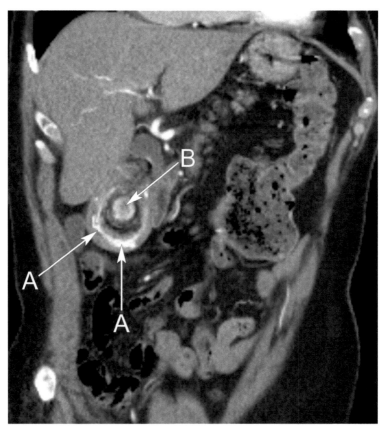

Fig. 7.6C Coronal postcontrast CT RUQ showing porcelain gallbladder. Note the curvilinear calcification in a thickened gallbladder wall (A) and stone in the gallbladder lumen (B). Stones and sludge can form a dense mixture in the gallbladder, and tumour can have a similar appearance.

LEARNING POINTS: PORCELAIN GALLBLADDER

- Calcification of the gallbladder wall, known as porcelain gallbladder owing to the brittle nature of the calcified gallbladder.
- Often detected on AXR as rim-like calcification in the RUQ.
- A CT or US scan should be performed to confirm that the calcification is in the wall of the gallbladder.
- Normally asymptomatic.
- Treated with cholecystectomy owing to the increased risk of gallbladder carcinoma.
- The differential diagnosis of RUQ calcification is gallstones, milk of calcium bile (bile that contains high levels of calcium salts), and calcified lesions in the kidney, pancreas, adrenal gland or liver.

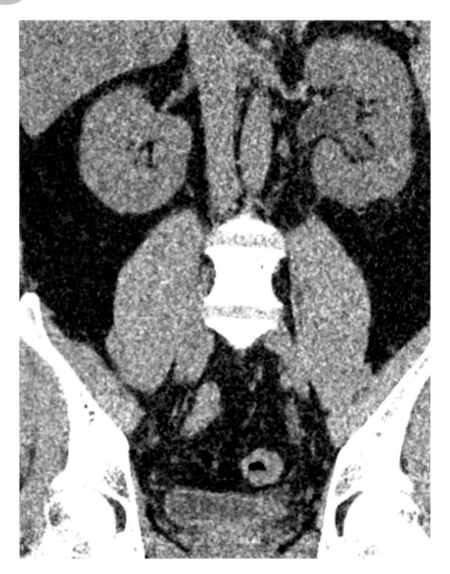

Fig. 7.7A Coronal unenhanced CT image at the level of the kidneys.

A 45-year-old male presents to the ED with sudden-onset severe left-sided loin pain radiating inferiorly and anteriorly to his groin. He describes the pain as colicky in nature.

On examination between attacks his abdomen is soft with no palpable masses but during the attacks it is not possible to examine him because he is rolling around and in pain. He is tachycardic at 100 bpm, BP 140/80 mmHg, and apyrexial. Urinalysis shows blood ++ but is negative for leucocytes, nitrites, and glucose. Routine blood tests are normal.

An unenhanced CT of the abdomen and pelvis is requested (CT KUB study) (**Figures 7.7A** and **7.7B**).

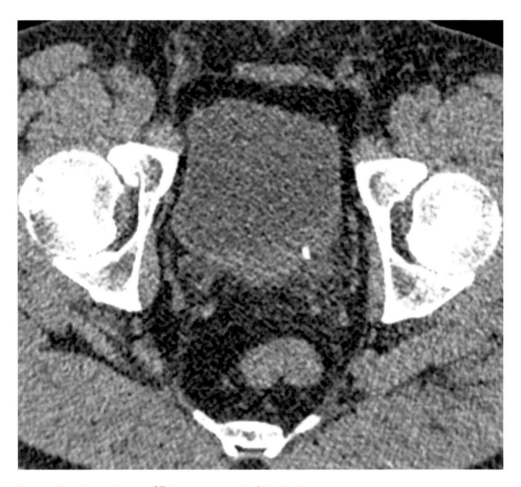

Fig. 7.7B Axial unenhanced CT image at the level of the bladder.

CASE 7.7: QUESTIONS

1 What is the diagnosis?
2 What key radiological findings do these CT images show?
3 What are the possible causes?
4 What are the potential complications?
5 How should this patient be managed?

CASE 7.7: ANSWERS

1 What is the diagnosis?

This patient has left renal colic as a result of an obstructing left ureteric calculus.

2 What key radiological findings do these CT images show?

The CT shows a 4 mm calculus at the left vesicoureteric junction (VUJ) with resultant left hydronephrosis and associated perinephric inflammatory change ('fat stranding'). (**Figures 7.7C** and **7.7D**). This stone is small and lies at the VUJ, therefore it is likely to pass spontaneously.

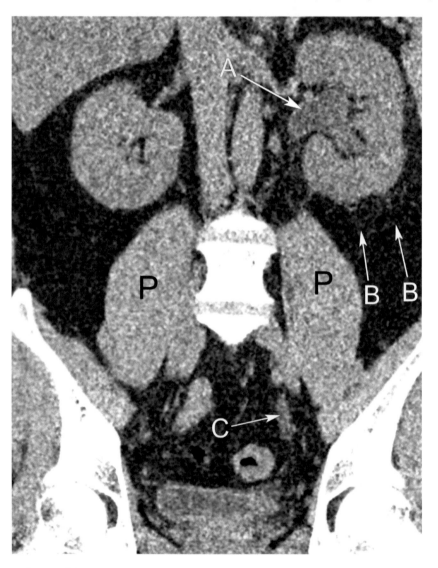

Fig. 7.7C Coronal CT image demonstrating moderate left hydronephrosis (A) with some inflammatory change in the perinephric fat (B). Note the dilated ureter in the pelvis (C). Iliopsoas muscles (P).

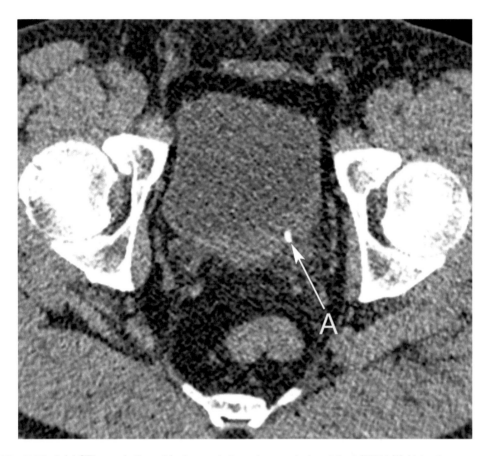

Fig. 7.7D Axial CT image in the pelvis demonstrates a 4 mm calculus at the left VUJ (A). Note: these scans are acquired with the patient prone; the calculus is, therefore, nondependent (it has not fallen anteriorly in the bladder with patient prone) indicating that it is lodged in the VUJ.

3 What are the possible causes?

The majority of renal calculi are idiopathic. Most stones are composed of calcium and are visible on unenhanced CT (if large enough, >4 mm, they may be visible on AXR). Causes of calcium stones are listed in *Table 7.7*.

Table 7.7 Common causes of calcium renal calculi

- Idiopathic hypercalciuria
- Hypercalcaemia (e.g. primary hyperparathyroidism)
- Low fluid intake
- Urinary tract malformations (e.g. horseshoe kidney)
- Recurrent urinary tract infections
- Prolonged bed rest

Other common types of renal calculi include uric acid (usually radiolucent), struvite, and cysteine-based stones.

4 What are the potential complications?

The complications associated with renal calculi are:

- Infection of the obstructed kidney and resultant septicaemia.
- Rupture of the renal pelvis.
- Renal impairment.
- Stone build up resulting in staghorn calculus and nonfunctioning kidney (**Figure 7.7E**).
- Bladder stones and associated complications including recurrent cystitis and urinary frequency.
- Chronic irritation of urothelium, squamous metaplasia, and malignancy.

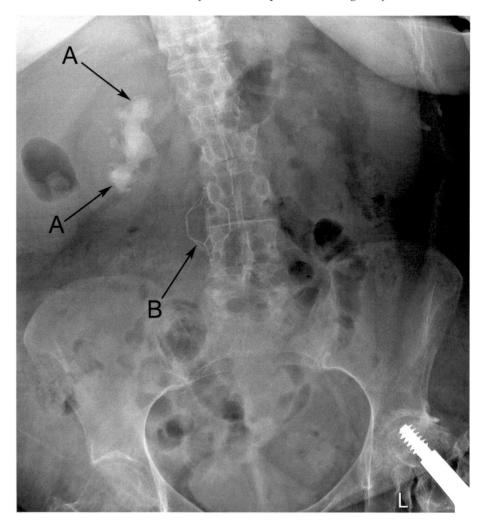

Fig. 7.7E Supine AXR in an elderly female patient demonstrating a large staghorn calculus of the right kidney (A). This patient also has an inferior vena caval filter *in situ* (B). Note the previous left dynamic hip screw.

5 How should this patient be managed?

Initial management of renal colic requires strong analgesia (e.g. NSAID or opiate). Most ureteric stones that are < 5 mm will pass spontaneously. Indications for intervention include:

- Ongoing pain.
- Sepsis.
- Failure for the stone to spontaneously pass.
- Larger impacted stones.

  If intervention is required then the options for management include:

- Extracorporeal shock wave lithotripsy (ESWL).
- Ureteroscopy and removal or *'in situ'* stone fragmentation.
- Percutaneous nephrostomy may be required to drain/relieve an obstructed or infected pelvicalyceal system.
- Open surgery.

LEARNING POINTS: RENAL COLIC

- Renal colic presents classically as intermittent severe loin to groin pain with haematuria.
- Unenhanced low-dose abdominal CT is the imaging technique of choice and may show extrarenal causes of pain in addition (e.g. appendicitis, diverticulitis).
- Look for opaque calculi within the kidneys, ureters, and bladder.
- Look for a dilated renal pelvicalyceal system or ureter to indicate urinary obstruction.
- Always check renal function (plasma urea, creatinine, and GFR) and for signs of infection.

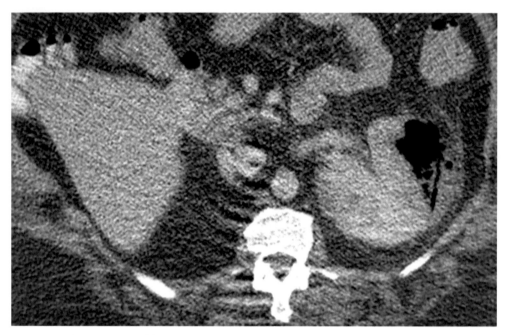

Fig. 7.8A Axial noncontrast CT image at the level of the left kidney.

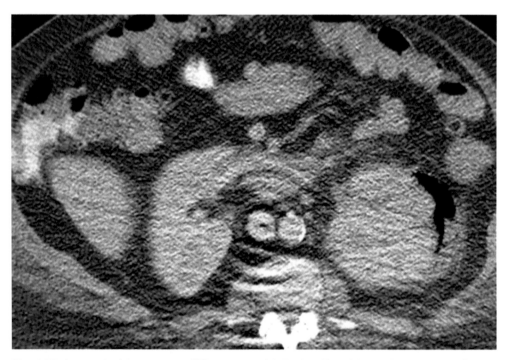

Fig. 7.8B A second axial noncontrast CT image, more inferior than Fig. 7.8A, but also at the level of the left kidney.

A 68-year-old female presents acutely unwell to the ED with fever and confusion. She is unable to give a coherent history. She is known to have type 2 diabetes. On examination she is haemodynamically unstable with the following observations: temperature 39.5°C, HR 130 bpm, respiratory rate 28 bpm, and BP 105/80 mmHg. She is hyperglycaemic on fingerprick testing. Urinalysis is positive for glucose, white cells, and nitrites. Cardiorespiratory examination is unremarkable but she is very tender in the left loin region with guarding. Bowel sounds are present. A CT KUB study is performed (**Figures 7.8A** and **7.8B**).

CASE 7.8: QUESTIONS

1 What do the CT images show?
2 What is the likely diagnosis?
3 How should the patient be managed?

CASE 7.8: ANSWERS

1 What do the CT images show?

The left kidney is enlarged and oedematous. There is an intraparenchymal cortical gas-containing crescenteric collection and associated inflammatory perinephric fat stranding (**Figures 7.8C** and **7.8D**). There is no evidence of hydronephrosis, stones or lymph node enlargement.

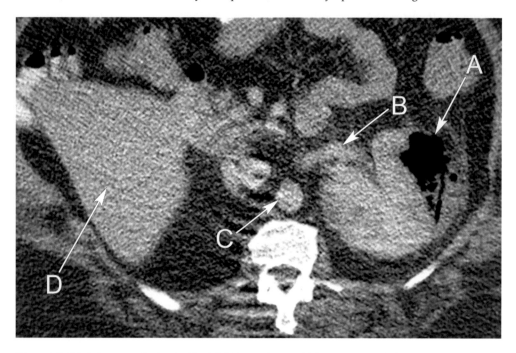

Fig. 7.8C CT abdomen at the level of the left kidney mid-pole. This shows gas within the left renal cortical parenchyma (A). Note the normal ureter (B), aorta (C), and right lobe liver (D).

2 What is the likely diagnosis?

The diagnosis is emphysematous pyelonephritis. This is a serious condition characterised by gas within the collecting system and renal parenchyma secondary to a urinary tract infection.

- The causative organism is usually *Escherichia coli* and patients are typically diabetic or immunocompromised.
- In contrast, gas confined to the collecting system, called emphysematous pyelitis, confers a more favourable prognosis.

3 How should the patient be managed?

ABCDE approach, IV access, routine bloods (including blood sugar, inflammatory markers, and renal function), blood cultures, and midstream urine for culture are also needed. The patient should be treated as per the local hospital sepsis pathway, including aggressive IV fluid and antibiotic therapy. The patient should be commenced on an insulin sliding scale with regular monitoring of blood glucose levels. This condition has a high mortality rate and the patient should be

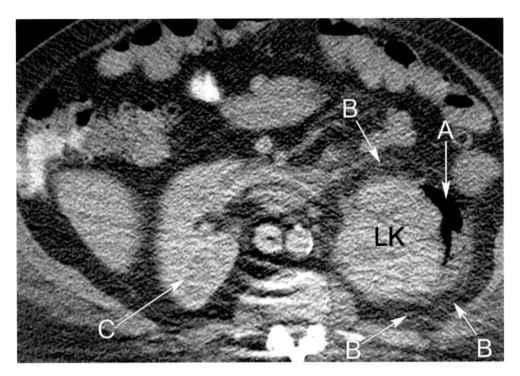

Fig. 7.8D CT abdomen at the level of the kidneys showing an enlarged left kidney (LK) with an intrasubstance crescenteric parenchymal gas collection (A) and perinephric fat stranding (B). Normal right kidney (C).

urgently referred to the urology team and diabetic physicians. Urgent percutaneous drainage of perinephric collections should be considered. Ultimately, nephrectomy may be required.

Emphysematous pyelonephritis is a condition with a high mortality and diabetics are predisposed. Infection may spread to/from the ureter and bladder (emphysematous cystitis). Urgent recognition and treatment is needed.

> **LEARNING POINTS: EMPHYSEMATOUS PYELONEPHRITIS**
>
> - Gas within the ureter or renal collecting system on AXR should raise the suspicion of emphysematous pyelonephritis.
> - The diagnosis is best demonstrated with CT, which may also show complications such as renal or extrarenal fluid collections.
> - Emphysematous pyelonephritis is a urological emergency and urgent specialist referral should be undertaken.

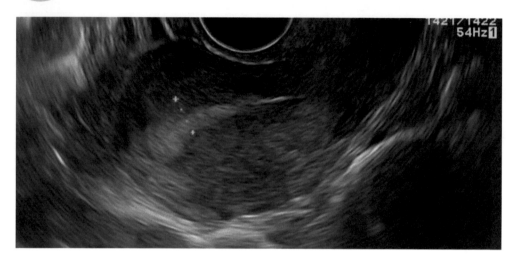

Fig. 7.9A Longitudinal US image of the uterus. The endometrial thickness has been measured (calipers).

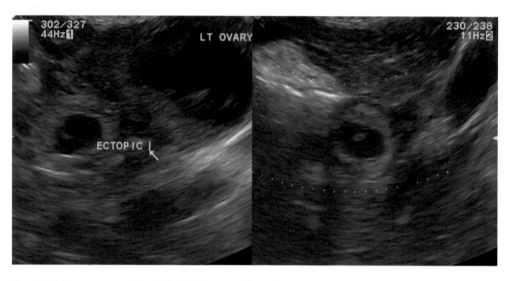

Fig. 7.9B Transverse and longitudinal US images of the left adnexa. The radiologist has labelled the left ovary and a suspected ectopic pregnancy.

A 24-year-old female presents to the ED with sudden-onset severe lower abdominal pain. She is sexually active and cannot remember the date of her last menstrual period (LMP).

On examination there is lower abdominal tenderness. Observations reveal pulse 120 bpm, BP 90/60 mmHg, and normal temperature. She is apyrexial. A urine HCG test is positive and her other blood results are normal.

An urgent transvaginal US is performed (**Figures 7.9A** and **7.9B**).

CASE 7.9: QUESTIONS

1 What is an ectopic pregnancy?
2 How do patients with ectopic pregnancy normally present?
3 What do the US images show?
4 How would you manage this patient?

CASE 7.9: ANSWERS

1 What is an ectopic pregnancy?

An ectopic pregnancy is when the embryo implants outside the uterus, most commonly in the Fallopian tube:

- It is often idiopathic; however, it is more common in patients who have damaged Fallopian tubes from previous pelvic inflammatory disease or previous tubal surgery.

2 How do patients with ectopic pregnancy normally present?

If a tubal ectopic causes rupture, then bleeding can be catastrophic and the patient presents with collapse and abdominal pain. This is a surgical emergency and laparoscopy is required:

- With increasing use of US, increasingly patients are diagnosed early and while asymptomatic. If a patient with a positive pregnancy test undergoes US that does not detect an intrauterine pregnancy it may be because:
  - The gestation is too early (<5 weeks).
  - There has been a complete miscarriage.
  - The pregnancy is ectopic.

3 What do the US images show?

The US images show an empty uterus with normal endometrial thickness. The left ovary contains a normal corpus luteum, which is sustaining the pregnancy. In the left adnexal region (in the left Fallopian tube) is a mass with a hyperechoic ring and internal material suggestive of a fetal pole.

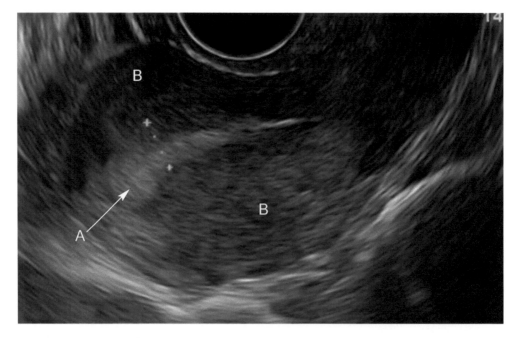

Fig. 7.9C Longitudinal US image of the uterus. Normal hyperechoic endometrium (A) and normal myometrium (B) are noted. There is no evidence of an intrauterine pregnancy.

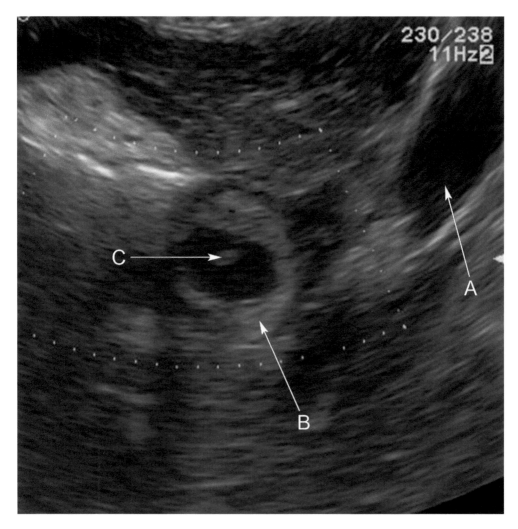

Fig. 7.9D Transverse US image of the left adnexal region. The normal left ovary containing a corpus luteum is noted (A). Medial to this (in the left Fallopian tube) is a round structure with a hyperechoic rim (B) containing echogenic material (C) in keeping with a fetal pole. Appearances are those of a left tubal ectopic pregnancy.

A heartbeat was present and according to fetal pole length the expected gestation is 6 weeks (**Figures 7.9C** and **7.9D**). Although not imaged, there was also a moderate volume of echogenic free fluid in the pelvis suggestive of blood.

4 How would you manage this patient?

Management of symptomatic patients with suspected ectopic pregnancy includes:

- Nil by mouth, IV access.
- FBC and cross match.
- Urine pregnancy test.
- Gynaecology referral on an urgent basis.

- Urgent US should be undertaken if appropriate/available. Do not let this delay surgical intervention if that is required (patient unstable, shocked).
- Laparoscopy or medical management if appropriate, i.e. asymptomatic patient and early gestation.
- Particular support must be given to these patients who not only have 'lost their baby' and had to undergo emergency surgery but also are likely to have reduced fertility in the future.

> **LEARNING POINTS: ECTOPIC PREGNANCY**
>
> - A pregnancy test (urine HCG) must be performed in all women of childbearing age who present with abdominal pain.
> - A urine HCG is almost always positive in patients with an ectopic pregnancy.
> - A transvaginal US will not always visualise an ectopic pregnancy (depending on the stage of gestation) but it should detect an intrauterine pregnancy.
> - Imaging should not delay intervention if that is required on clinical grounds.

Case 7.10

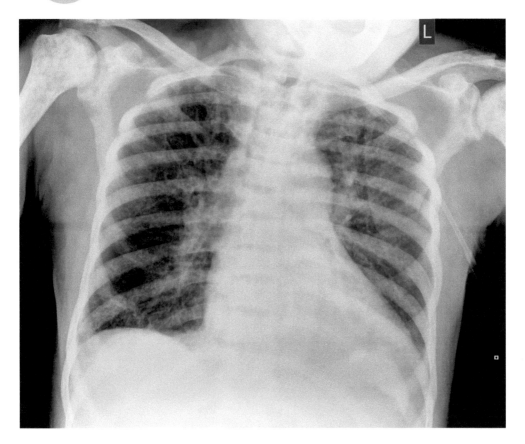

Fig. 7.10A Erect CXR.

A 27-year-old Afro-Caribbean male presents to the ED by ambulance, with generalised severe and nonspecific chest and abdominal pain. On examination, he is febrile 37.5°C, with HR 130 per min, BP 90/65 mmHg, respiratory rate 29 bpm, and oxygen saturations of 94% on 2 litres of oxygen by mask. A CXR is performed as part of his investigations (**Figure 7.10A**).

CASE 7.10: QUESTIONS

1 What does the CXR show?
2 What underlying medical condition is this patient likely to have?
3 How should the patient be managed?

CASE 7.10: ANSWERS

1 What does the CXR show?

There are a number of key findings in the CXR (**Figure 7.10B**):

- Diffusely increased bone density in keeping with bony sclerosis.
- Sclerotic (dense) and partially collapsed humeral heads bilaterally indicating avascular necrosis ('snowcap' appearance).
- Calcified spleen in the LUQ.

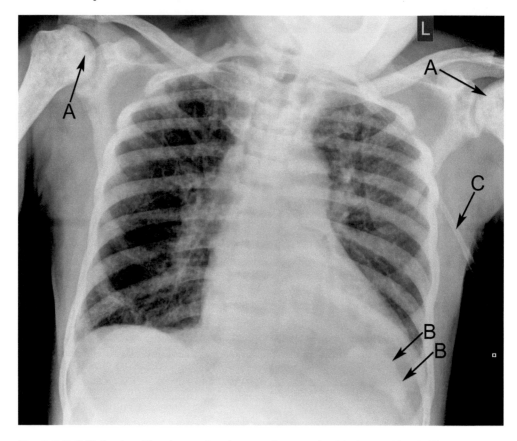

Fig. 7.10B CXR showing diffuse bony sclerosis, avascular necrosis of the humeral heads (A), and a calcified atrophic spleen (B) in keeping with sickle cell disease. Note the oxygen tubing (C).

2 What underlying medical condition is this patient likely to have?

The combination of bony sclerosis, avascular necrosis, and calcified spleen in a young patient suggests an underlying diagnosis of sickle cell disease. He is likely to have a painful sickle crisis; infection commonly precipitates a painful crisis. The spleen is particularly prone to vaso-occlusion and damage. Vaso-occlusion in blood vessels causes bone infarcts, pain, and progressive bony sclerosis. As the spleen is progressively damaged it atrophies and over time will calcify. Hyposplenism predisposes individuals to infection with certain bacteria, including *Streptococcus pneumoniae*, non-typhi *Salmonella* spp. and *Haemophilius influenzae* type b.

- Sickle cell disease is a genetic autosomal recessive condition particularly common in people of African descent, in which a mutated form of haemoglobin causes RBCs to become sickle-shaped in conditions of stress or hypoxia. The abnormal RBCs are viscous and fragile, have a reduced lifespan, and adhere very easily to endothelium leading to chronic haemolytic anaemia plus vaso-occlusion with pain and distal organ damage.

3 How should the patient be managed?

The abnormal observations mean that this patient is unstable, therefore a structured ABCDE approach is essential. In an OSCE situation you will gain marks if you say you would seek senior help. A blood gas may provide key information while waiting for formal blood results. An ECG should also be performed, especially in view of the patient's tachycardia. He will need opiate analgesia, oxygen, fluid resuscitation, monitoring, and antibiotics (after blood, urine and sputum cultures) if there is any suggestion of infection. Urgent haematology review is needed.

In the long term, management of sickle cell disease is focussed on treating anaemia, pain, and vaso-occlusive crises. Prevention of further complications, such as infection, is also important, therefore people with sickle cell disease who are hyposplenic are offered additional vaccinations.

LEARNING POINTS: SICKLE CELL DISEASE

- Inherited condition common in people of African descent.
- Diagnosis by haemoglobin electrophoresis.
- Causes anaemia and vaso-occlusive crises, which may be triggered by dehydration, hypoxaemia, and temperature changes.
- Initially causes splenic enlargement followed by repeated infarction leading to atrophy and calcification.
- Increased risk of infections due to autosplenectomy, particularly encapsulated bacteria.
- CXR appearances include bony sclerosis, avascular necrosis, H-shaped vertebrae (due to endplate infarction and collapse (**Figure 7.10C**), pulmonary infarcts and pneumonia, calcified spleen, and osteomyelitis.

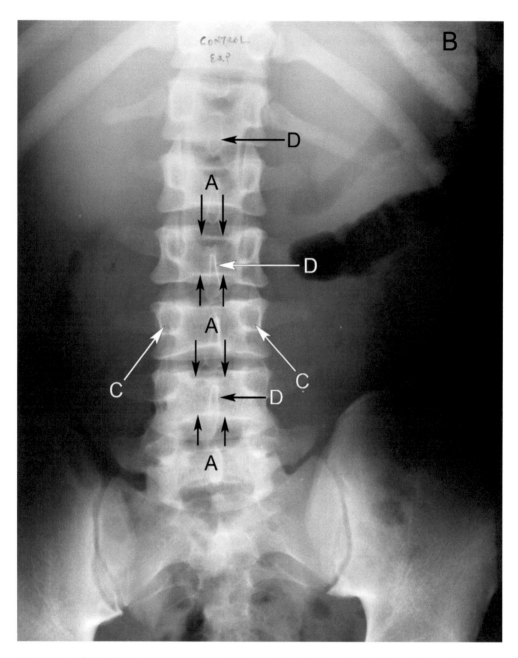

Fig. 7.10C AP view of the lumbar spine in a sickle-cell patient. He has classical 'H' vertebrae with endplate depressions (A). Note the calcified and hypoplastic spleen (B). The endplates are particularly prone to ischaemic damage as they are a 'watershed' area of blood supply, and with progressive vaso-occlusive events they soften and collapse causing the 'H' appearance. The vertebral pedicles (C) and spinous processes (D) are also shown.

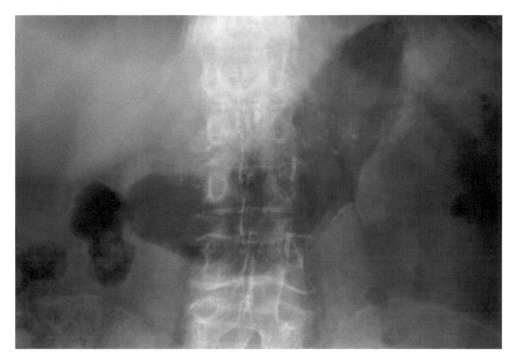

Fig. 7.11A Supine AXR, with a magnified view of the epigastric region.

A 45-year-old male presents to the ED with a 48-hour history of severe upper abdominal pain radiating to his back. He has a long history of alcohol misuse and has seen his GP several times over the past 4 years with recurrent abdominal pains.

On examination, he is pale, looks malnourished, and is tender in the epigastrium. No abdominal masses are palpable and he is not jaundiced. Observations reveal he is apyrexial, has oxygen saturations 99% on air, HR 95 bpm, and BP 115/85 mmHg.

An AXR is performed (**Figure 7.11A**). Blood test results are:

Hb	108 g/L (130–180 g/L)	ALT	143 IU/L (0–41 IU/L)
MCV	90 fL (80–100 fL)	AST	214 IU/L (0–40 IU/L)
Platelets	400 × 10⁹/L (150–450 × 10⁹/L)	ALP	110 IU/L (40–129 IU/L)
INR	1.2 (0.8–1.2)	Bilirubin	20 micromol/L (0–21 micromol/L)
Sodium	136 mmol/L (135–146 mmol/L)	Amylase	300 IU/L (28–100 IU/L)
Potassium	3.3 mmol/L (3.2–5.1 mmol/L)	GGT	469 IU/L (10–71 IU/L)
Urea	2.0 mmol/L (1.7–8.3 mmol/L)	Albumin	31 g/L (34–48 g/L)
Creatinine	120 micromol/L (62–106 micromol/L)	CRP	73 mg/L (0–5 mg/L)

CASE 7.11: QUESTIONS

1 What does the AXR show?
2 What does this abnormality represent and what are the causes of this condition?
3 What findings should be specifically looked for on clinical examination?
4 How should the patient be managed?

CASE 7.11: ANSWERS

1 What does the AXR show?

Diffuse punctate epigastric calcification is present in the region of the pancreas on AXR (**Figure 7.11B**).

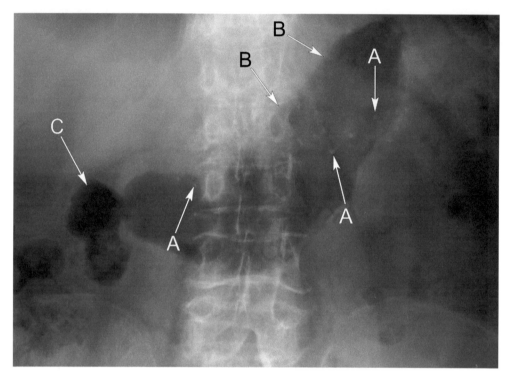

Fig. 7.11B AXR showing diffuse punctate pancreatic calcification (A). Note the air-filled stomach (B) and duodenum (C).

2 What does this abnormality represent and what are the causes of this condition?

Pancreatic calcification is caused by chronic pancreatitis in the vast majority of cases. Repeated episodes of inflammation cause progressive fibrotic destruction of pancreatic glandular tissue and over time it loses function and calcifies. Most cases of chronic pancreatitis are related to long-term alcohol misuse but some are idiopathic or secondary to autoimmune pancreatitis.

3 What findings should be specifically looked for on clinical examination?

Given the alcohol history, it is important to look for signs of chronic liver disease such as:

- Clubbing.
- Jaundice.
- Spider naevi.
- Ascites.
- Muscular atrophy.

- Gynaecomastia.
- Palmar erythema.
- Encephalopathy.
- Hepatomegaly.

4 How should the patient be managed?

The patient will require further investigation to confirm position and distribution of pancreatic calcification. CT (**Figure 7.11C**) will also help exclude pancreatic carcinoma, which may complicate this condition (more commonly in smokers). MRCP can be helpful in some cases to confirm changes of pancreatic atrophy and duct dilatation with calculus formation. The organ damage is irreversible so there is no specific treatment for chronic pancreatitis, other than pain control and lifestyle modification, particularly reducing alcohol intake. If the organ damage is sufficiently severe the patient may develop diabetes, which will need to be tested for and treated. Patients may also have diarrhoea and malabsorption resulting from lack of pancreatic enzymes, and enzyme supplements can help. Patients with chronic pancreatitis have an increased risk of developing pancreatic cancer: there is up to a 5% increase of malignancy over a 20-year period.

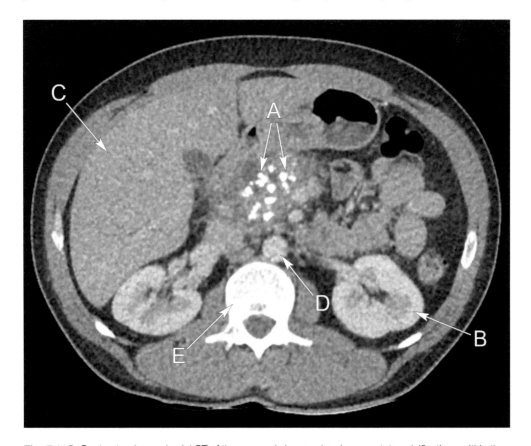

Fig. 7.11C Contrast-enhanced axial CT of the upper abdomen showing punctate calcifications within the pancreatic head (A). Normal left kidney (B), right lobe of liver (C), aorta containing contrast (D), and lumbar vertebra (E).

LEARNING POINTS: CHRONIC PANCREATITIS

- Associated with recurrent epigastric abdominal pain radiating to the back.
- Mainly affects men.
- Causes include chronic alcohol misuse and, less commonly, autoimmune pancreatitis. Some cases are idiopathic.
- No specific treatment other than pain control and lifestyle modification.
- Chronic inflammation leads to pancreatic calcification and dysfunction over time.
- Increased risk of diabetes and pancreatic cancer.

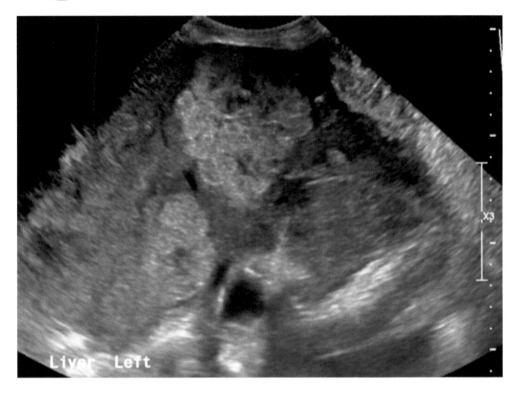

Fig. 7.12A Liver US, section through the left lobe of liver.

A 65-year-old male presents to his GP with malaise and RUQ abdominal discomfort. He has a 20 pack-year smoking history but no other relevant medical history. On examination he has a palpable, tender, and irregular liver edge. He is noted to have deranged liver function tests and mild anaemia. A liver US is performed (**Figure 7.12A**).

CASE 7.12: QUESTIONS

1 What does the US show?
2 What are the possible causes?
3 What investigation should be carried out next?
4 How should the patient be managed?

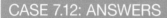

CASE 7.12: ANSWERS

1 What does the US show?

The grey-scale image (**Figure 7.12B**) shows multiple well-defined hyperechoic liver lesions. The liver contour is smooth and there are no imaging features of hepatic cirrhosis. The liver capsule and smooth liver surface are seen anteriorly.

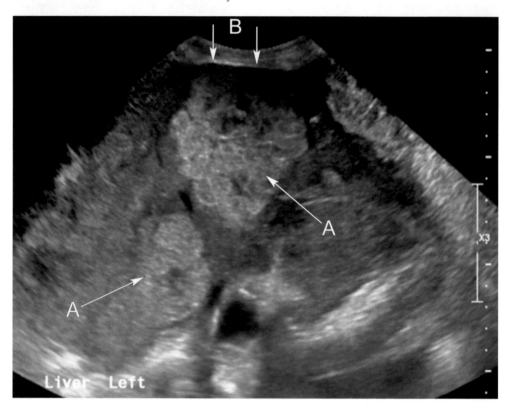

Fig. 7.12B Liver US showing hyperechoic (brighter than liver) liver lesions (arrows A) and liver capsule/anterior margin (arrows B).

2 What are the possible causes?

There are several possible causes for multiple solid liver lesions (including benign lesions such as haemangiomata, focal nodular hyperplasia, and adenomata). The latter two are more common in young females. However, in an older patient the most likely cause is hepatic metastases. Patients may be asymptomatic at presentation. Alternatively, if there is a high tumour burden, patients may present with abdominal, liver capsular pain or features of hepatic decompensation such as jaundice and ascites.

3 What investigation should be carried out next?

A CT chest, abdomen (**Figure 7.12C**), and pelvis with contrast should be performed in order to identify and stage the primary malignancy.

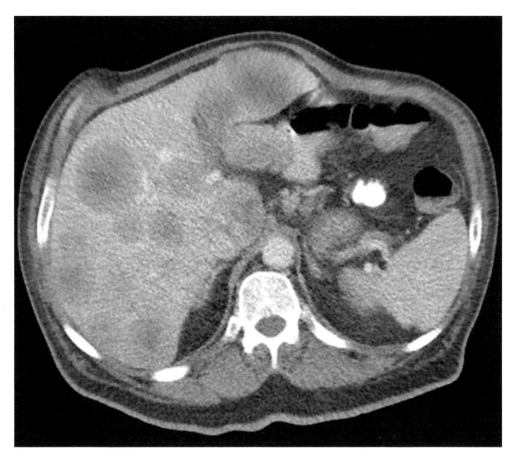

Fig. 7.12C Contrast-enhanced CT abdomen through the liver showing multiple hypodense liver metastases throughout both hepatic lobes.

4 How should the patient be managed?

The patient should be discussed at the appropriate MDT meeting where further treatment options can be discussed. Histology can be obtained via US-guided biopsy of one of the liver lesions in order to confirm the diagnosis if the primary site is not apparent or suitable for biopsy. The diagnosis in this patient was caecal carcinoma; this lesion was demonstrated on CT (**Figure 7.12D**) and biopsied colonoscopically.

Tumours that metastasise to the liver include:

- GI tract (colon, stomach) and pancreas.
- Breast.
- Lung.
- Melanoma.
- Kidney.
- Ovaries.

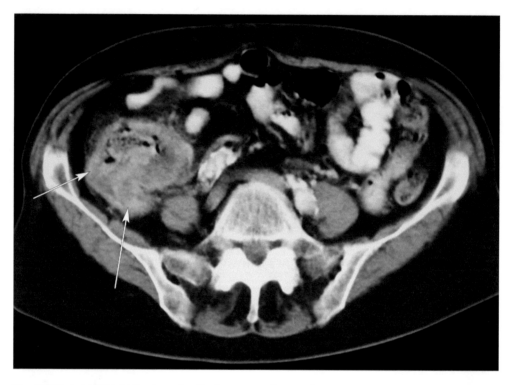

Fig. 7.12D Axial CT right iliac fossa level in the same patient confirms a caecal mass consistent with likely caecal carcinoma (arrows). This was confirmed on colonoscopic biopsy.

LEARNING POINTS: LIVER METASTASES

- The most common cause of multiple solid liver lesions in an older patient is metastases.
- Patients are often asymptomatic or have few symptoms and the diagnosis is often made while investigating abnormal liver function tests.
- The site of the primary tumour should be sought. Many different tumours metastasise to the liver; however, the commonest types are colorectal, pancreatic, oesophageal, breast, and lung cancer.

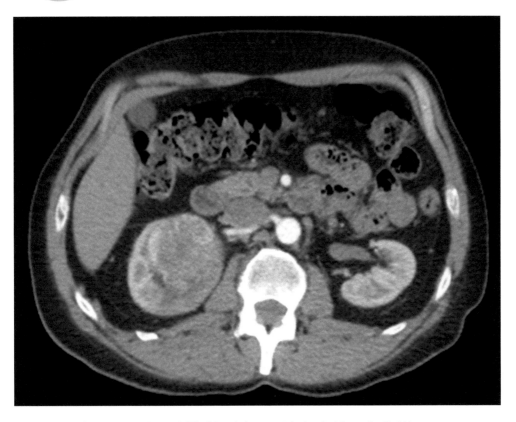

Fig. 7.13A Axial contrast-enhanced CT of the abdomen at the level of the patient's kidneys.

A 45-year-old male is referred by his GP for an US for a suspected gall stone. Incidental note is made of a solid lesion arising from his right kidney. He is asymptomatic. His bloods, in particular his renal function, are normal.

A CT is arranged for further characterisation (**Figure 7.13A**).

CASE 7.13: QUESTIONS

1 What does the CT show?
2 How may this condition present?
3 How should this patient be treated?

CASE 7.13: ANSWERS

1 What does the CT show?

A heterogeneously enhancing mass arising from the interpolar region of the right kidney. There is a solitary enlarged aortocaval lymph node (**Figure 7.13B**). The appearances are consistent with likely right renal cell carcinoma (RCC, adenocarcinoma) and aortocaval nodal metastasis.

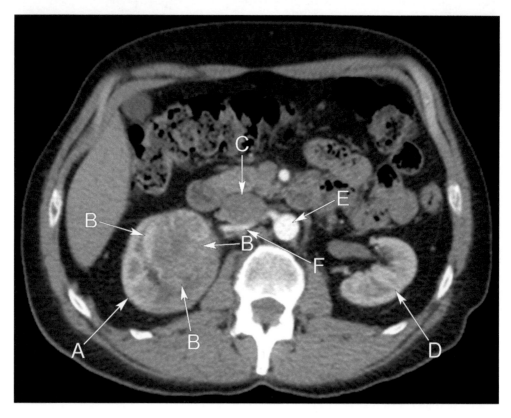

Fig. 7.13B Axial CT scan demonstrating the right kidney (A) containing a solid and heterogeneously enhancing mass (B) measuring 3.5 cm. In addition there is an enlarged aortocaval lymph node (C), suggestive of nodal metastasis. Note the normal left kidney (D), abdominal aorta (E), and inferior vena cava (F) compressed by the node.

2 How may this condition present?

Although this lesion was picked up incidentally, patients are often symptomatic. They may present with:

- Haematuria.
- Loin pain.
- Mass in the flank.
- Malaise.
- Weight loss.

- Fever (RCC is a cause of pyrexia of unknown origin).
- Polycythaemia, hypercalcaemia, and thrombocytosis are associated paraneoplastic syndromes.

As a general rule, the larger the tumour the more likely the patient is to be symptomatic (**Figure 7.13C** – the patient presented with constitutional symptoms, polycythaemia, and a left loin mass). Smoking, obesity, and hypertension are significant risk factors for RCC, and this tumour type is more common in men >65 years of age.

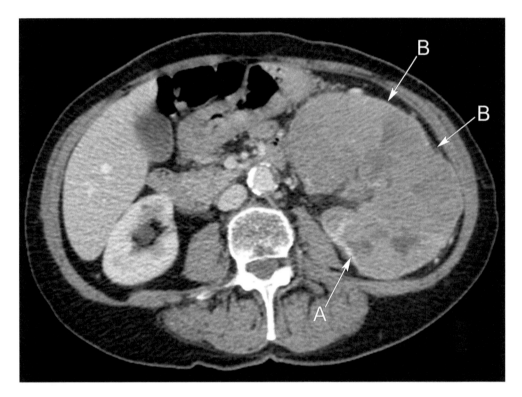

Fig. 7.13C Axial postcontrast renal CT scan. Only a small amount of the left renal cortex is visible (A), it is largely replaced by a huge left RCC (B), and this had metastasised to the lungs at the time of diagnosis.

3 How should this patient be treated?

Treatment depends on the stage at presentation. All patients require full staging of the chest and urinary tract with CT and MDT discussion. PET scanning may be helpful in complex cases. RCC has a tendency to involve the renal vein and then to metastasise haematogenously; lung metastases are most common. There may be involvement of regional lymph nodes. Surgery is the treatment of choice for localised disease; regional involved lymph nodes can also be removed if there are no distant metastases.

- The presenting patient in this case should be considered for a nephrectomy, although the left kidney must be scrutinised to make sure there is not a contralateral tumour. A PET/CT scan will help to establish if there is disease in the aortocaval lymph node, which may affect treatment. Many tumours are resistant to chemotherapy and radiotherapy, and immunotherapy may be helpful (interferon, interleukin-2).

- Smaller tumours at the upper or lower pole can be considered for 'nephron-sparing' partial nephrectomy surgery.
- If the patient is not fit for surgery then image-guided tumour ablation could be considered.
- The second patient in the case may need to be considered for surgery for symptom control.

LEARNING POINTS: RENAL CELL CARCINOMA

- RCC is the most common type of malignant renal tumour.
- It classically presents with loin pain and haematuria but may be diagnosed in the asymptomatic patient on incidental imaging.
- Contrast-enhanced CT of the chest, abdomen, and pelvis is needed for staging.
- The patient should be discussed urgently at the local urology MDT meeting and treatment options discussed.

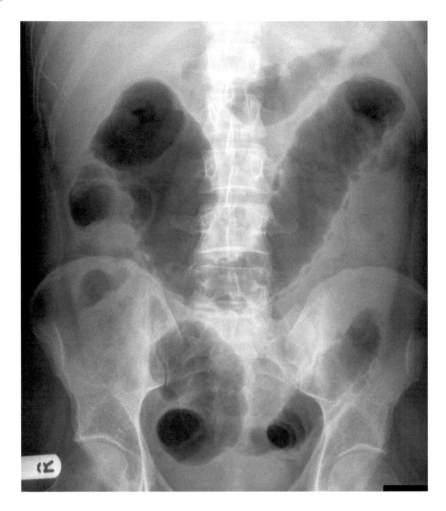

Fig. 7.14
Supine AXR.

A 22-year-old male presents to the ED with a 1-week history of worsening abdominal pain and distension. He also describes increasing loose bowel motions containing dark and altered blood over the past month and he feels unwell with episodes of shivering and sweats.

On examination he looks pale, tachycardic 100 bpm, BP 105/65 mmHg, and pyrexial at 37.8°C. His abdomen is distended and generally tender with guarding in the upper abdomen. Bowel sounds are barely audible. An AXR has been undertaken (**Figure 7.14A**).

CASE 7.14: QUESTIONS

1 What three key radiological findings are demonstrated?
2 What is the likely diagnosis?
3 Would you arrange any other imaging?
4 How should this patient be managed?

CASE 7.14: ANSWERS

1 What three key radiological findings are demonstrated?

The AXR (**Figure 7.14B**) demonstrates:

- Dilatation of the transverse colon (>6 cm maximum transverse dimension).
- Mucosal oedema causing mural and haustral thickening of the transverse colon.
- Air within the thickened wall of the transverse colon (pneumatosis coli).

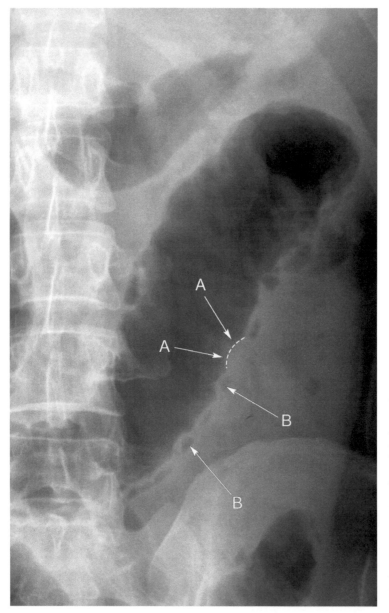

Fig. 7.14B Cropped and enlarged section of the same AXR showing the abnormal distal transverse colon, which is pathologically dilated. Note the pronounced thickening of the bowel wall with oedema of the haustra (A). The haustral thickening gives the classical radiological appearance of 'thumb printing', i.e. one could imagine a thumb imprint causing the impression. The other important finding is air within the thickened wall, termed pneumatosis coli (B).

2 What is the likely diagnosis?

The likely diagnosis in this patient is acute toxic colitis with dilatation of the transverse colon, also known as toxic megacolon. Toxic megacolon may involve all or parts of the colon and is a complication of several colitides:

- Most commonly associated with inflammatory bowel disease, ulcerative colitis > Crohn's disease.
- Infective, and a number of organisms are associated, including salmonella, shigella, campylobacter and cytomegalovirus in HIV. Toxic megacolon as a complication of *Clostridium difficile* pseudo membranous colitis is also increasingly recognised.
- Other causes include irradiation and ischaemia.
- There are recognised and diagnostic criteria for toxic megacolon, which include:
  - Radiological evidence of colonic dilatation (usually >6 cm).
  - Fever, tachycardia, leucocytosis, and anaemia.
  - Evidence of dehydration or shock.

The pathogenesis of toxic megacolon, however, remains unclear.

3 Would you arrange any other imaging?

These patients are at high risk of bowel perforation. Sepsis and shock are the other key complications. At presentation an erect CXR should be undertaken to exclude free intraperitoneal air. The use of other imaging will depend on the condition of the patient. If not seriously unwell, CT can be valuable to provide further information on the distribution of disease, potential ischaemic bowel, and to look for occult free intraperitoneal air. Seriously unwell and peritonitic patients may need to go straight to theatre.

4 How should this patient be managed?

The initial management involves an ABCDE assessment. Patients require IV access, rehydration, routine bloods including cross-match, and urgent discussion with senior surgical, gastroenterological, and anaesthetic colleagues. It is essential in OSCE scenarios to emphasise the initial resuscitation of the patient, monitoring, and baseline investigation, and indicate that senior advice would be sought. All these statements will gain marks and need to be stated even if they seem obvious.

- In this patient the presentation is highly suggestive of underlying inflammatory bowel disease. The patient failed to respond to initial IV steroids and antibiotics, and following senior review underwent a subtotal colectomy with end ileostomy formation. The final diagnosis histologically was Crohn's disease. An AXR of toxic megacolon in a patient with ulcerative colitis is shown in **Figure 7.14C**.

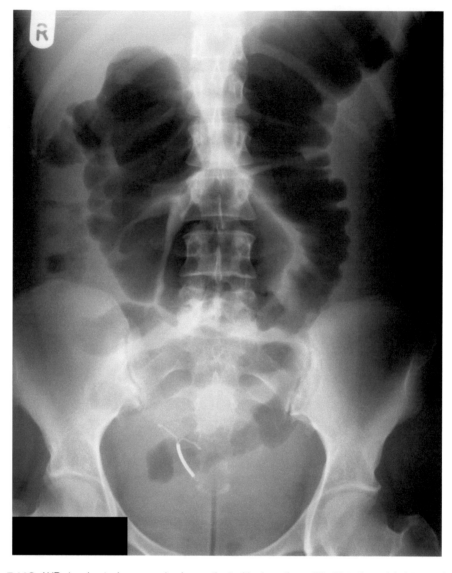

Fig. 7.14C AXR showing toxic megacolon in a patient with ulcerative colitis. Note the pelvic intrauterine contraceptive device (IUCD).

LEARNING POINTS: PNEUMATOSIS COLI

- This term refers to gas in the bowel wall.
- The pathogenesis is poorly understood.
- In adults most cases are asymptomatic, and there is an association with COPD.
- When associated with diseases leading to bowel necrosis (such as toxic megacolon) the presence of pneumatosis coli is an ominous finding and associated with a high mortality.
- Pneumatosis coli does also occur in neonates, usually secondary to necrotising enterocolitis.

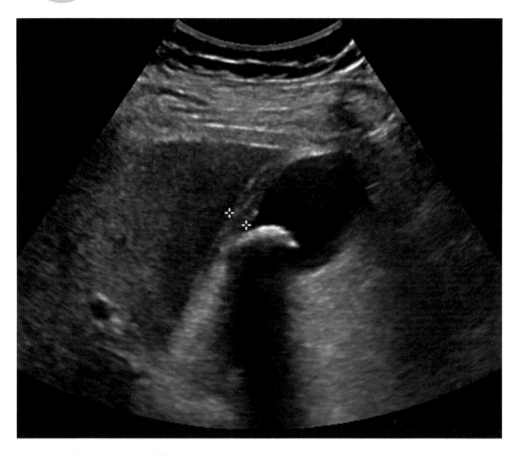

Fig. 7.15A Upper abdominal US showing the liver and gallbladder.

A 42-year-old female presents to the ED acutely unwell with a 1-day history of fever, vomiting, and severe RUQ abdominal pain. She has no relevant past medical history but has a raised BMI of 28 kg/m². Baseline observations: temperature 38.5°C, HR 120 bpm, respiratory rate 20 bpm, and BP 130/80 mmHg. On examination she appears dehydrated and has a positive Murphy's sign on palpation of the right upper abdominal quadrant. An abdominal US is performed (**Figure 7.15A**). She has raised WCC and inflammatory markers.

CASE 7.15: QUESTIONS

1 What does the US show?
2 What additional findings should be looked for on US?
3 How should the patient be managed?

CASE 7.15: ANSWERS

1 What does the US show?

The abdominal US image shows a large echobright (hyperechoic) calculus at the gallbladder neck (**Figure 7.15B**). There is posterior acoustic shadowing as the US waves cannot penetrate the dense calculi and are reflected back towards the US probe (a characteristic imaging finding in both gallbladder and renal calculi). The gallbladder wall is thickened and inflamed, confirming the clinical diagnosis of acute cholecystitis. Note the positive Murphy's sign, gallbladder tenderness on palpation; this sign may also be elicited with the US probe.

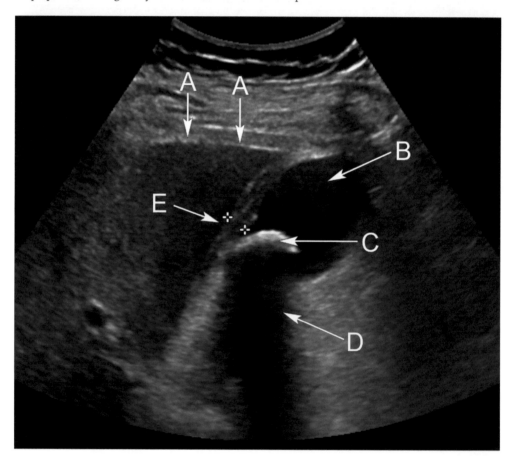

Fig. 7.15B Upper abdominal US showing the liver capsule anteriorly (A), gallbladder lumen (B), gallstone (C), and posterior acoustic shadow (D). The gallbladder wall is thickened (E, callipers).

2 What additional findings should be looked for on US?

It is important sonographically to look for a dilated common bile duct (CBD) and assess for the presence of an obstructing stone (choledocholithiasis). In the context of sepsis this would imply a diagnosis of acute cholangitis and would alter the patient's management, as the patient may then need to undergo ERCP (endoscopic retrograde cholangiopancreatography), which involves

CBD cannulation via endoscopy and stone retrieval. MRCP is often used to visualise the bile ducts noninvasively. US is very accurate at demonstrating the gallbladder and upper CBD but often, owing to pain or bowel gas, the distal bile duct is usually not well seen. MRCP is needed to exclude an intraductal calculus, particularly if US demonstrates CBD dilatation or if derangement in liver function tests persists. CT is the technique of choice in acutely ill patients with suspected gallbladder empyema or gallbladder perforation (**Figure 7.15C**).

Gallstones are extremely common, with a prevalence of approximately 10–15% in the adult population. However, only 1–4% of individuals are symptomatic. Gallstones are more common in middle-aged female Caucasians. Risk factors include obesity, pregnancy, hypercholesterolaemia, family history, and diabetes. Patients may present with biliary colic (pain following eating) owing to temporary obstruction of the cystic duct. Prolonged obstruction may result in inflammation of the gallbladder wall (acute cholecystitis). Complications of acute cholecystitis include gallbladder necrosis, gangrene, perforation, and abscess formation/empyema (**Figure 7.15C**).

Other complications of gallstones include:

- Chronic cholecystitis (gallbladder wall may calcify, 'porcelain' gallbladder).
- Increased risk of gallbladder cancer, particularly in 'porcelain' gallbladder.
- Gallstone ileus.
- Stone in CBD leading to cholangitis, obstructive jaundice, pancreatitis.

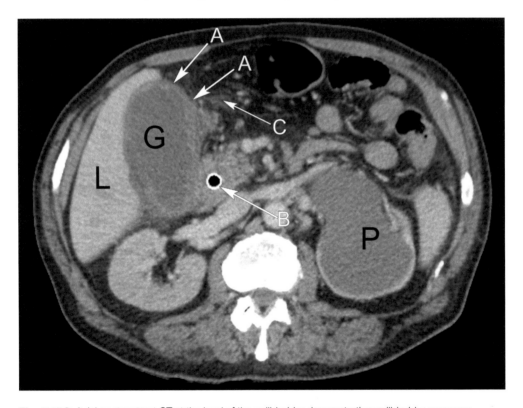

Fig. 7.15C Axial postcontrast CT at the level of the gallbladder demonstrating gallbladder empyema. The gallbladder (G) is distended with a thickened wall (A) and contains material of mixed density. The right lobe of liver (L), incidental chronic left pelviureteric junction obstruction (P), and indwelling common bile duct stent (B) are seen. Note the inflammatory changes in the mesenteric fat adjacent to the gallbladder (C).

3 How should the patient be managed?

The patient should be referred to the upper GI surgery team. The patient's acute management should include being placed nil by mouth, IV fluid resuscitation, IV antibiotic treatment, and analgesia (remember opiates can worsen pain with spasm of the sphincter of Oddi).

After resolution of the acute episode, an elective cholecystectomy is performed some weeks later. The reason for delay in surgery is to allow for inflammation of the gallbladder to resolve, which is thought to result in reduced operative morbidity and reduced need for conversion from a laparoscopic to an open approach. MRCP can also then be performed to exclude any further CBD stones. However, not all surgeons agree with this approach, some preferring 'hot' surgical intervention during the acute episode.

LEARNING POINTS: ACUTE CHOLECYSTITIS

- Acute cholecystitis is a surgical emergency and the diagnosis should be considered in patients with fever, vomiting, and RUQ pain. Remember the ABCDE concept and to call for senior advice.
- The initial diagnostic imaging test of choice is US, which may show gallstones and gallbladder wall thickening. MRCP is used to demonstrate common duct stones when indicated.
- Complications of acute cholecystitis include gallbladder necrosis, perforation, and empyema.

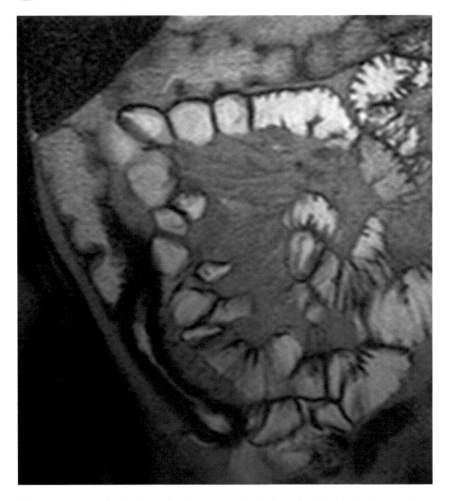

Fig. 7.16A Coronal T2-weighted image from MRI small bowel through the right iliac fossa region.

A 23-year-old male presents to gastroenterology outpatients with a 3-month history of intermittent abdominal pain and diarrhoea. He also reports unintentional weight loss of 15 kg over the preceding months but has no relevant past medical history. On direct questioning he has also experienced joint pains and itching of both eyes. On examination he has a low-grade fever. Blood tests reveal the following abnormalities:

WCC	13 × 10⁹/L (4.0–11.0 × 10⁹/L)	CRP	120 mg/L (<5 mg/L)

A small bowel MRI is performed (**Figure 7.16A**).

CASE 7.16: QUESTIONS

1 What does the MRI small bowel show?
2 What is the likely diagnosis?

3 How should the patient be managed?
4 What are the complications of this disease?

CASE 7.16: ANSWERS

1 What does the MRI small bowel show?

There is a long segment of terminal ileal thickening and stricturing (**Figure 7.16B**) when compared with the remaining visualised small bowel (where wall thickness does not exceed the upper normal limit of 3 mm). There is also mild increased bowel wall signal within the thickened segment, in keeping with oedema, indicating active inflammation. There is luminal narrowing, which was shown to persist on all sequences, in keeping with a stricture. Post-IV contrast images show increased enhancement of the thickened terminal ileum (**Figure 7.16C**), confirming the diagnosis of terminal ileitis.

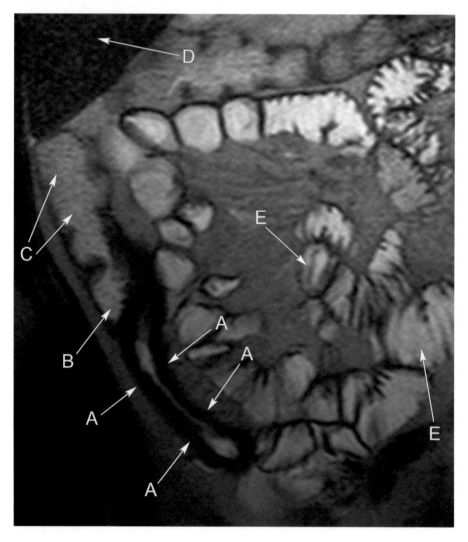

Fig. 7.16B Coronal T2-weighted image from MRI small bowel. The MRI confirms diffuse stricturing of a thick-walled terminal ileum (A). Note: caecum (B), ascending colon (C), right lobe liver (D), and normal ileal loops (E).

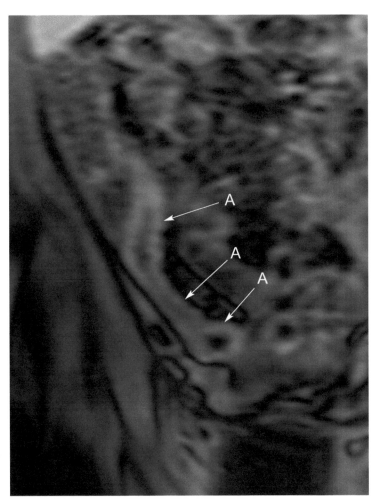

Fig. 7.16C
T1 fat-saturated post-gadolinium coronal image showing thickening and enhancement of the terminal ileum (arrows A).

2 What is the likely diagnosis?

The most likely diagnosis is inflammatory bowel disease, most likely Crohn's disease with this distribution. The large bowel appeared unremarkable (images not shown although normal caecum and ascending colon can be seen). However, it should be remembered that backwash ileitis may occur in patients with ulcerative colitis. The differential diagnosis of terminal ileitis also includes TB; however, the caecum is usually affected in this condition and there are usually intra-abdominal necrotic lymph nodes. Atypical infection, for example amoebiasis and typhilitis owing to chemotherapy, should not be included in the differential diagnosis in this particular patient as there is no relevant history of travel/immunocompromise or treatment for cancer.

3 How should the patient be managed?

The patient should be managed by the gastroenterology team with discussion at the inflammatory bowel disease MDT meeting. In addition:

- The diagnosis of Crohn's disease can be confirmed with colonoscopy, terminal ileoscopy, and terminal ileal biopsy.

- Treatment is with steroids and appropriate immunosuppressive agents (e.g. azathioprine) or immunomodulatory therapies (e.g. infliximab), as directed by the gastroenterology team, with appropriate monitoring.
- Surgery may be considered in the event of future complications, for example SBO caused by fibrotic strictures or following abscess or fistula formation.

4 What are the complications of this disease?

Crohn's disease is an inflammatory disorder of the GI tract that most often affects the terminal ileum but may affect any part of the tract from mouth to anus. It has a multifactorial aetiology where autoimmune and genetic factors are thought to play important roles. Patients typically present in the second to third decades of life although there is a second peak of presentation in the seventh decade. Typical presenting symptoms include abdominal pain and weight loss but non-GI manifestations, such as arthralgia and episcleritis, may also be observed. Imaging may reveal small bowel inflammation (typically affecting the terminal ileum) with characteristic features including transmural inflammation, skip lesions, and strictures.

Complications of Crohn's disease include SBO owing to strictures, fistulae (between small bowel loops, small bowel and large bowel, and between the bowel and the skin), and abscess formation. Perianal disease is also typical of Crohn's disease. Patients are also at increased risk of small bowel cancer and lymphoma.

MRI small bowel is the most sensitive imaging test for the diagnosis of small bowel Crohn's disease and is preferable in young patients as it does not involve ionising radiation. However, CT is an excellent alternative in patients presenting with an acute abdomen (possible megacolon, perforation, abscess). This is because CT is more readily available in most centres and is quick to perform (therefore better tolerated by acutely unwell patients).

Early diagnosis and aggressive medical therapy has been shown to improve prognosis in patients with Crohn's disease.

Extraintestinal complications of Crohn's disease include:

- Skin – erythema nodosum, pyoderma gangrenosum.
- Joints – sacroiliitis, ankylosing spondylitis.
- Eyes – uveitis, episcleritis.
- Liver – hepatitis, sclerosing cholangitis, cirrhosis, gallbladder carcinoma.

Note: this patient also had eye and joint symptoms.

LEARNING POINTS: CROHN'S DISEASE

- Crohn's disease is the most common cause of terminal ileitis.
- Small bowel MRI is the most sensitive imaging test and may show bowel wall thickening and increased enhancement, strictures, and complications (e.g. fistulae and abscesses). However, terminal ileal biopsy is the reference standard diagnostic test.
- CT abdomen and pelvis should be considered in patients presenting with a surgical acute abdomen to look for complications of megacolon, perforation, and abscess.
- Local complications of Crohn's disease include strictures, abscesses, and fistulae.

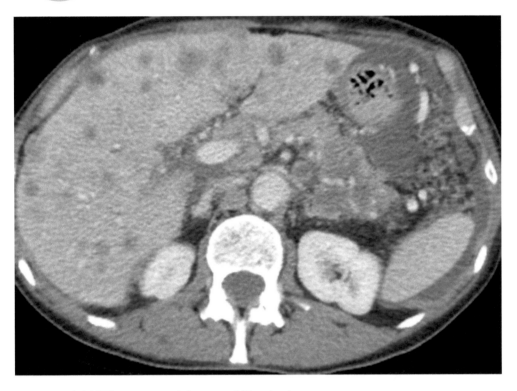

Fig. 7.17A Axial CT image upper abdomen post IV contrast.

A 65-year-old man presents to his GP with upper abdominal pain radiating to his back and malaise. On direct questioning he says he has lost one stone in weight over 6 weeks. He has no other medical complaints but gives a 20 pack-year history of smoking and consumes approximately four bottles of wine per week. On examination he is haemodynamically stable but appears cachectic and has pale sclerae. He is not jaundiced. His abdomen is nontender; however, he has a palpable liver edge and is tender in the epigastrium.

CXR and AXR are unremarkable. CT of the abdomen and pelvis is undertaken (**Figure 7.17A**). Blood investigations reveal the following abnormalities:

Hb	90 g/L (130–180 g/L)	ALT	90 IU/L (<41 IU/L)
Bilirubin	50 micromol/L (<21 micromol/L)	ALP	200 IU/L (40–129 IU/L)

CASE 7.17: QUESTIONS

1 What does the image show?
2 What is the diagnosis?
3 How should the patient be managed?

CASE 7.17: ANSWERS

1 What does the CXR show?

The CT image shows a large low-density mass in the pancreatic tail, multiple hypovascular liver metastases, and a necrotic peripancreatic lymph node (**Figure 7.17B**). There is also LUQ ascites and peritoneal stranding as well as nodularity anterior to the spleen.

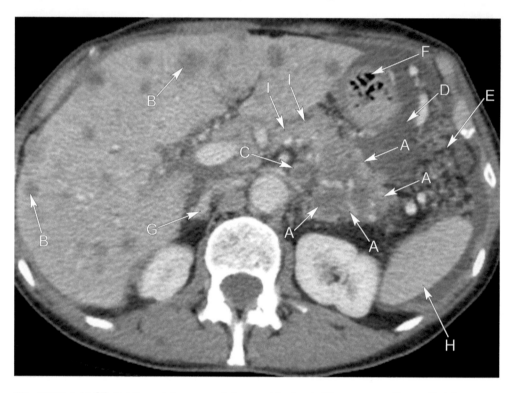

Fig. 7.17B Axial CT slice through the upper abdomen at the level of the pancreas. Pancreatic tail mass (A), liver metastases (B), necrotic peripancreatic lymph node (C) and ascites (D). Infiltration of the mesenteric fat is present (E). Note the stomach (F), right adrenal (G), spleen (H), and also normal pancreatic body (I). The pancreatic tumour encases adjacent vessels.

2 What is the diagnosis?

The diagnosis is pancreatic cancer with hepatic, nodal, and peritoneal metastases. Pancreatic carcinoma is an adenocarcinoma, with high mortality owing to frequently inoperable disease at presentation. Increasing age, smoking, obesity, and diabetes are risk factors as well as alcohol excess and chronic pancreatitis.

- Note that the mass is in the pancreatic tail and, therefore, has not caused biliary obstruction, hence the patient did not present with jaundice. More commonly the tumour will occur in the pancreatic head and block the common bile duct causing biliary duct dilatation and painless jaundice.

3 How should the patient be managed?

The patient should be admitted urgently to hospital for management of his pain, for diagnosis, and for discussion of treatment options:

- ABCDE approach.
- CT chest to complete staging.

The patient should also be referred urgently to the hepatobiliary MDT for surgical and oncological opinion. The diagnosis of metastatic pancreatic carcinoma was diagnosed on percutaneous US-guided liver biopsy. In this case surgery was not an option owing to the multiple hepatic metastases and peritoneal disease. The patient was referred for palliative chemotherapy. His prognosis is extremely poor.

LEARNING POINTS: PANCREATIC CANCER

- Pancreatic cancer is a common cause of painless jaundice caused by biliary obstruction.
- Risk factors include smoking and alcohol excess.
- CT may demonstrate the primary tumour and metastatic disease, including liver, nodal, lung, and peritoneal metastases, as well as relationship of the primary tumour to the mesenteric vessels.
- Patients often present with irresectable disease.
- Factors affecting suitability for surgery include relationship of the tumour with the mesenteric vessels, presence of metastatic disease, and patient fitness for surgery.

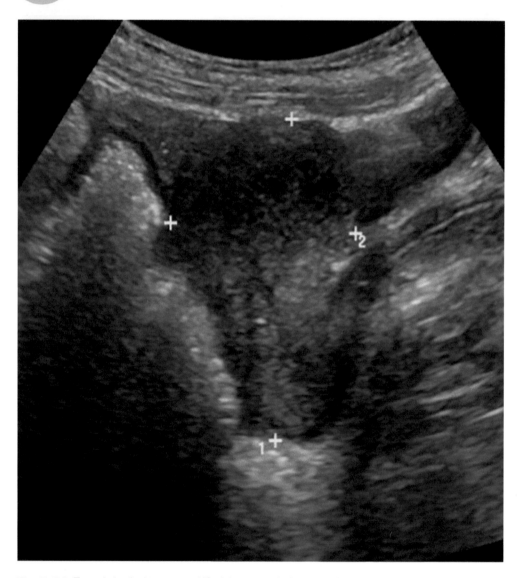

Fig. 7.18A Transabdominal transverse US of the uterus (delineated with calipers).

A 44-year-old female presents to her GP with a 6-month history of menorrhagia and dysmenor-rhea. On examination a firm suprapubic mass is palpable. Blood tests reveal a slightly low Hb at 118 (125–165 g/L) but blood parameters are otherwise normal.

The GP suspects a diagnosis of uterine fibroids and requests a pelvic US (**Figures 7.18A** and **7.18B**).

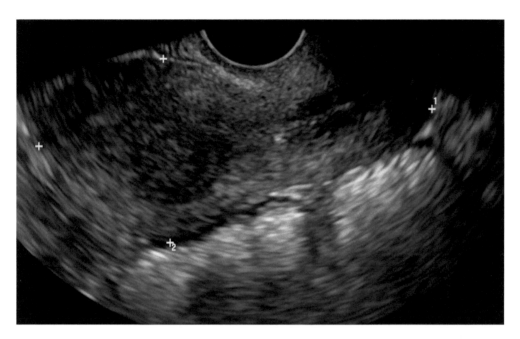

Fig. 7.18B Transvaginal US of the uterus in longitudinal section (delineated with calipers).

CASE 7.18: QUESTIONS

1 What are fibroids?
2 What does the US show?
3 What other imaging is available for suspected fibroids?
4 What are the potential complications of fibroids?
5 How are fibroids managed?

CASE 7.18: ANSWERS

1 What are fibroids?

Fibroids (also known as leiomyomata) are benign tumours of the myometrium. They are more common in Afro-Caribbean women and in women approaching the menopause. They may compress the endometrial cavity (submucosal fibroids) and cause symptoms of menorrhagia and dysmenorrhea, or arise from the surface of the uterus (serosal fibroids) and be asymptomatic. Fibroids may also be 'pedunculated', arising from the uterine surface as a pedunculated mass.

Fibroids can vary in size from a few millimeters to a massive tumour occupying the abdomen. Their growth is oestrogen-dependent and they therefore tend to increase in size during pregnancy and regress after the menopause.

Patients with fibroids may be asymptomatic or present with:

- Abnormal vaginal bleeding.
- Pain.
- Infertility.
- Palpable pelvic mass.
- Pressure effects.

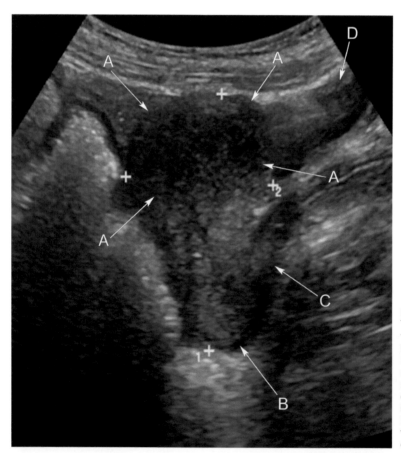

Fig. 7.18C Transabdominal transverse US image of the uterus. Fundal low-density (hypoechoic) fibroid noted (A). The endometrial cavity is not visualised. Note: the cervix (B), vagina (C), and empty collapsed bladder (D).

2 What does the US show?

The US demonstrates a fibroid at the fundus of the uterus compressing the superior aspect of the endometrial cavity (**Figures 7.18C** and **7.18D**).

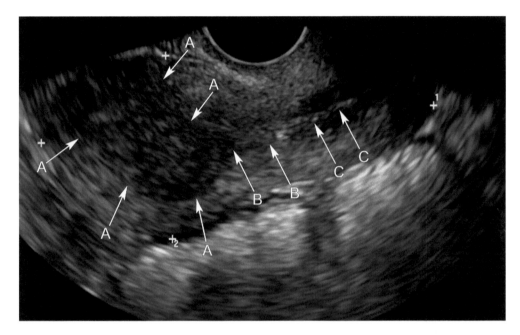

Fig. 7.18D Transvaginal US image of the uterus in longitudinal section. Note: the fundal fibroid (A) compressing and distorting the endometrial cavity. Uterine cervix (B), vagina (C).

3 What other imaging is available for suspected fibroids?

US is the workhorse for the diagnosis of fibroids. It is essential to acquire transabdominal and transvaginal views to ensure full visualisation and assessment of the extent of the fibroids (the transvaginal US probe only has a sound penetration depth of around 4 cm, which will underestimate large fibroids).

Where there is doubt about the diagnosis or if further treatment planning is required, an MRI scan will provide further information (**Figure 7.18E**).

CT will demonstrate fibroids as a soft tissue density mass in the pelvis but does not provide good anatomical detail and it can be difficult to differentiate uterine fibroids from adnexal lesions. There is also a significant associated radiation dose.

4 What are the potential complications of fibroids?

Complications of fibroids include:

- Menorrhagia and subsequent anaemia.
- Torsion of a pedunculated fibroid.
- Degeneration (can be associated with pain).
- Malignancy (leiomyosarcoma). This is rare, but if the fibroid is growing rapidly, in particular after menopause, then malignancy should be considered.

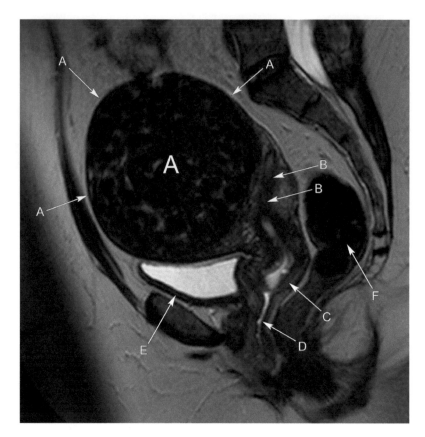

Fig. 7.18E Sagittal T2-weighted MRI image of the female pelvis. A large fundal fibroid is noted (A), which is displacing the endometrium posteriorly (B). Note the cervix (C), vagina (D), bladder (E), and rectum (F).

5 How are fibroids managed?

Treatment options for fibroids depend on their size and location, the extent of symptoms, the age of the patient, and patient wishes. They include:

- Myomectomy.
- Hormone administration.
- Hysterectomy (in a patient not wishing to preserve her fertility).
- Uterine artery embolisation (radiological procedure involving uterine artery catheterisation via the femoral artery and embolisation of feeding vessels).

LEARNING POINTS: UTERINE FIBROIDS

- Uterine fibroids are commonly asymptomatic but can cause menorrhagia and dysmenorrhea if submucosal.
- Transabdominal and transvaginal US are required for complete initial assessment.
- MRI may be used as an adjunct in complex cases and for pretreatment planning.
- Treatment options include myomectomy, hysterectomy, hormone replacement, and uterine artery embolisation.

Case 7.19

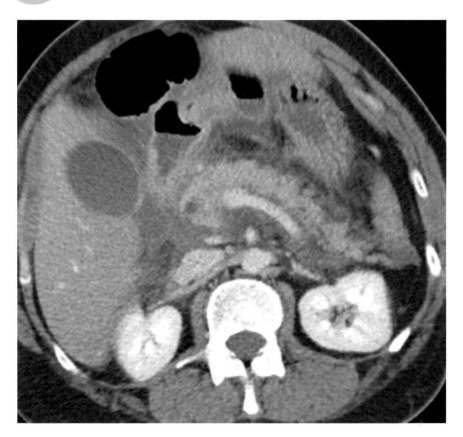

Fig. 7.19A Axial CT abdomen at the epigastric level post IV contrast.

A 35-year-old male presents to the ED with 2 days of severe central abdominal pain and vomiting. The pain radiates to the back and is mildly relieved by sitting forwards. He has no relevant past medical history, takes no regular medications and is a nonsmoker. He drinks 50 units of alcohol per week. On examination he appears unwell and is haemodynamically unstable with the following observations: HR 130 bpm, respiratory rate 24 bpm, BP 100/80 mmHg, and temperature 38°C. He has central abdominal guarding to palpation. Blood tests reveal the following abnormalities:

WCC	20 × 10⁹/L (4–11 × 10⁹/L)	Urea	14 mmol/L (1.7–8.3 mmol/L)
CRP	200 mg/L (<5 mg/L)	Creatinine	150 micromol/L (62–106 micromol/L)

ABG reveals a metabolic acidosis. CT of the abdomen is arranged (**Figure 7.19A**).

CASE 7.19: QUESTIONS

1 What does the imaging show and what is the diagnosis? What other blood tests might help?
2 How should the patient be managed?
3 What are the underlying causes of this condition?
4 What are the complications of this condition?

CASE 7.19: ANSWERS

1 What does the imaging show and what is the diagnosis? What other blood tests might help?

There is fluid and soft tissue density inflammatory fat stranding surrounding the pancreas, with loss of the normal dark fat density (**Figures 7.19B** and **7.19C**), in keeping with acute pancreatitis. Additional findings include:

- The pancreas enhances normally with no low-density gas areas to suggest necrosis, no focal abscess.
- The splenic vein enhances normally and is patent.
- The gallbladder is thin walled and contains no gallstones (on this image).
- The CBD is not dilated.

Serum amylase and serum lipase would be helpful. Both are raised in acute pancreatitis, and a mild to moderate increase in amylase can also be seen in other abdominal inflammation disorders, and when pancreatitis is subacute. Lipase is more specific to alcohol-related pancreatitis.

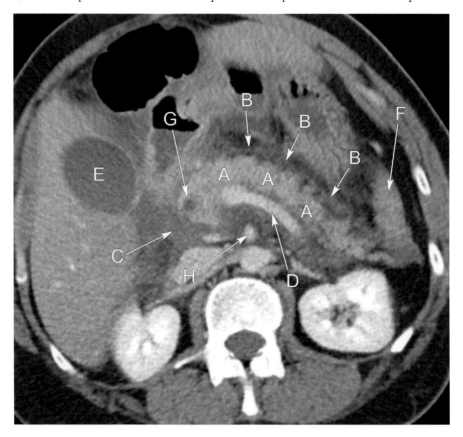

Fig. 7.19B Axial CT abdomen post IV contrast at the level of the pancreas. The pancreas (A) appears swollen and there is diffuse soft tissue attenuation around the pancreas (B) with fluid also present (C). The splenic vein appears patent (D) and the gallbladder appears distended but thin walled (E). Note: spleen (F), distal nondilated common bile duct (G), and patent superior mesenteric artery (H).

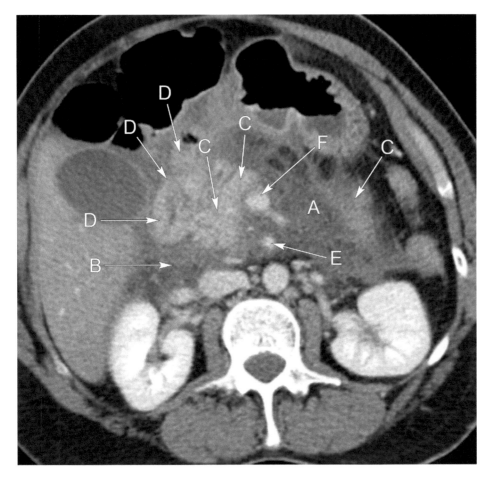

Fig. 7.19C More caudal axial CT abdomen in the same patient. There is extensive fluid surrounding the pancreas (A). There is also extensive inflammatory change in the peripancreatic fat (B). Note: swollen pancreatic tissue, head and tail (C), duodenum second part (D), superior mesenteric artery (E), and vein (F).

2 How should the patient be managed?

The patient should be kept nil-by-mouth and managed supportively on the high dependency unit with IV fluid resuscitation, prophylactic antibiotics to be considered, and adequate analgesia. Additionally:

- A NG tube should be sited in order to prevent vomitus and abdominal distension, and aspiration pneumonia (**Figure 7.19D**).
- Fluid balance and blood gases should be monitored (the patient may need a urinary catheter and central venous access).
- The underlying cause of pancreatitis should be investigated and complications managed as appropriate.
- Abdominal US has a higher sensitivity than CT for detection of gallstones in the gallbladder and should be considered if the underlying cause is unknown, Consider MRCP for suspected CBD stones when patient condition allows.

3 What are the underlying causes of this condition?

The commonest causes of acute pancreatitis are CBD gallstones and alcohol (alcohol in this case).
Less common causes include:

- Iatrogenic (e.g. post ERCP).
- Medications (e.g. steroids, azathioprine).
- Autoimmune.
- Hyperlipidaemia.
- Viral (e.g. mumps, Coxsackie B).
- Miscellaneous (e.g. trauma).
- Idiopathic.

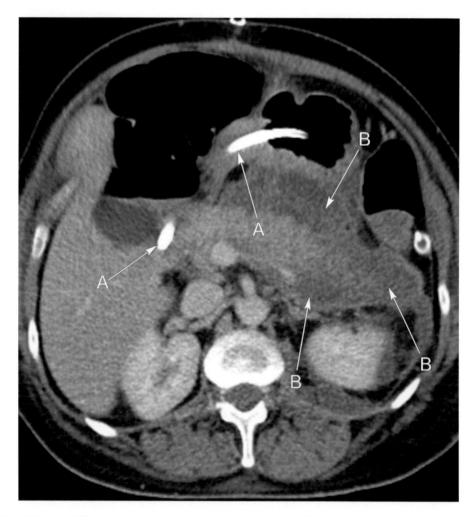

Fig. 7.19D Axial CT abdomen in the same patient 1 week later. A NG tube has been inserted (A). There is now a peripancreatic fluid collection (B). These are common in the early stages of acute pancreatitis but may progress into a pseudocyst. Pseudocysts have a rim of granulation tissue and form approximately 6 weeks after the acute episode. These can be drained via a percutaneous, endoscopic or surgical approach.

4 What are the complications of this condition?

Complications of acute pancreatitis include:

- Pancreatic infection, abscess, and necrosis.
- Peripancreatic fluid collection and late stage pseudocyst formation (**Figure 7.19D**).
- Splenic vein thrombosis.
- Splenic artery pseudoaneurysm.
- Acute respiratory distress syndrome.
- Cullen's sign (periumbilical bruising) and Grey Turner's sign (flank bruising) are both clinical signs indicative of severe pancreatitis and suggest a poor prognosis.

LEARNING POINTS: ACUTE PANCREATITIS

- Epigastric pain radiating to the back and relieved on sitting forwards is the typical presentation of acute pancreatitis.
- The commonest causes are gallstones and alcohol excess.
- CT may show pancreatic oedema, peripancreatic inflammation, and complications, e.g. pancreatic necrosis, collection, and pseudocyst.
- Patients should be treated supportively with fluid resuscitation, analgesia, and prophylactic antibiotics and may benefit from nasojejunal/NG tube.
- Patients may be septic and should be closely monitored in a high dependency environment, and close liaison with specialist regional unit is recommended.

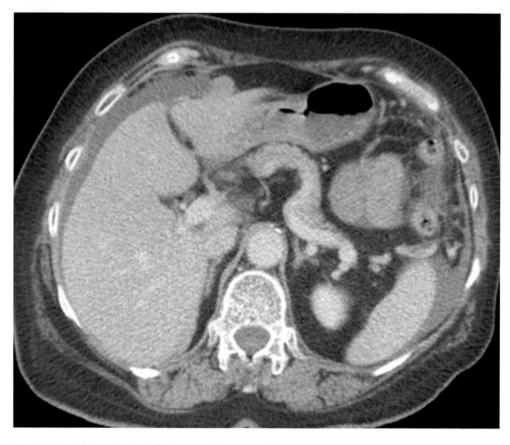

Fig. 7.20A Axial postcontrast CT image of the upper abdomen.

A 63-year-old female presents to her GP with a 6-month history of abdominal distension, nausea, and bloating. Clinical examination and routine blood tests are normal but her serum CA125 is raised, at 1,988 units/mL (0–35 units/mL).

The GP refers the patient to the gynaecology oncology department who arrange a CT scan of the chest, abdomen, and pelvis (**Figures 7.20A, 7.20B,** and **7.20C**). She is subsequently discussed at the MDT meeting.

CASE 7.20: QUESTIONS

1 What abnormalities do these CT images show?
2 What is the differential diagnosis?
3 How is this disease diagnosed and staged?
4 What complications is this patient at risk of?

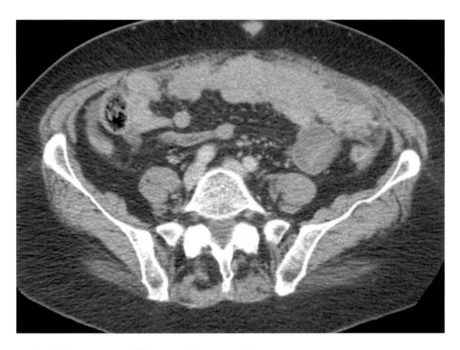

Fig. 7.20B Axial postcontrast CT image of the upper pelvis.

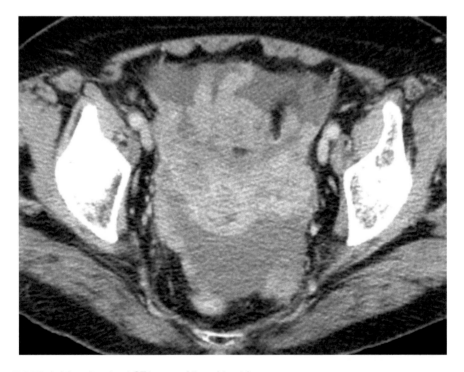

Fig. 7.20C Axial postcontrast CT image of the mid pelvis.

CASE 7.20 ANSWERS

1 What abnormalities do these CT images show?

The CT demonstrates ascites and peritoneal metastases. There is stranding and thickening of the anterior omentum ('omental cake'), with pelvic peritoneal nodular thickening and enhancement, and a pelvic mass (**Figures 7.20D, 7.20E,** and **7.20F**).

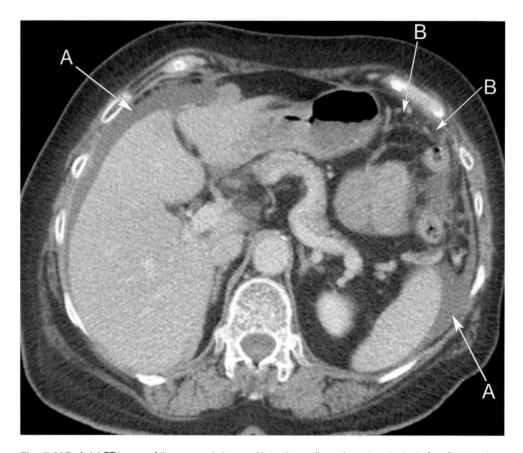

Fig. 7.20D Axial CT image of the upper abdomen. Note: the perihepatic and perisplenic free fluid (ascites) (A), and the ill-defined soft tissue and nodular infiltration in the LUQ (B). This is peritoneal metastatic disease.

2 What is the differential diagnosis?

Metastatic primary ovarian cancer is the most likely diagnosis. The differential diagnoses are:

- Metastases from breast, stomach or colon carcinoma; lobular breast cancer in particular can cause this pattern of disease. Ovarian metastases are also known as Krukenberg tumours and comprise 5–10% of all ovarian tumours; they are signet-ring adenocarcinomas.
- Peritoneal mesothelioma.
- Peritoneal tuberculosis.

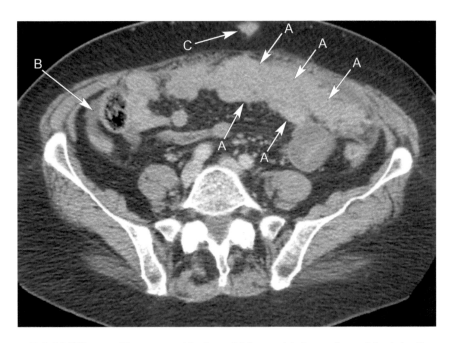

Fig. 7.20E Axial CT image of the upper pelvis shows thick omental disease ('omental cake' – A). In addition there is a trace of free fluid in the right paracolic gutter (B) and a subcutaneous tumour deposit can be seen near the umbilicus (C).

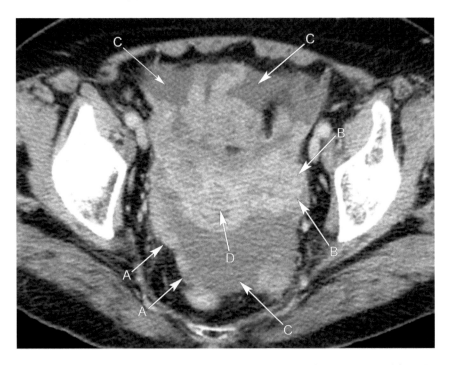

Fig. 7.20F Axial CT image of the mid pelvis shows nodular thickening of the peritoneum (A), a left adnexal mass, and likely ovarian primary malignancy (B) and ascites (C). Normal uterus (D).

Malignant spread in ovarian cancer can occur via:

- Intraperitoneal seeding and direct invasion (most commonly).
- Haematogenous dissemination.
- Lymphatic dissemination (rare).

As a result, if a patient presents with an indeterminate cystic ovarian lesion, biopsy is not recommended because if malignant it can rupture and leak, causing peritoneal seeding and upstaging the tumour.

3 How is this disease diagnosed and staged?

The diagnosis may be acquired as a result of surgical excision of a complex ovarian mass. If disease is more advanced, ascitic tap and cytology or percutaneous biopsy of omental tumour may be used. Currently, depending on the extent of disease at presentation, patients will either undergo early surgical debulking followed by chemotherapy, or primary chemotherapy (for more advanced disease).

If the patient undergoes surgical debulking then biopsy for histological diagnosis and staging is often performed at the time of surgery.

If the patient undergoes primary chemotherapy then histology is acquired via a radiological-guided biopsy procedure (such as US-guided omental biopsy) and the CT scan is relied on for radiological staging.

4 What complications is this patient at risk of?

Complications of peritoneal disease may require treatment for palliation and include:

- Bowel obstruction as a result of serosal surface deposits. Serosal infiltration of the liver and splenic capsules may also be observed.
- Malignant ascites (requiring repeated drainage). This is best done under US guidance as thick omental disease should be avoided during the drain insertion.

LEARNING POINTS: OVARIAN CARCINOMA

- Ovarian carcinoma is often clinically silent and asymptomatic, and patients, therefore, typically present late with more advanced disease.
- In the UK there is currently no screening programme for ovarian cancer. High-risk patients may undergo annual CA125 estimation and pelvic US.
- Imaging features of primary ovarian malignancy include: rapid growth of an observed ovarian lesion, abdominal ascites, and an ovarian mass with complex (part solid, part cystic) appearance with increased vascularity on US/CT of the solid component.

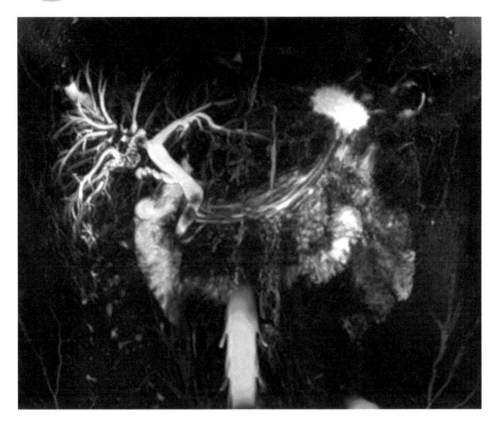

Fig. 7.21A Maximum intensity projection (MIP) coronal T2-weighted image from MRCP of the upper abdomen.

A 42-year-old Caucasian female presents acutely to the ED with a 2-day history of fevers and RUQ pain. Her partner notes that she has developed a yellowish discolouration of the skin. She has a past surgical history of laparoscopic cholecystectomy. Clinical examination reveals a temperature of 39°C, HR 120 bpm, BP 100/80 mmHg, respiratory rate 24 bpm, and oxygen saturation 98% on room air. There is a yellowish discolouration of her sclera and skin. She has severe RUQ pain on superficial and deep palpation that radiates to the right shoulder tip. Her salient abnormal blood results are:

WCC	15 × 10⁹/L (4.0–11.0 × 10⁹/L)	Bilirubin	150 micromol/L (<21 micromol/L)
CRP	180 mg/L (<5 mg/L)	ALP	300 IU/L (35–104 IU/L)

Initial US obtains poor quality views owing to bowel gas but suggests intrahepatic biliary tree dilatation. MRCP is performed (**Figure 7.21A**).

CASE 7.21: QUESTIONS

1 What does the MRCP show?
2 What is the diagnosis?

3 How should the patient be managed?

CASE 7.21: ANSWERS

1 What does the MRCP show?

The intra- and extrahepatic biliary tree is dilated owing to two large obstructing calculi within the distal common bile duct (CBD) (**Figure 7.21B**).

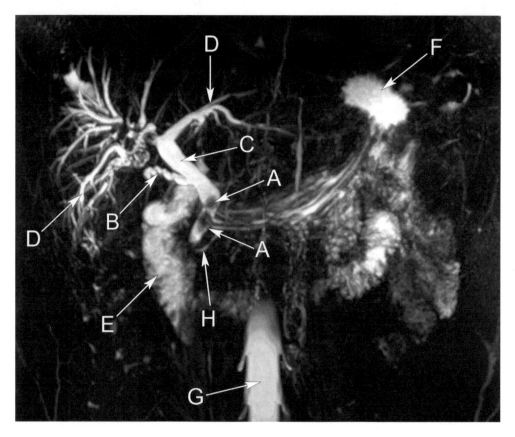

Fig. 7.21B MIP coronal image from an MRCP. These images are highly fluid sensitive so that fluid appears bright/high signal. Obstructing calculi within the dilated CBD are seen as low signal filling defects (A). The cystic duct (B) and CBD (C) are also dilated. Note cholecystectomy. The intrahepatic ducts are dilated (D), normal duodenum (E), stomach (F), cerebrospinal fluid in the spinal canal (G) and normal pancreatic duct (H).

2 What is the diagnosis?

Choledocholithiasis with secondary ascending cholangitis, i.e. stones within the biliary tree, resulting in biliary obstruction and subsequent infection.

3 How should the patient be managed?

Ascending cholangitis is a surgical emergency:

- The patient is septic and should be treated with IV fluids and antibiotics, analgesia, and careful monitoring of fluid balance. ABCDE approach, monitoring, routine investigations to include blood cultures, and senior discussion.
- Urgent ERCP should be performed, the CBD stones retrieved, and the obstruction relieved. A CBD stent may need to be sited if there is a stricture.

LEARNING POINTS: CHOLEDOCHOLITHIASIS

- Choledocholithiasis is the commonest cause of painful obstructive jaundice.
- US abdomen is usually performed in the first instance to look for biliary dilatation; however, MRCP is the most sensitive imaging test and can add detail about the number of stones, level of obstruction, and alternative pathologies (e.g. biliary strictures).
- ERCP is the definitive treatment.
- If the patient is septic this should be managed as an emergency.

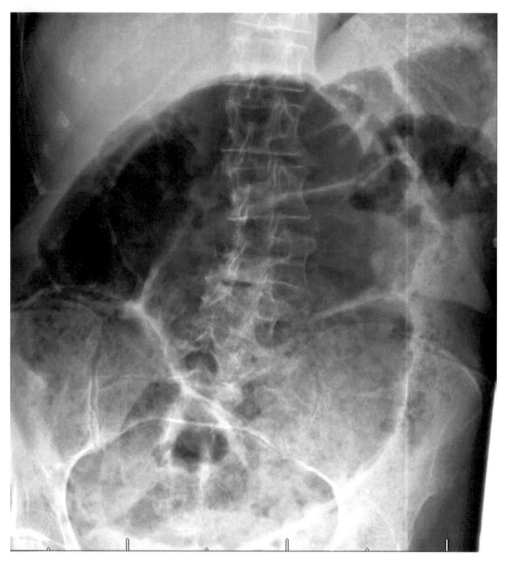

Fig. 7.22A Supine AXR.

A 60-year-old male presents to the ED with a 5-day history of colicky abdominal pain and vomiting. He has been unable to eat or drink for the past 24 hours. He has no relevant past medical history but had a previous laparotomy many years ago for appendicitis with localised perforation. Clinical examination reveals cool peripheries, a prolonged capillary refill time of 4 seconds, tachycardia (HR 120 bpm), and mild hypotension (BP 110/80 mmHg). He is apyrexial. Abdominal examination reveals marked distension, generalised discomfort to palpation, and tinkling bowel sounds on auscultation. Routine bloods reveal a mild leukocytosis and elevated CRP. Supine AXR is performed (**Figure 7.22A**). Erect CXR is unremarkable.

CASE 7.22: QUESTIONS

1 What does the AXR show and what is the diagnosis?
2 What further imaging could be performed?
3 How should the patient be managed?

CASE 7.22: ANSWERS

1 What does the AXR show and what is the diagnosis?

There is a very dilated colonic loop, which arises from the right-sided abdomen (**Figure 7.22B**). The dilated colonic loop displays haustral markings. The large bowel is otherwise nondilated. There is no free intra-abdominal gas. This gas-filled bowel loop is massively dilated, 12–15 cm at least, and also contains haustra, which partially traverse the bowel lumen. This lesion is large bowel at this size and in this position, and the configuration is consistent with a dilated caecum, secondary to caecal volvulus – the 'kidney bean' sign.

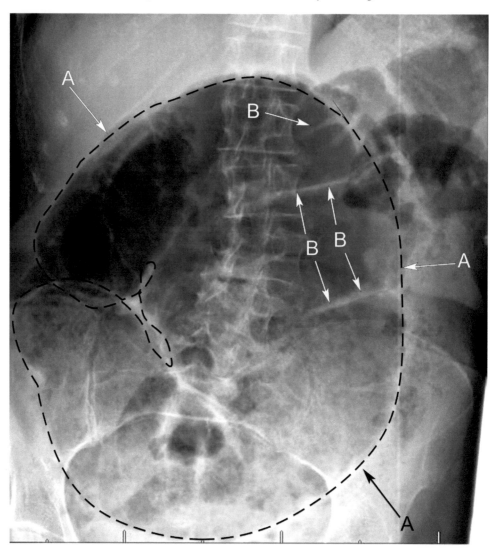

Fig. 7.22B Annotated AXR. Note: massive distension of the caecum (loop outlined: A) and presence of haustrations (B), which do not fully traverse the bowel lumen. A loop this large cannot be small bowel, and is most likely caecum in this position and with this configuration.

2 What further imaging could be performed?

CT abdomen and pelvis could be performed if there is diagnostic doubt or concern regarding complications of caecal volvulus, e.g. bowel ischaemia or perforation (**Figure 7.22C**).

- CT further demonstrates a dilated bowel loop within the right-sided abdomen in the approximate position of the caecum.
- CT may show a change in large bowel calibre and twist of the mesentery at the caecal level.

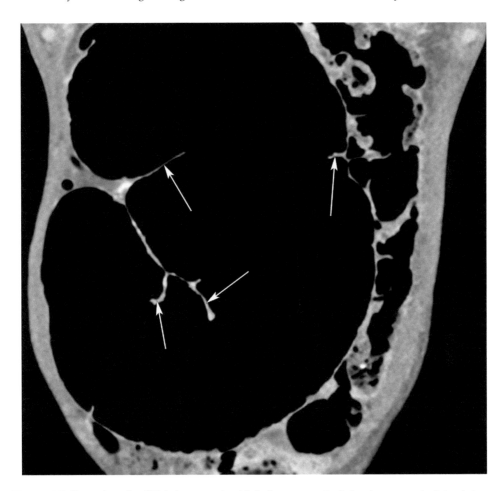

Fig. 7.22C Coronal section CT abdomen and pelvis in the same patient showing a grossly distended bowel loop within the right abdomen in the approximate position of the caecum. Note the massive distension and haustration (arrows).

3 How should the patient be managed?

The patient should be managed supportively with nil by mouth, IV fluids, and NG tube ('drip and suck'). Also:

- Erect CXR to look for perforation (CT is more sensitive).
- General/colorectal surgery referral urgently.

- Surgical options include laparotomy with (usually) right hemicolectomy; in some patients caecopexy (the caecum is fixed to the abdominal wall) or caecostomy (stoma between caecum and abdominal wall) may be considered.
- If the patient is unfit for surgery, colonoscopic decompression may be attempted.

The term volvulus means twisting of the bowel/mesentery on its vascular pedicle.

- Caecal volvulus tends to occur in younger patients than sigmoid volvulus and accounts for 10–20% of cases of large bowel volvulus.
- Patients either have a congenital defect in peritoneal fixation or have an acquired predisposition, e.g. as a result of previous abdominal surgery, or a pelvic mass.
- The caecum may rotate in the transverse plane (dilated loop appears in RLQ) or may twist and invert (dilated loop in LUQ).
- Complications include bowel infarction and perforation.

LEARNING POINTS: THE ILEOCAECAL VALVE

- If competent, this will prevent caecal decompression and these patients will present acutely with closed-loop caecal obstruction and secondary small bowel dilatation: high risk of perforation.
- If valve is incompetent (in elderly), this will allow intermittent caecal decompression and a more subacute presentation.

LEARNING POINTS: CAECAL VOLVULUS

- Caecal volvulus is an uncommon cause of LBO.
- AXR shows a dilated large bowel loop within the right lower abdominal quadrant or sometimes in the LUQ.
- Erect CXR should be performed to look for perforation.
- Patients are usually managed surgically.
- Complications include bowel ischaemia and perforation.

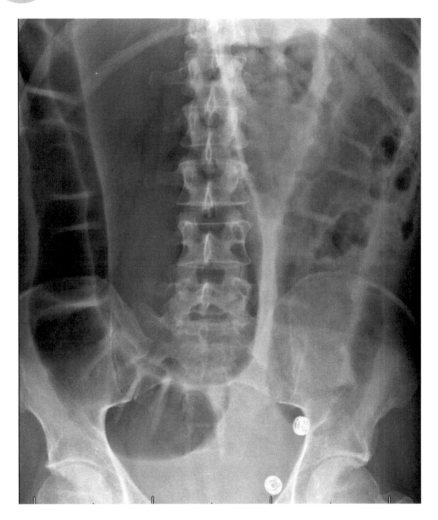

Fig. 7.23A Supine AXR.

A 72-year-old female presents to the ED with a 10-day history of worsening generalised colicky abdominal pain and vomiting. She has not opened her bowels for 4 days and is now unable to pass flatus. She is afebrile, mildly tachycardic (HR 110 bpm), and mildly tachypnoeic (respiratory rate 24 bpm). Her BP is 160/90 mmHg. Clinical examination reveals a grossly distended abdomen, generalised tenderness to abdominal palpation, and tinkling bowel sounds. Blood tests reveal a mild leukocytosis and mildly elevated CRP. Supine AXR is performed (**Figure 7.23A**).

CASE 7.23: QUESTIONS

1 What does the AXR show and what is the diagnosis?
2 What further imaging would you recommend?
3 How should the patient be managed?

CASE 7.23: ANSWERS

1 What does the AXR show and what is the diagnosis?

There is a grossly dilated loop of large bowel arising from the pelvis with an inverted U shape (**Figure 7.23B**).

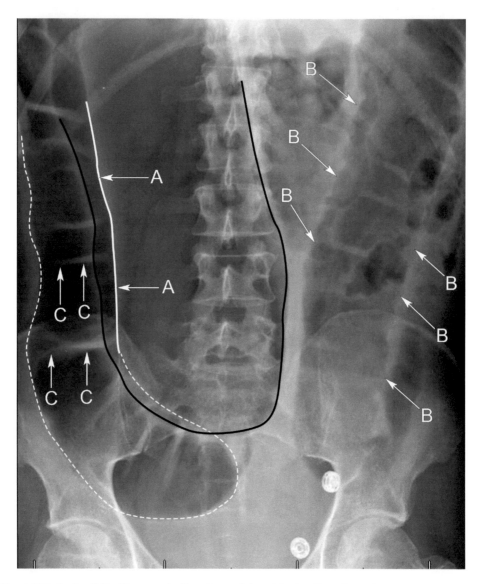

Fig. 7.23B Supine AXR with a grossly dilated loop of sigmoid colon. The afferent (dotted white line) and efferent (solid black line) loops are outlined, converging into the pelvis, with summation overlap line (solid white line, A) evident. The dilated left proximal colon is shown (B). Haustrations can be seen in one of the sigmoid loops. Note: in places, these appear to almost traverse the bowel lumen (C) and are not to be confused with valvulae conniventes. (The two round densities in the lower right part of the XR are buttons on the patient's gown.)

The dilated loop:

- Extends above the level of T10 vertebra. Note: the upper abdomen is not included in the field of view and a repeat film to show the upper abdomen/diaphragm and an erect CXR (perforation) would also be appropriate.
- Has a 'coffee bean' appearance.
- Has visible haustral markings.
- The dilated sigmoid loops converge into the pelvis (convergence sign) and also overlap (summation line).

The more proximal large bowel is also dilated. These are all features of sigmoid volvulus. The term volvulus means twisting of the bowel and mesentery on its vascular pedicle.

2 What further imaging would you recommend?

CT abdomen and pelvis with contrast is performed when there is diagnostic doubt or concern regarding complications of sigmoid volvulus, e.g. bowel ischaemia or perforation:

- CT better demonstrates the degree and level of bowel obstruction and may demonstrate pneumoperitoneum (intraperitoneal free gas).
- At the transition point (where the bowel changes in calibre) the mesenteric vessels and fat have a whorled appearance, the site of volvulus (**Figure 7.23C**).

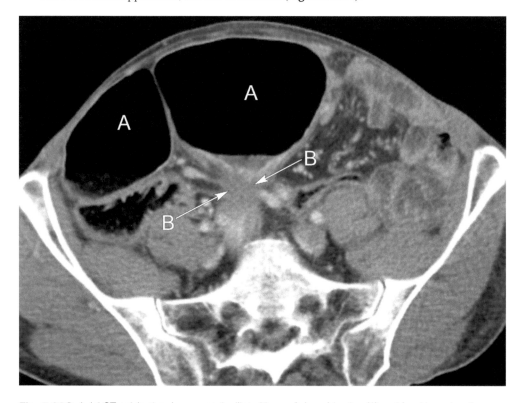

Fig. 7.23C Axial CT pelvis showing a grossly dilated loop of sigmoid colon (A) and focal bowel wall thickening with fat/vessel distortion of the mesentery at the transition point (B) at the site of bowel twist. There is no evidence of perforation on this image.

3 How should the patient be managed?

The patient should be managed supportively with nil by mouth, IV fluids, and NG tube ('drip and suck'):

- Erect CXR should be performed to look for perforation.
- General/colorectal surgery referral urgently.
- Insertion of flatus tube to decompress the large bowel, curative in the short term in 90% of patients, indicated in the absence of perforation/peritonism.
- If flatus tube fails then surgical management, with fixation of the bowel or sigmoid colectomy, may be required.

Sigmoid volvulus:

- Sigmoid volvulus is more common in elderly patients and is caused by redundant mesenteric colonic attachment allowing the bowel to mobilise and twist. It is often recurrent. There is an association with large bowel pathology, sigmoid carcinoma in particular.
- The commonest sites of large bowel volvulus are at the sigmoid colon (80% cases of volvulus) and caecum (20%).
- Complications include bowel infarction and perforation.

> **LEARNING POINTS: SIGMOID VOLVULUS**
>
> - Sigmoid volvulus is the commonest form of large bowel volvulus.
> - AXR shows a grossly dilated large bowel loop arising from the pelvis with inverted U shape.
> - The dilated loop has a coffee bean appearance.
> - Erect CXR should be performed to look for perforation.
> - Patients are managed supportively and with flatus tube, unless there is evidence of necrosis or perforation (when surgery is indicated).
> - Complications include bowel ischaemia and perforation.

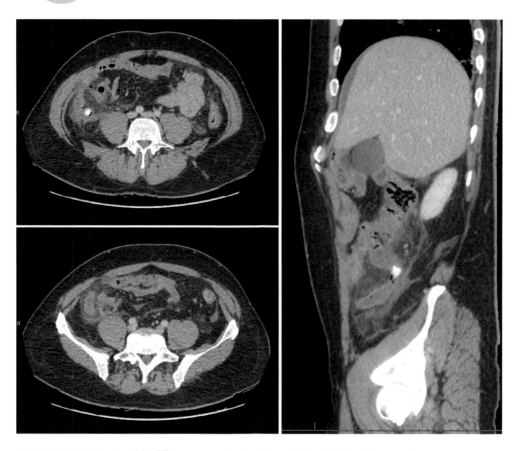

Fig. 7.24A Axial and sagittal CT images postcontrast through the right iliac fossa region.

A 32-year-old male presents to the ED with a 48-hour history of abdominal pain that has localised to the right iliac fossa (RIF). On examination, there is tenderness and guarding in the RIF, tachycardia at 120 bpm, BP is normal, and he is pyrexial at 38.2°C.

A CT scan of the abdomen and pelvis is arranged (**Figure 7.24A**). This comprises a selection of axial and also sagittal CT images through the right iliac fossa.

CASE 7.24: QUESTIONS

1 How would you describe the CT appearances?
2 What is the diagnosis and differential diagnosis?
3 What other imaging modalities may be helpful?
4 How is this condition usually treated?
5 What are the potential complications of this condition?

CASE 7.24: ANSWERS

1 How would you describe the CT appearances?

The CT demonstrates a dilated appendix with a distended lumen and a thickened wall. There is periappendiceal inflammation (with stranding of the surrounding fat). An appendicolith (focus of calcification) is noted at the neck of the appendix and there is a locule of free gas in keeping with localised perforation (**Figure 7.24B**).

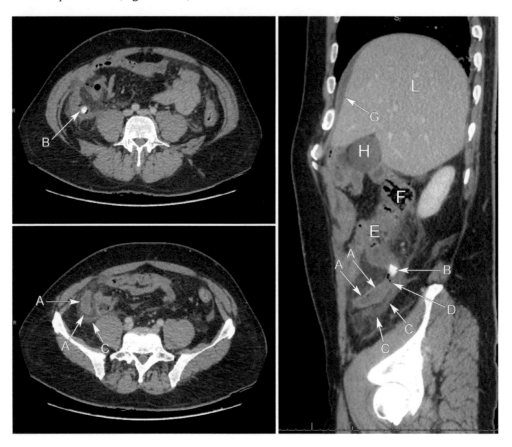

Fig. 7.24B A selection of CT images demonstrating a dilated and thick-walled appendix (A). There is a calcified appendicolith (B) seen at the appendix neck. Note: inflammatory changes/fluid in the surrounding periappendicular fat (C) and bubbles of air secondary to infection (D), caecum (E) and ascending colon (F), free fluid around the liver (G), gallbladder (H), and liver (L).

2 What is the diagnosis and differential diagnosis?

This patient has acute appendicitis. Conditions that may mimic acute appendicitis include:

- Nonspecific mesenteric lymphadenitis.
- Terminal ileitis (due to Crohn's disease or *Yersinia* infection).
- Inflamed Meckel's diverticulum.

In female patients consider:

- Acute salpingitis.
- Ovarian cyst accident.
- Ovarian torsion.

3 What other imaging modalities may be helpful?

AXR is rarely helpful and therefore not routinely performed. Occasionally, however, a calcified appendicolith can be detected in the RIF, if not obscured by overlying bowel gas. This is therefore a review area to check in the acute abdomen (**Figure 7.24C**).

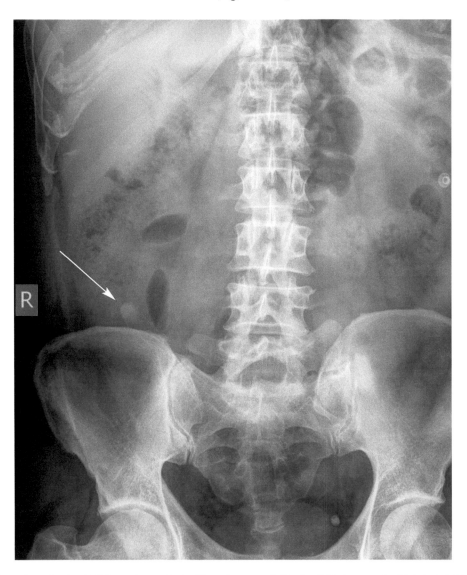

Fig. 7.24C Supine AXR in another patient with acute appendicitis. A calcified appendicolith is just visible (arrow) in the right iliac fossa. This finding is subtle and will be readily obscured by overlying bowel gas.

US is a useful diagnostic test in some cases, as it is effective at identifying appendiceal inflammation, particularly in thin patients. US should be considered the initial diagnostic choice for children and young women as it is nonionizing and is accurate in making the diagnosis of acute appendicitis if the appendix can be visualised. In patients who are very tender, where there is bowel gas or in obese/larger patients, US is less accurate and CT is usually needed. Appendicitis also occurs in elderly patients but many present in a more nonspecific way and CT is usually needed for more general assessment in older adults and the elderly.

4 How is this condition usually treated?

Treatment is with urgent open or laparoscopic appendicectomy.

5 What are the potential complications of this condition?

The potential complications of acute appendicitis include:

- Gangrene and perforation.
- Localised abscess formation.
- Generalised peritonitis.
- Treatment is usually surgical.

LEARNING POINTS: ACUTE APPENDICITIS

- Appendicitis classically presents with periumbilical pain that localises to the RIF with associated fever, nausea, and vomiting. A classical presentation is, however, less common in the elderly.
- US is the investigation of choice in younger patients although CT has a greater sensitivity and specificity, and is increasingly used first line, especially in older patients, to confirm the diagnosis and exclude mimics.
- Complications include perforation and abscess.
- Treatment is usually surgical.

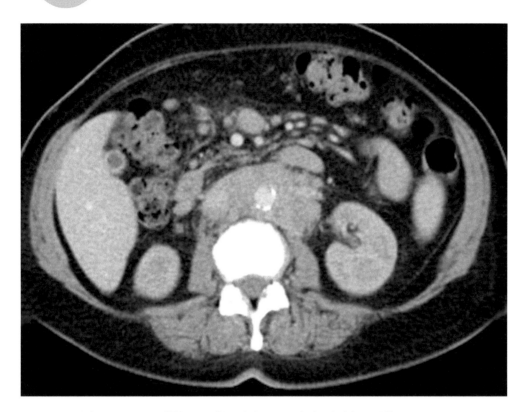

Fig. 7.25A Axial postcontrast CT image of the abdomen at the level of the umbilicus.

A 52-year-old male presents to his GP with nonspecific symptoms of fatigue and malaise. He reports a history of recent unintentional weight loss and night sweats. On examination the GP notes enlarged painless cervical, axillary, and inguinal lymphadenopathy. Observations are normal.

The GP requests routine bloods and finds that the patient is pancytopenic. He refers to haematology for further investigation. A CT scan is performed (**Figure 7.25A**).

CASE 7.25: QUESTIONS

1 What does the CT show?
2 What are the causes of generalised lymphadenopathy?
3 How could the diagnosis be made?
4 What are the other causes for the CT abnormality?

CASE 7.25: ANSWERS

1 What does the CT show?

The CT demonstrates a soft tissue retroperitoneal mass that is encasing the aorta. These appearances are typical for lymphadenopathy as a result of non-Hodgkin lymphoma (NHL) (**Figure 7.25B**).

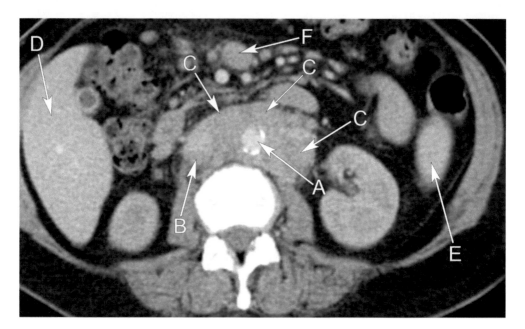

Fig. 7.25B Axial CT image demonstrating the calcified aorta (A) and inferior vena cava (B) surrounded by a soft tissue density nodal mass (C). Nodal disease in lymphoma typically encases but does not invade the vessels. Note the liver (D), spleen tip (not enlarged, E), and a pathological mesenteric node (F).

2 What are the causes of generalised lymphadenopathy?

Causes of generalised lymphadenopathy include:

- Lymphoma.
- Leukaemia (chronic lymphatic leukaemia, acute lymphoblastic leukaemia).
- Glandular fever.
- Acquired immune deficiency syndrome (AIDS).
- Chronic infection (such as TB).
- Connective tissue disorders (systemic lupus erythematosus, sarcoid).

3 How could the diagnosis be made?

As the patient also has palpable cervical, axillary, and inguinal lymphadenopathy, an US-guided core biopsy of an enlarged peripheral node is likely to give the diagnosis. Bone marrow aspiration and trephine biopsy will confirm bone marrow involvement if required. CT-guided para-aortic node biopsy would be feasible but is more invasive.

4 What are the other causes for the CT abnormality?

Causes of a retroperitoneal mass are listed in *Table 7.25*.

Table 7.25 Causes of a retroperitoneal mass

Nodal disease	Primary retroperitoneal tumour
Neoplastic	
Testicular tumour	Liposarcoma
Renal cell carcinoma	Leiomyosarcoma
Lymphoma	Rhabdomyosarcoma
Post-transplant lymphoproliferative disease	
Non-neoplastic	
Retroperitoneal fibrosis	
Extramedullary haematopoiesis	
Lipoma	
Peripheral nerve sheath tumour (neurofibroma)	
Psoas abscess	
Haematoma (aneurysm leak, warfarin complication, trauma)	

NHL also typically presents with both mediastinal and abdominal para-aortic lymphadenopathy (see **Figures 7.25C** and **7.25D**).

> **LEARNING POINTS: RETROPERITONEAL MASS**
>
> - A thorough clinical examination is essential in a patient presenting with lymphadenopathy and will expedite the diagnosis.
> - Encasement of the aorta on CT is typical for lymphadenopathy as a result of lymphoma.
> - In a male patient with retroperitoneal nodes, ensure the testicles are examined clinically. US of the testes and testicular tumour markers may also be helpful.

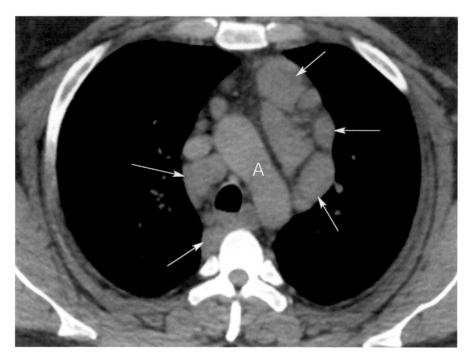

Fig. 7.25C Axial postcontrast CT image in another patient with NHL at the level of the aortic arch (A). Note the widespread enlarged mediastinal lymph nodes (arrows).

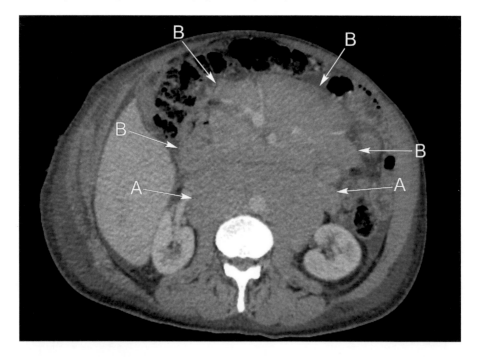

Fig. 7.25D Axial postcontrast CT image in the same patient as in Figure 7.25C at the level of the kidneys. This demonstrates massive para-aortic (A) and mesenteric (B) lymphadenopathy.

Case 7.26

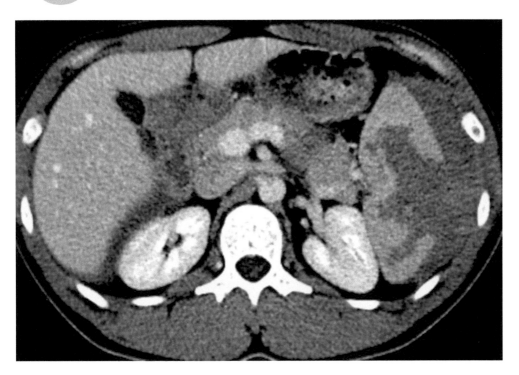

Fig. 7.26A Axial postcontrast CT image of the upper abdomen.

A 25-year-old male is brought to the ED by ambulance following a RTA in which he was knocked off his bicycle. He has a GCS of 13; however, witnesses report loss of consciousness at the scene. He complains of severe left-sided chest and abdominal pain. He is visibly short of breath. On examination his HR is 110 bpm, respiratory rate 32 bpm, and BP 100/80 mmHg. Respiration is asymmetrical, there is hyper-resonance to percussion over the left chest wall, and left-sided breath sounds are reduced. There is LUQ bruising and guarding to palpation, and bowel sounds are quiet. He has no spinal tenderness but his cervical spine is immobilised.

A portable CXR shows a moderate left-sided pneumothorax, not under tension, which was treated initially with pleural aspiration with view to insertion of a chest drain. He then proceeded to CT of the head, spine, chest, abdomen, and pelvis. An image of the upper abdomen is included (**Figure 7.26A**).

CASE 7.26: QUESTIONS

1. What does the CT abdomen show?
2. What is the diagnosis?
3. How should the patient be managed?

CASE 7.26: ANSWERS

1 What does the CT abdomen show?

There is rupture of the spleen with a large intraparenchymal and subcapsular haematoma. Low density within the pancreatic tail suggests a further site of damage with haematoma and laceration. There is also haemoperitoneum with blood in the hepatorenal space (**Figure 7.26B**).

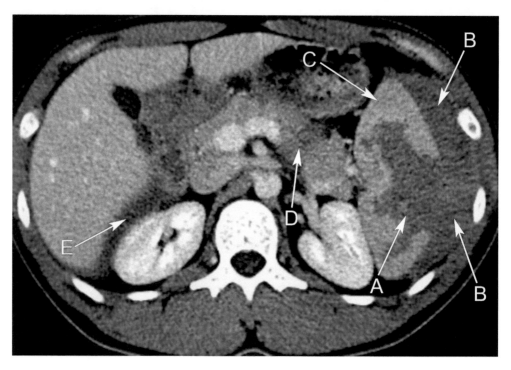

Fig. 7.26B Axial portal venous (mildly delayed imaging post injection of contrast) enhanced CT image of the upper abdomen. There is splenic rupture with large intraparenchymal (A) and subcapsular (B) haematoma. Normal splenic enhancement (C), pancreatic tail haematoma (D), and blood in the hepatorenal space (E) (Morrison's pouch). Visualised kidneys and liver appear normal.

2 What is the diagnosis?

Major thoracoabdominal trauma with splenic rupture and pancreatic haematoma with possible laceration:

- Initial arterial phase contrast imaging showed multiple high-density foci within the spleen indicative of contrast extravasation owing to active arterial bleeding (**Figure 7.26C**).
- While this is a serious injury, the splenic hilar vessels remain intact with splenic perfusion apparent, which is an important radiological finding. There is a grading system for splenic trauma (American Association for the Surgery of Trauma – AAST) ranging from grade 1 (subcapsular haematoma <10%, capsular laceration <1 cm) through to grade 5 (spleen shattered, splenic hilar vessel damage). This patient has a grade 3

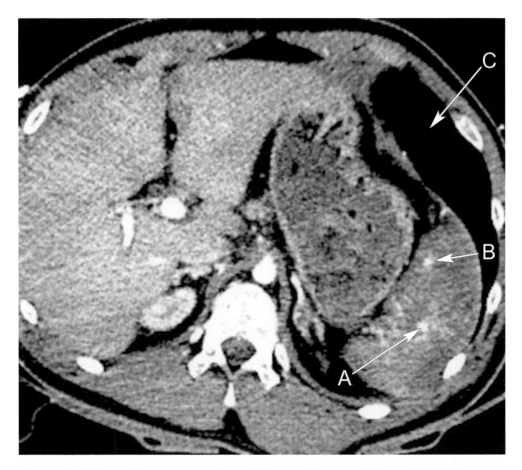

Fig. 7.26C Axial arterial phase contrast enhanced CT image of the upper abdomen. High-density contrast blushes (A and B) indicate sites of active haemorrhage. The residual left lung base pneumothorax is also seen (C).

injury (large intraparenchymal and subcapsular haematomas but no evidence of major devascularisation). Further treatment (conservative versus embolisation versus surgery) is based on the haemodynamic and clinical condition of the patient in combination with imaging findings.

3 How should the patient be managed?

The patient should be managed initially via an ABCDE approach with early involvement of the entire trauma team. Remember the patient must be haemodynamically stable and safely self-ventilating or intubated prior to CT transfer:

- Management of his breathing involves decompressing (draining) the pneumothorax. Management of circulation involved aggressive fluid resuscitation, ABG, full routine bloods, and group and save. Early transfusion with group O-negative blood may be required.

- The patient should be urgently referred to the on-call surgical/interventional radiology team. Injury severity is graded according to extent/depth of the laceration/haematoma, and disruption of the vascular pedicle denotes a severe injury. Severe splenic injuries with active haemorrhage may require urgent embolisation or surgery. Less severe injuries, however, are managed conservatively owing to the important immunological function of the spleen.

> **LEARNING POINTS: MAJOR ABDOMINAL TRAUMA, SPLENIC INJURY**
>
> - Trauma patients should be managed via an ABCDE approach, i.e. pneumothorax before circulatory shock.
> - CT imaging should be undertaken as soon as the patient is stabilised if immediate surgery is not warranted.
> - Splenic injury is seen in up to 45% of patients with blunt abdominal trauma and necessitates urgent surgical referral.

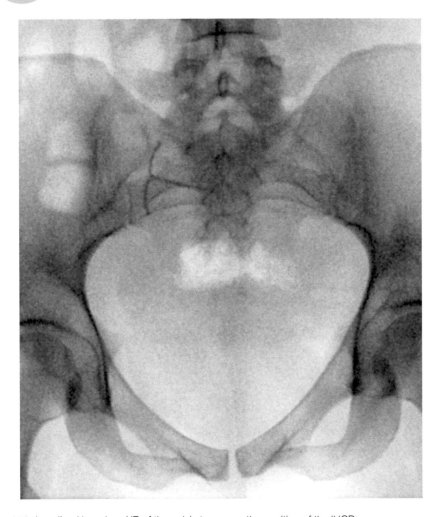

Fig. 7.27A Localised low-dose XR of the pelvis to assess the position of the IUCD.

A 37-year-old female has a Mirena IUCD *in situ* but cannot feel the threads. She is asymptomatic with no lower abdominal pain. She does not recall the device being expelled vaginally.

She undergoes transvaginal US having been referred by her GP to confirm the coil has not migrated but the US does not demonstrate an IUCD in the endometrial cavity.

As the device is metal, she undergoes low-dose localised XR of the pelvis to assess its position (**Figure 7.27A**).

CASE 7.27: QUESTIONS

1 Can you see the device? What has happened?
2 What other causes of 'lost threads' are there?
3 What advice should you give this patient?

CASE 7.27: ANSWERS

1 Can you see the device and what has happened?

The IUCD is projected over the right sacral ala (**Figure 7.27B**). The device has perforated through the myometrium and migrated outside of the uterus. This has been clinically 'silent' but patients may present with nonspecific lower abdominal pain and, rarely, peritoneal sepsis.

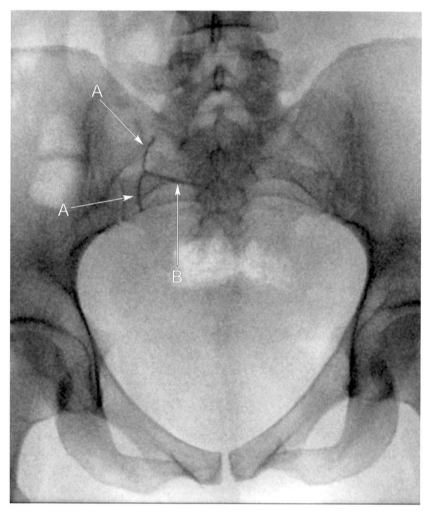

Fig. 7.27B The displaced coil is projected over the right sacral ala. Note the 'T'-shaped configuration of the device (A) with the stem labelled (B).

2 What other causes of 'lost threads' are there?

The threads may be coiled in the cervix or they may have been cut too short. Often threads are lost after a medical procedure such as a colposcopy

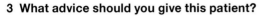

3 What advice should you give this patient?

The patient requires referral to gynaecology for consideration of laparoscopic removal of the device. She should be advised that in the interim she should use alternative methods of contraception.

LEARNING POINTS: MISPLACED INTRAUTERINE CONTRACEPTIVE DEVICE

- US is the preferred modality for demonstrating an IUCD.
- If it cannot be visualised, a pelvic XR is performed initially, and if this is unhelpful full AXR or sometimes CT may be needed.
- An IUCD lying lateral to the midline suggests that it is displaced.

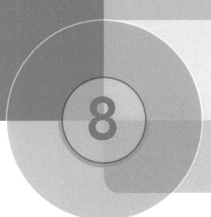

Musculoskeletal cases

EDWARD SELLON AND
ANDREW SNODDON

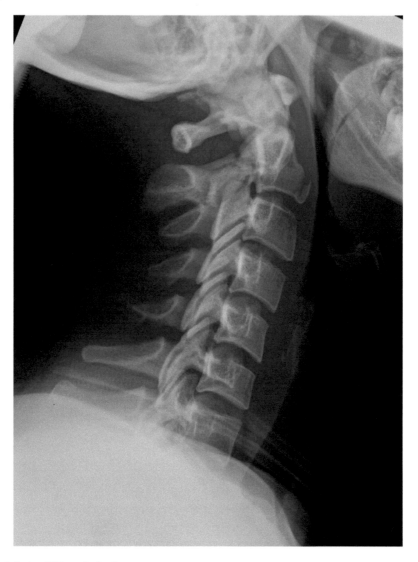

Fig. 8.1A Lateral XR cervical spine.

A 35-year-old male is brought by ambulance to the regional trauma centre following a fall down a flight of stairs. The patient reports pain throughout his cervical spine.

On examination the patient has bony tenderness over the upper cervical spine. Neurological examination is normal. The neck is immobilised in a collar to enable safe transfer to the radiology department. An XR of the cervical spine is arranged (**Figure 8.1A**).

CASE 8.1: QUESTIONS

1 What features are seen on the XR?
2 What is your technique for interpreting a cervical spine XR?
3 What further imaging could be performed?
4 How would you manage a suspected cervical spine fracture?

CASE 8.1: ANSWERS

1 What features are seen on the XR?

There are multiple fractures of the C2 vertebra (**Figure 8.1B**). These include a displaced fracture of the anterior inferior corner of the vertebral body and bilateral fractures of the pedicles/pars interarticularis. This is a so-called 'Hangman's' fracture (a hyperextension injury) with bilateral pedicular fractures of C2, an unstable and potentially lethal injury. Immobilisation of the cervical spine and urgent discussion with seniors is required.

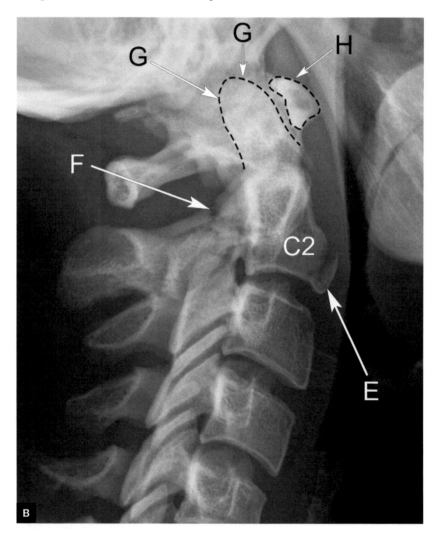

Figs. 8.1B, C Lateral XR of the cervical spine (**8.1B**) with C2 fractures involving the anterior inferior corner of the body (E) and through the pedicles (F). Note the normal alignment lines (see lines A–D, **8.1C**), normal odontoid peg (G), and anterior arch atlas (H). Alignment lines are nondisrupted in this patient and only minor soft tissue swelling is also present. C2 and C7 vertebrae are labelled. Note the C7/T1 junction is not visualised clearly and also how difficult this serious fracture is to diagnose on XR, with minimal soft tissue swelling and no malalignment.

2 What is your technique for interpreting a cervical spine XR?

Evaluation of the cervical spine XR in trauma involves searching for malalignment, cortical fracture, and soft tissue swelling.

- The standard radiographic views are the lateral, AP, and peg views. Remember to review all of these. You are very unlikely to be asked to report a cervical spine XR in an exam at finals but you do need to understand the principles. You would always ask for senior help and would not 'clear' a spine XR on your own (you should not do this as a FY1/FY2 either!).
- Check for adequate spinal coverage. You must be able to see from the craniocervical junction down to T1 on the lateral view for the XR to be adequate. In this case C7 is labelled but not well seen. C7/T1 is where most fracture/dislocations occur and must be clearly visualised on XR to ensure normal alignment.
- Check for vertebral alignment on the lateral view (**Figure 8.1C**). Review the anterior vertebral line (A – the line of the anterior longitudinal ligament), the posterior vertebral line (B – the line of the posterior vertebral ligament), and the spinolaminar line (the line formed by the anterior margin of the spinous processes – C) plus line D (tips of spinous processes). These lines should be continuous, without any steps.

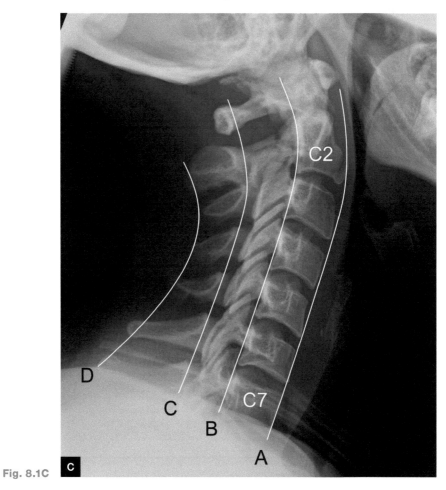

Fig. 8.1C

- Check the outline of each bone for fractures.
- Check the disc spaces. These should be approximately equal in height.
- Check the prevertebral soft tissues for haematoma and swelling:
  - In adults, above C4, the prevertebral soft tissues should measure less than one-third of the width of the vertebral body. Below C4 these should measure less than the width of the vertebral body.
- There are many patterns of cervical spine fracture and these are usually classified according to the mechanism of injury (i.e. excess flexion, extension, or rotation).

3 What further imaging could be performed?

CT is the best first-line investigation for the cervical spine in the context of trauma, particularly in the elderly or following high energy trauma. CT can be followed by MRI if there is neural compromise. The cervical spine should first be immobilised and then senior help sought to assist with the patient transfer onto the scanner.

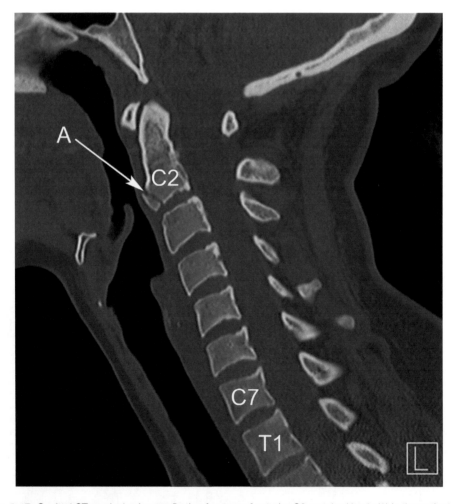

Fig. 8.1D Sagittal CT cervical spine confirming fracture of anterior C2 vertebral body (A) in the patient from **Figure 8.1B**. C2 and C7/T1 normal alignment are labelled.

- CT may be required following XR if:
  - The XR is inadequate (not showing the top of T1).
  - The XR shows an abnormality that requires further evaluation.
  - The XR is normal despite strong clinical suspicion of fracture.
- CT should be used as the first-line investigation instead of XR if:
  - There is abnormal neurology, (prior to arranging an MRI).
  - There is a high energy mechanism of injury.
  - The patient is elderly (>65 years).
  - The patient has a head injury requiring a CT brain and also has a suspected cervical spine injury.
  - The patient is being scanned for multi-region trauma (polytrauma).
- CT provides excellent spatial resolution and bone detail. It can also help to further evaluate the soft tissues (**Figures 8.1D** and **8.1E**).
- MRI provides excellent soft tissue contrast resolution, providing a detailed assessment of the ligamentous structures in the neck and also the spinal cord.

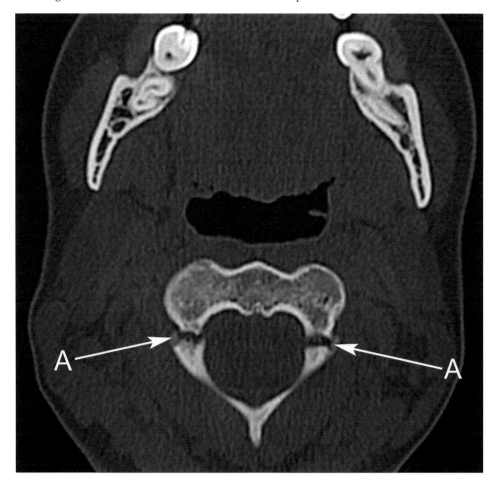

Fig. 8.1E Axial CT cervical spine (same patient as in Figure 8.1D) confirming bilateral pars interarticularis/pedicle fracture of C2 (A).

4 How would you manage a suspected cervical spine fracture?

Management may be conservative or surgical depending on type/stability of fracture and condition of the patient.

- Conservative management may be chosen for stable cervical spine fractures, and may take the form of a collar or brace.
- Surgical management may be used in patients with neurological injuries or unstable cervical spine fractures, to stabilise the cervical spine and improve alignment before bone healing will occur.

LEARNING POINTS: CERVICAL SPINE FRACTURE

- Ensure that the spine has been adequately immobilised before you request imaging.
- Always seek senior advice early and do not feel pressurised to 'clear' cervical spine XRs as a foundation doctor.
- Make sure that the XR is adequate and that you have seen all the required views before making comment.
- Avoid 'satisfaction of search'. Once you have seen one abnormality, carry on looking for others!
- If there is high clinical suspicion of fracture, CT should be performed regardless of XR findings.

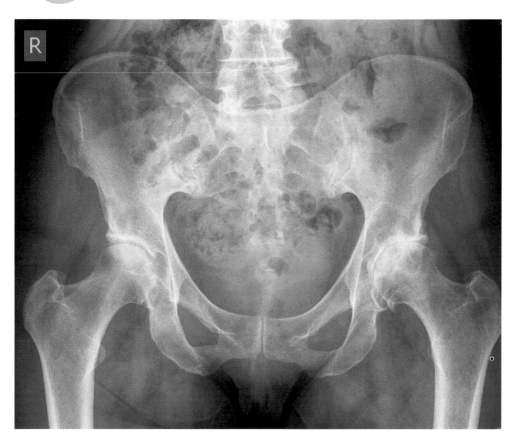

Fig. 8.2A XR of the pelvis.

A 72-year-old female presents to the orthopaedic outpatient clinic with a 12-month history of progressive left hip pain and stiffness. She notes her symptoms are worse after exercise. No significant discomfort is present in her right hip.

On examination there is a reduced range of movement and crepitus in the left hip joint. A normal range of movement is demonstrated in the right hip.

An XR of the pelvis is obtained (**Figure 8.2A**).

CASE 8.2: QUESTIONS

1 What are the XR findings?
2 What is the diagnosis?
3 What is the difference between primary and secondary forms of this condition?
4 How should this patient be managed?

CASE 8.2: ANSWERS

1 What are the XR findings?

XR of the pelvis shows the following changes around the left hip joint (**Figure 8.2B**):

- **L**oss of joint space.
- **O**steophyte formation.
- **S**ubchondral cyst formation.
- **S**ubchondral sclerosis.

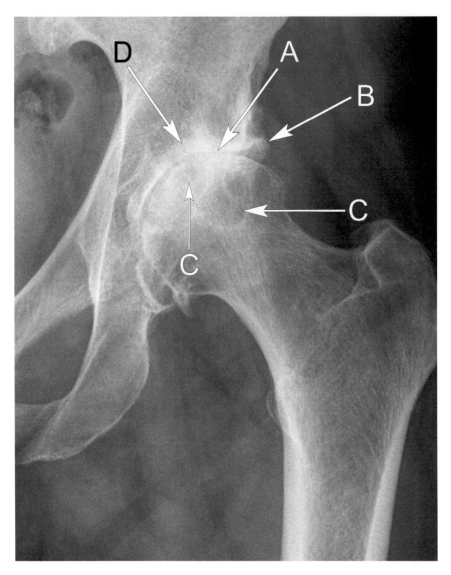

Fig. 8.2B XR left hip. Loss of joint space (A), marginal osteophyte (B), subchondral cyst formation (C), and subchondral sclerosis (D).

2 What is the diagnosis?

Severe osteoarthritis (OA) of the left hip joint:

- The classic XR features are listed above and form the mnemonic 'LOSS'.
- Classification is usually subjective using mild, moderate or severe. During clinical placements take the opportunity to review XRs that demonstrate the full spectrum of disease.
- OA is usually bilateral and commonly affects the large weight-bearing joints. Always remember to review the contralateral side.
- The Kellgren-Lawrence scoring tool (*Table 8.2*) is useful to know about but need not be learnt for the exam.

Table 8.2 Kellgren-Lawrence scoring tool

Grade 1	Minor joint space narrowing and osteophyte formation
Grade 2	Definite osteophyte formation and possible joint space narrowing
Grade 3	Multiple osteophytes, definite joint space narrowing, sclerosis, and possible bony deformity
Grade 4	Large osteophytes, marked joint space narrowing, severe sclerosis, and definite bony deformity

3 What is the difference between primary and secondary forms of this condition?

Primary (idiopathic) OA mainly affects the hips, knees, and hands (base of thumb and distal interphalangeal joints). The aetiology is unknown; however, it is more common in women and a hereditary link has been proposed.

Secondary OA occurs as a result of previous joint damage, for example cartilage injury, fracture, neuropathy (such as diabetic neuropathy leading to Charcot joint), and congenital or acquired deformity.

4 How should this patient be managed?

It is important to note that XR findings do not necessarily correlate with clinical findings. Management should, therefore, be tailored to the level of pain and disability. Management options are physical, medical, and surgical:

- Physiotherapy to improve strength and mobility.
- Medical therapy includes analgesia and anti-inflammatory medication. Intra-articular injections are sometimes used.
- Surgical management options include joint replacement once conservative measures have failed (**Figure 8.2C**, overleaf).

LEARNING POINTS: OSTEOARTHRITIS

- The classical features of OA are loss of joint space, osteophyte formation, subchondral cyst formation, and sclerosis ('LOSS').
- Common joints affected include weight-bearing joints, such as the hip and knee, and small joints of the hand, e.g. 1st carpometacarpal and distal interphalangeal joints.
- Remember to comment on both hips if presented with an XR of the pelvis.
- Symptoms may not correlate well with XR findings. Management options include physical, medical, and surgical approaches.

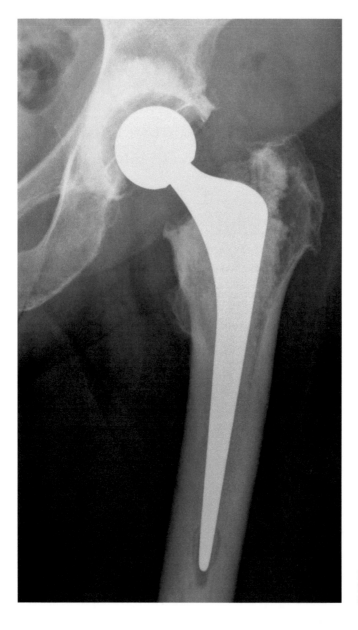

Fig. 8.2C Cemented total hip replacement in the same patient as in **Figure 8.2A**.

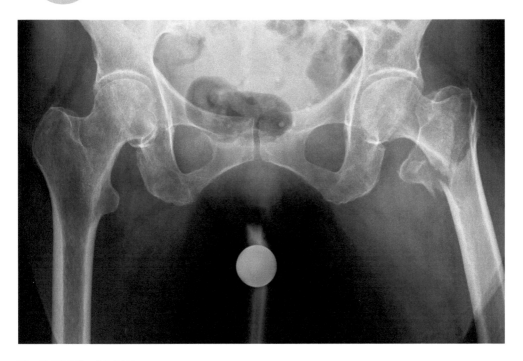

Fig. 8.3A XR pelvis/hips.

A 70-year-old female presents to the ED with an acute episode of pain in her left groin, radiating to the thigh following a fall down four steps. She has a history of hypertension but is otherwise fit and well.

On examination there is tenderness over the left hip, with a very limited range of movement. The left leg appears shortened and externally rotated. She is not able to weight bear. An XR of the pelvis and left hip is arranged (**Figure 8.3A**).

CASE 8.3: QUESTIONS

1 What is the XR diagnosis?
2 How can this condition be classified?
3 How should this patient be managed?
4 What important complications should be considered?

CASE 8.3: ANSWERS

1 What is the XR diagnosis?

There is a displaced extracapsular, intertrochanteric fracture of the left neck of femur, with impaction and shortening (**Figure 8.3B**). Ideally, as with all suspected fractures, the joint should be demonstrated in two orthogonal planes (AP and lateral), although lateral views may be technically difficult owing to pain.

2. How can this condition be classified?

Neck of femur fractures are classified according to their anatomical position along the neck but are also broadly split into intracapsular and extracapsular fractures as this affects management (**Figure 8.3B** shows line of capsule insertion).

- The distinction between intracapsular and extracapsular femoral neck fractures is important because of the impact on blood supply to the femoral head and the risk of subsequent femoral head avascular necrosis (AVN). Blood supply to the femoral head is from retinacular vessels, which pass along the femoral neck, receiving blood supply from the circumflex femoral arteries – some arterial supply is also via the ligamentum teres. These vessels are all at risk

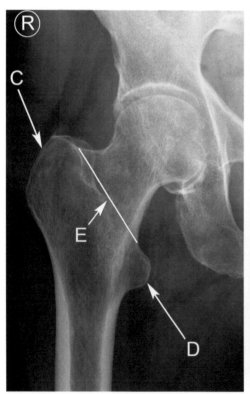
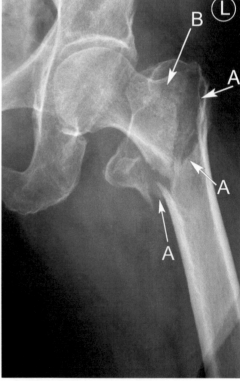

Fig. 8.3B Cropped XRs of the left hip (right image) and normal right hip (left image). There is an extracapsular, intertrochanteric fracture of the left neck of the femur (A) with impaction, angulation, and shortening (B). Normal right hip: greater trochanter (C), lesser trochanter (D), intertrochanteric line (E, site of hip capsular insertion).

from intracapsular fractures. Displaced intracapsular neck fractures require replacement of the femoral head with hemiarthroplasty, whereas extracapsular and nondisplaced intracapsular fractures can usually be safely managed with a dynamic hip screw (DHS).

- Garden classification of intracapsular fractures:
  - *Type I:* Incomplete, undisplaced.
  - *Type II:* Complete, undisplaced.
  - *Type III:* Complete, incompletely displaced.
  - *Type IV:* Complete, completely displaced.
- Remember the rhyme '*1, 2 Dynamic Hip Screw; 3 and 4 Austin Moore*' (the Austin Moore is an uncemented hemiarthroplasty).

3 How should this patient be managed?

In this patient the extracapsular fracture can be managed with open reduction and internal fixation using a DHS (**Figure 8.3C**). If there is evidence of osteoporosis this should also be treated medically.

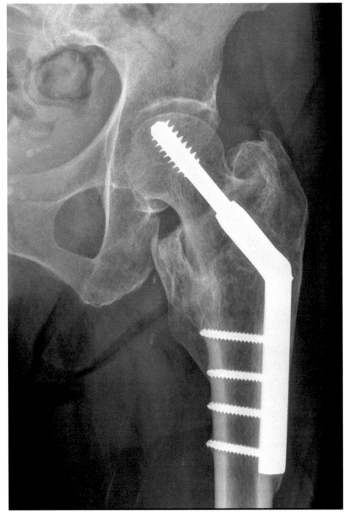

Fig. 8.3C XR left hip with DHS and satisfactory alignment, and remodelling across the fracture site.

- It is particularly important not to overlook an undisplaced intracapsular fracture, as if these are missed they will extend and displace, requiring hemiarthroplasty. If caught early, (Garden type 1 or 2), screw and plate fixation will suffice (**Figure 8.3D**).
- If the XR appears normal but there is continued clinical suspicion (i.e. the patient is still unable to weight bear), then cross-sectional imaging is recommended. CT may be sufficient but MRI is the reference standard investigation.

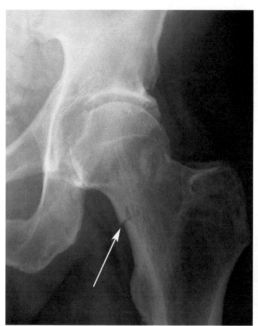 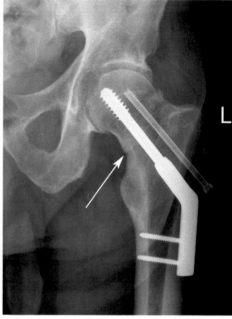

Fig. 8.3D XR left hip with a transcervical, intracapsular fracture, before (left) and after surgical fixation with a DHS (right). This fracture is subtle. Note the medial cortical breach (arrow).

4 What important complications should be considered?

Mortality risk increases after a hip fracture and there is evidence that this correlates with the length of hospital stay. Long periods of immobility may predispose to venous thromboembolism or pressure sores. Surgical complications include fracture, nonunion or malunion, avascular necrosis, fat embolus, and infection of the prosthesis metalwork.

LEARNING POINTS: HIP FRACTURES

- XRs of the pelvis and affected hip are usually sufficient to make the diagnosis.
- CT or MRI are useful in the context of a normal XR but high clinical suspicion.
- '1, 2 Dynamic Hip Screw; 3 and 4 Austin Moore' guides the management of intracapsular fractures.
- Mortality risk increases following a hip fracture; therefore, careful medical as well as surgical management is required.
- Prevention is important: home assessments to reduce risk of fall, hip pads, and osteoporosis screening and treatment in those at risk.

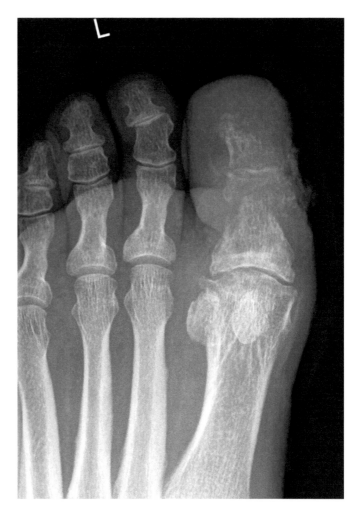

Fig. 8.4A AP XR of left big toe.

A 72-year-old tablet-controlled diabetic male presents to the ED with a 3-week history of pain over his left big toe, increasing in severity over the last 2 days. He is feverish and struggling to weight bear. He lives alone and has had problems with diabetic control.

On examination there is an ulcer adjacent to the medial aspect of the distal interphalangeal joint of his left big toe, with surrounding soft tissue swelling, erythema, and tenderness. He is pyrexial at 39.1°C and inflammatory markers are elevated, with blood tests showing:

WCC 15.6 × 10⁹/L (4–11 × 10⁹/L)   Neutrophils 12.5 × 10⁹/L (2–7.5 × 10⁹/L)   CRP 154 mg/L (<5 mg/L)

An XR of the big toe is arranged (**Figure 8.4.A**).

CASE 8.4: QUESTIONS

1 What features are seen on the XR?
2 What is the diagnosis?

3 What further investigations may be helpful?
4 How should this patient be managed?

CASE 8.4: ANSWERS

1 What features are seen on the XR?

The left big toe XR demonstrates multiple sites of bone destruction at the hallux involving the distal (A) and proximal (B) phalanges (**Figure 8.4B**).

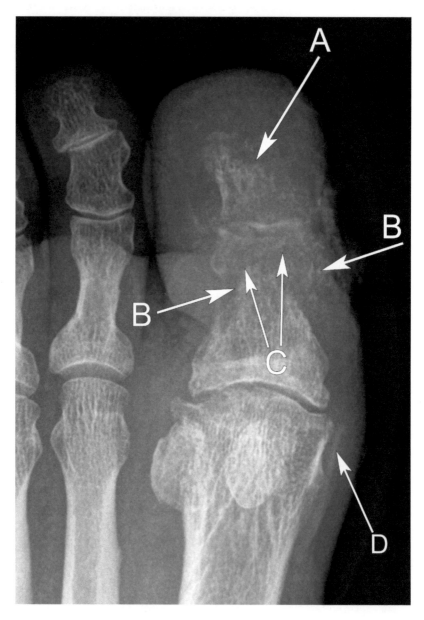

Fig. 8.4B XR left hallux (big toe) demonstrating bony destruction of the distal (A) and proximal (B) phalanx of the left hallux. There is a pathological fracture of the distal proximal phalanx (C). Note: marked overlying soft tissue swelling and also vascular calcification (D).

2 What is the diagnosis?

The history and XR appearances are typical of osteomyelitis, in this case secondary to underlying diabetes mellitus.

- Osteomyelitis or bone infection can occur secondary to haematogenous or direct spread of infection. In diabetes it is often secondary to direct spread from a pressure ulcer.
- The most common causative organism is *Staphylococcus aureus*.
- *Salmonella* infection is associated with sickle cell anaemia patients.
- In the early stages of osteomyelitis the XR may be normal. Soft tissue swelling and obliteration of fat planes are early signs. Bone destruction is a late feature (**Figure 8.4C**).
- Management involves IV antibiotics, debridement of large abscesses, and surgery for progressive disease.

Also look carefully for evidence of gas in the soft tissues, which may be secondary to gas-forming organisms, and vascular calcification is common in diabetics (**Figure 8.4B**).

3 What further investigations may be helpful?

In addition to inflammatory markers, blood cultures and wound swabs can help to isolate an organism. A bone biopsy may be necessary in some cases. MRI is also useful to further delineate the extent of bone and soft tissue involvement (**Figure 8.4D**). The loss of high fat signal intensity in the bone marrow on T1 imaging is highly specific for infection.

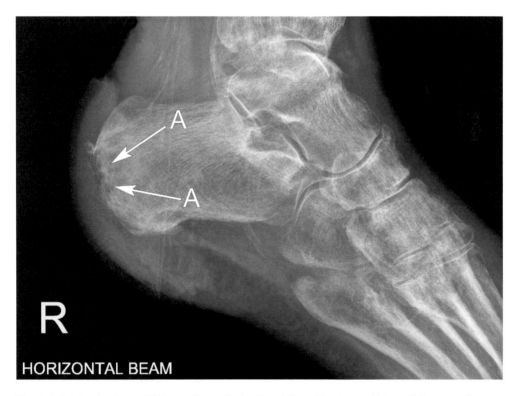

Fig. 8.4C Lateral calcaneal XR in another patient with an infected heel ulcer. Note: soft tissue swelling and calcaneal cortical destruction (A).

Local complications of infection include:

- Adjacent abscess in soft tissue.
- Sinus or fistula.
- Pathological fracture.
- Extension into an adjacent joint, leading to septic arthritis.
- Deformity or subsequent growth disturbance.
- Progression to chronic osteomyelitis.
- Systemic infection, e.g. septicaemia.

4 How should this patient be managed?

The patient will need a combination of surgical debridement of the ulcer and IV antibiotics guided by the causative organism. Longer term, he will need help with diabetic control and a podiatric assessment.

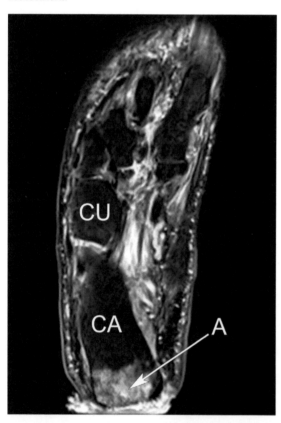

Fig. 8.4D A fat suppressed MR image (this sequence highlights fluid as bright/white) in this patient showing high signal oedema with loss of fat marrow signal in the dorsal calcaneus (A) consistent with infection deep to the ulcer. Calcaneus (CA), cuboid (CU).

LEARNING POINTS: DIABETIC FOOT/OSTEOMYELITIS

- Osteomyelitis may occur secondary to haematogenous or direct spread of infection.
- XR is usually normal in the early stages. Bone destruction is a late sign.
- MRI can help to delineate the extent of bone and soft tissue infection.
- Antibiotic therapy should be guided by the results of bone or tissue biopsy and microbiology assessment.

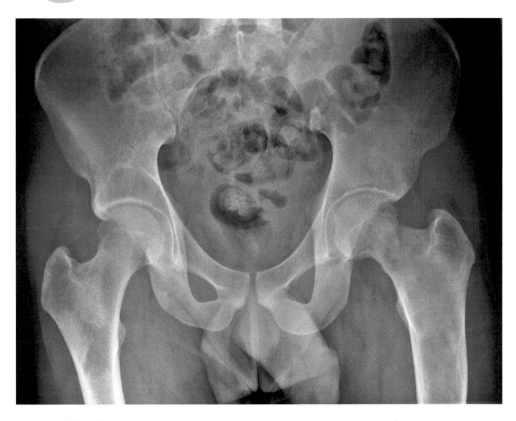

Fig. 8.5A XR pelvis.

A 25-year-old male presents to the ED with acute on chronic pain in his left hip exacerbated by a minor fall from standing on the way to work. There is no relevant past medical history.

On examination there is tenderness over the left hip and limited range of movement. XR of the pelvis and left hip is arranged (**Figure 8.5A**).

CASE 8.5: QUESTIONS

1 What features are seen on the XR?
2 What is the cause for the hip pain?
3 What conditions can cause lytic bone lesions?
4 What further investigations may be indicated?
5 How should this patient be managed?

CASE 8.5: ANSWERS

1 What features are seen on the XR?

XR of the pelvis (**Figure 8.5B**) shows:

- A subcapital fracture through the left neck of femur, passing through a lucent (dark) lesion within the femoral neck. The fracture is intracapsular and undisplaced.
- Further abnormal lucent lesions are noted within the left and right proximal femoral diaphyses. Note the inferior extent of the left femoral diaphyseal lesion is not included in the field of view and additional radiographic views of the more distal femur should be performed.
- A pathological fracture is a fracture occurring through an area of abnormal bone. This can be due to a focal abnormality or a generalised, diffuse process. The underlying abnormality may be benign or malignant.
- The term 'lucent' refers to a bone lesion where the cortex or marrow is replaced with less dense material and therefore appears dark or radiolucent; sclerotic implies replacement with more dense material. Associated bone destruction in relation to a lucent lesion suggests an aggressive process and these type of lesions are termed 'lytic'.

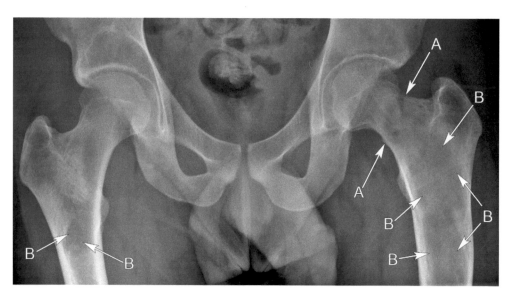

Fig. 8.5B XR pelvis with a pathological impacted, undisplaced subcapital fracture of the left femoral neck (A) and bilateral lucent bone lesions (B).

2 What is the cause for the hip pain?

In the above case, the multifocal lucent lesions are due to fibrous dysplasia (confirmed on biopsy), a benign disorder in which normal bone is replaced with fibrous tissue causing deformity and pain. It produces a 'ground-glass matrix' appearance to the bone, expansion, remodelling, and often endosteal scalloping. The affected bone is weak and, therefore, susceptible to pathological fractures. Fibrous dysplasia is not a condition for finals but pathological fracture and lucent/lytic lesions might occur in the exam.

3 What conditions can cause lytic bone lesions?

There are many conditions, benign and malignant, that can cause lucent or lytic bone lesions. The XR appearances should be correlated with the clinical details and the patient's age. The important aggressive conditions to consider are metastases and myeloma (in an adult), and infection (all ages). Examples of lytic lesions and myeloma are included elsewhere in this book.

Factors aiding in the diagnosis of malignant bone tumours from benign lesions are:

- Zone of transition from normal to abnormal bone: a sharp, discrete, and narrow zone is associated with slow growing benign lesions, whereas less well-defined lesions are associated with fast growing aggressive processes.
- Location: lesions often arise in specific bones and regions of bones. Say if the lesion is epiphyseal, metaphyseal or diaphyseal and if it is central, eccentric or cortical.
- Periosteal reaction: a thick, wavy periosteal reaction is more often associated with slow growth, benign disease. A lamellated (onion-skin), amorphous or sunburst pattern is more aggressive.
- Age of the patient: specific lesions tend to occur at specific ages. Metastases and myeloma are rare under 40 years old.

4 What further investigations may be indicated?

A dedicated XR series of the lesion is usually sufficient. CT and MRI are sometimes also used, however, to further examine the nature of the underlying bone lesion (**Figure 8.5C**). If metastases are suspected, a staging CT of the chest, abdomen, and pelvis should be performed to look for the primary tumour together with a radionuclide bone scan to evaluate the entire skeleton. An image-guided bone biopsy may also be required. If myeloma is suspected, serum electrophoresis and urine Bence Jones protein are checked, and either an XR or MRI skeletal survey is performed.

5 How should this patient be managed?

The patient is at risk of further fractures and, given the large volume of bone affected, surgical fixation with an intramedullary nail is required (**Figure 8.5D**). Prophylactic internal fixation of the contralateral side may also be indicated if imaging confirms large volume lesions.

LEARNING POINTS: PATHOLOGICAL FRACTURE, LYTIC LESION

- A pathological fracture is a fracture through abnormally weakened bone.
- Suspect an underlying lesion if the fracture does not fit the mechanism of injury.
- Scrutinise for any abnormality in bone texture around the fracture. Lytic lesions can be single, multiple or diffuse.
- In patients over the age of 40 years, think of metastases and myeloma.
- In younger patients think of Ewing's sarcoma, osteosarcoma. Also, consider infection in patients of all ages.
- Management includes obtaining a dedicated XR series of the lesion, keeping the patient nonweight bearing with adequate analgesia, and seeking an orthopaedic opinion.

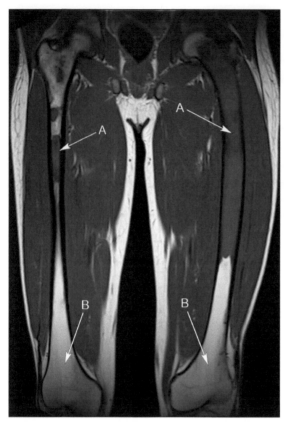

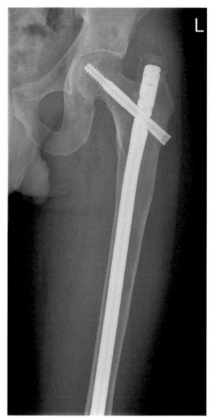

Fig. 8.5C Coronal T1-weighted MRI of both femurs in the same patient as in Figure 8.5A showing loss of the normal bright fat signal in both proximal femurs (A) due to fibrous dysplasia lesions. Normal fat-containing bone marrow is seen distally (B).

Fig. 8.5D XR left hip showing an intramedullary nail passing through the large lucent area of expanded medulla, and 'ground-glass matrix', which is typical for fibrous dysplasia.

Case 8.6

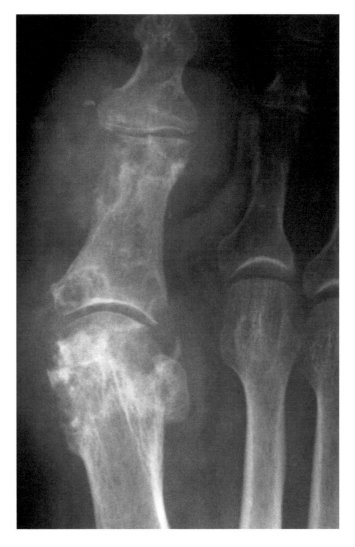

Fig. 8.6A XR right hallux.

A 55-year-old male presents to his GP with an acute episode of pain in his right great toe. There is no history of trauma. He has self-managed previous similar episodes with over the counter anti-inflammatories.

On examination the great toe is hot, swollen, and erythematous. He is afebrile. The toe is exquisitely tender on palpation over the metatarsophalangeal (MTP) and interphalangeal (IP) joints. No other joint swelling is identified.

An XR of the right hallux is arranged (**Figure 8.6A**).

CASE 8.6: QUESTIONS

1 What features are seen on the XR?
2 What is the diagnosis?

3 What further investigations may be ordered?
4 How should this patient be managed?

CASE 8.6: ANSWERS

1 What features are seen on the XR?

XR of the right hallux shows (**Figure 8.6B**):

- Marked soft tissue swelling around the MTP and IP joints.
- Multiple eccentric periarticular erosions on both sides of the MTP and IP joints, some with overhanging sclerotic margins.
- Bone density and joint spaces are preserved.

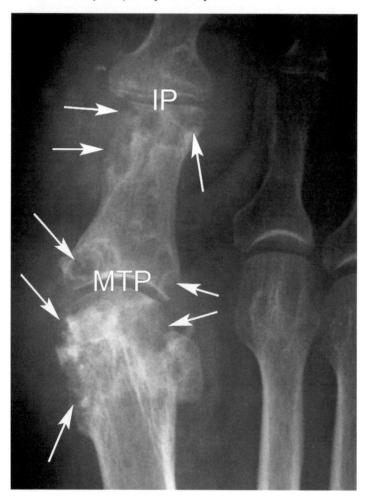

Fig. 8.6B XR right hallux. Soft tissue swelling around the MTP and IP joints. Periarticular erosions are present with thin sclerotic overlying edges (arrows). Note the preserved joint spaces and bone density.

2 What is the diagnosis?

The history and XR are typical for gout. When considering any hot and tender joint, however, the differentials also include septic arthritis and calcium pyrophosphate deposition (CPPD) or 'pseudogout'.

- Gout is a common arthritis caused by hyperuricaemia and deposition of monosodium urate crystals within joints and overlying soft tissues.

- The hands and feet are most commonly involved (particularly the hallux MTP joint) but knee, hip, and sacroiliac joint involvement is not uncommon. Associated soft tissue changes that may be seen on XR include bursitis (olecranon or prepatellar) and dense tophi (soft tissue deposition of urate crystals).
- Septic arthritis is characterised by a joint effusion, juxta-articular osteoporosis, and destruction of cartilage and bone on both sides of the joint. Early in the disease the XR is normal but later you may see bone and joint destruction.
- CPPD (often referred to as pseudogout when it results in acute pain and swelling) shares many XR features with OA, including loss of joint space and subchondral sclerosis. A key feature is chondrocalcinosis (calcification within cartilaginous structures). Commonly affected areas are the 1st and 2nd metacarpophalangeal (MCP) joints of the hand and the triangular fibrocartilage complex (TFCC) of the wrist (**Figure 8.6C**).

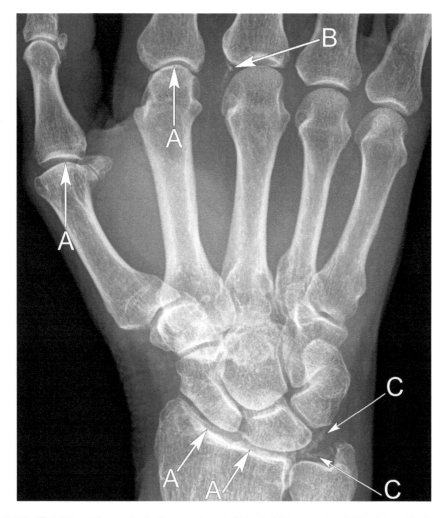

Fig. 8.6C XR right hand in a patient with pseudogout. There is joint space loss in the 1st and 2nd MCP joints and at the radiocarpal joint (A). Chondrocalcinosis is present in the 3rd MCP joint (B) and the triangular fibrocartilage complex of the wrist (C).

3 What further investigations may be ordered?

Other helpful investigations in suspected gout include:

- Serum urate levels and inflammatory markers (e.g. CRP), all of which are usually elevated.
- Microscopic examination of synovial fluid from an affected joint. This will demonstrate needle-shaped urate crystals with negative birefringence under polarised light. In CPPD, microscopy demonstrates rhomboid-shaped crystals with positive birefringence.
- A recent alternative to joint aspiration (usually under US guidance) and microscopy is dual-energy CT. This subtracts the soft tissues and leaves behind only residue of calcific or monosodium urate attenuation (density) (**Figure 8.6D**).

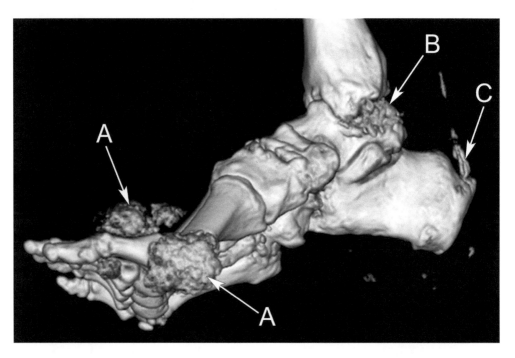

Fig. 8.6D Dual-energy CT showing urate crystal deposition around the MTP and IP joints of the right foot (A). Further deposition can be seen in the ankle joint (B) and Achilles tendon (C).

4 How should this patient be managed?

Management of an acute attack of gout is symptomatic with cool packs, NSAIDs, and either colchicine or steroids.

Preventive intervention aimed at lowering serum urate levels includes dietary advice (avoidance of beer, spirits, red meat, and seafood), weight loss, and allopurinol therapy (remember starting allopurinol therapy may precipitate a further acute episode). Strict management of comorbidities, such as renal disease, cardiovascular disease, and diabetes mellitus, is also important.

LEARNING POINTS: GOUT

- XR findings in gout include demarcated periarticular erosions with sclerotic, overhanging edges. Also, preserved joint space and bone mineral density.
- Soft tissue changes include calcified periarticular tophi and bursitis.
- In any hot swollen joint also consider septic arthritis and CPPD.
- US-guided aspiration of joint fluid for microscopy or dual energy CT can confirm the diagnosis.
- In discussing management, think: symptom relief, prevention strategy, and comorbidities.

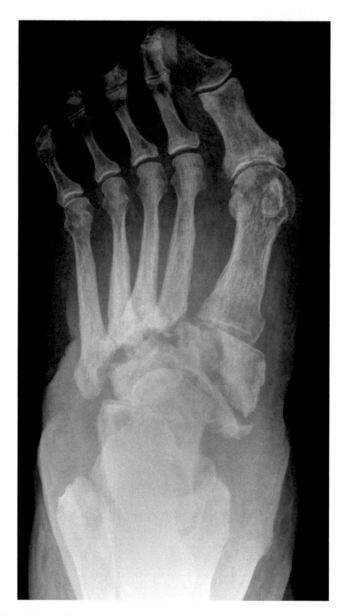

Fig. 8.7A AP view of the left foot.

A 79-year-old male visits his diabetic outpatient clinic with a 6-month history of swelling and pain in the left foot. For the last week he has been unable to weight bear on this side. He is reviewed by the Specialist Registrar who makes note of a long history of diabetes and several related complications including severe renal impairment and diabetic retinopathy.

Examination reveals a swollen left foot, the overlying skin is erythematous, and it feels hot. The skin is intact. There is loss of sensation to light touch around the ankle and foot, and the tarsal joint feels loose when moved. The patient is apyrexial. Reviewing the patient's blood tests

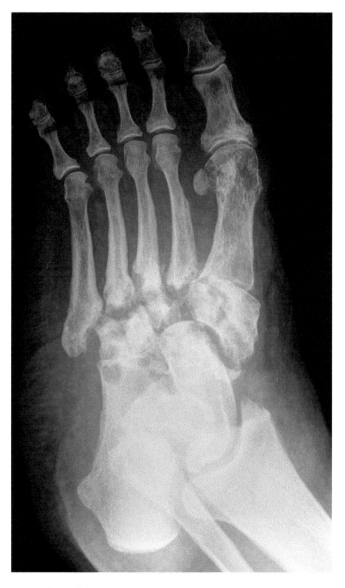

Fig. 8.7B Oblique view of the left foot.

you notice that the last HbA1c was 50 mmol/mol (target range in diabetes mellitus 42–48 mmol/mol). You arrange a new set of bloods including a FBC, renal profile, and repeat HbA1c. You also request an XR of the foot (**Figures 8.7A** and **8.7B**).

CASE 8.7: QUESTIONS

1 What is the most likely diagnosis and differential diagnosis?
2 What do the XRs show?
3 Is any further imaging indicated?
4 How might this patient be managed?

CASE 8.7: ANSWERS

1 What is the most likely diagnosis and differential diagnosis?

A neuropathic (Charcot) joint best fits the clinical findings. It is important, however, to exclude infection (i.e. septic arthritis and osteomyelitis).

2 What do the XRs show?

They show joint destruction. There are findings of bone sclerosis and fragmentation in the tarsus with subluxations evident. There are small foci of calcification projected over the joint in keeping with loose joint debris. There is also soft tissue swelling (**Figure 8.7C**).

These findings are characteristic of a neuropathic joint (Charcot joint). The neuropathy causes repetitive joint damage and is usually secondary to diabetes.

The D's of a neuropathic (Charcot) joint:

- **D**estruction of the articular cartilage.
- **D**egeneration (joint space loss).
- **D**ebris (loose bodies).

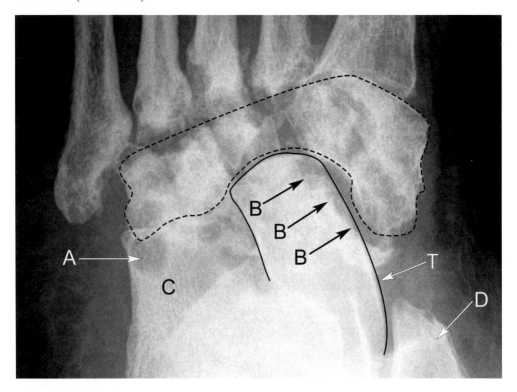

Fig. 8.7C Magnified XR of the left tarsus demonstrating the classical features of a neuropathic Charcot joint. There is soft tissue swelling overlying the tarsus with extensive destruction, fragmentation, and subluxation of the tarsal bones. The normal anatomy is disrupted with the normal tarsal bones hard to identify. The calcaneus is seen (C) and talus outline is shown (T). The normal cuboid (lateral), cuneiforms, and navicular are not well delineated and are fragmented and subluxed – the outline of these bones is traced by a dotted line. Note: subchondral cyst formation (A) and also evidence of bone erosion (B). Tip of medial malleolus is just seen (D).

- **D**islocation.
- **D**istension of the joint (i.e. effusion).
- **D**ensity of bone normal for the patient.

Diabetic neuropathy affects weight-bearing joints, most commonly the ankle or foot. Other causes of neuropathic joint include neurosyphilis (tend to have knee involvement) and syringo-myelia of the spinal cord (may demonstrate shoulder deformity).

3 Is any further imaging indicated?

A MRI scan may be helpful if there is clinical suspicion of infection. It is not always possible to differentiate between the two diagnoses on imaging findings alone. In osteomyelitis, however, there is usually a more focal pattern of bone destruction that often relates to an overlying skin ulcer. There may also be fluid collection or air in soft tissues.

CT is used to further characterise the extent of joint destruction and to help plan surgical management (**Figure 8.7D**). Subchondral cysts and loose bodies make a neuropathic joint a more probable diagnosis in this case than septic arthritis and osteomyelitis.

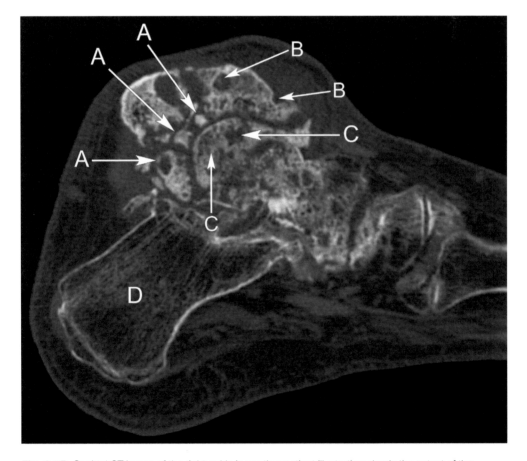

Fig. 8.7D Sagittal CT image of the right ankle in another patient illustrating clearly the extent of the abnormality. The articular surface of the distal tibia is fragmented (A) and there are numerous subchondral cysts (B). Note: also sclerosis and cyst formation of articulating talus (C). Calcaneus (D).

4 How might this patient be managed?

In most cases management is conservative once infection is excluded. However, surgery may be considered in order to facilitate ambulation (for example if adapted footwear is otherwise impossible) or to reduce a deformity that is at risk of ulceration and infection. Addressing diabetic control is also important.

> **LEARNING POINTS: NEUROPATHIC (CHARCOT) JOINT**
>
> - A neuropathic (Charcot) joint is most commonly seen as a complication of chronic and poorly controlled diabetes.
> - The location of the neuropathic joint gives a clue as to the underlying pathology. The ankle and foot are most commonly affected by diabetes.
> - Remember the '6 × Ds' of the Charcot joint.
> - Coexistence of osteomyelitis is common.

Case 8.8

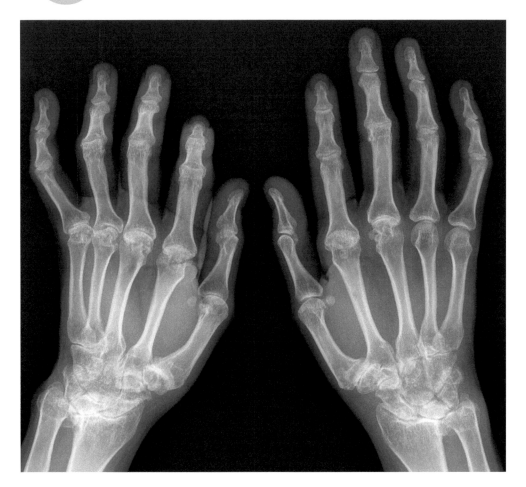

Fig. 8.8A XR of both hands and wrists.

A 47-year-old female presents to her GP with longstanding pain, morning stiffness, and swelling in the joints of the wrists and hands. On examination, there is muscle wastage of the small muscles of the hand and soft tissue swelling over the wrists, MCP, and proximal interphalangeal (PIP) joints. There is reduced movement at the wrist and a deformity in alignment of the little fingers.

An XR of both hands and wrists is obtained (**Figure 8.8A**).

CASE 8.8: QUESTIONS

1 What does the XR show?
2 What is the diagnosis?
3 What are the typical radiological features of this condition?
4 What are the diagnostic criteria?
5 How would you manage this patient?

CASE 8.8: ANSWERS

1 What does the XR show?

There is a bilateral symmetrical, polyarthropathy of the wrists and hands. There is periarticular soft tissue swelling over the wrists, MCP, and PIP joints (particularly in the 2–4th fingers). These joints display joint space narrowing, marginal erosions, and juxta-articular osteoporosis. There are ulnar subluxations at the 5th MCP joints. Severe secondary degenerative change is noted at the radiocarpal and thumb carpometacarpal (CMC) joints (**Figure 8.8B**).

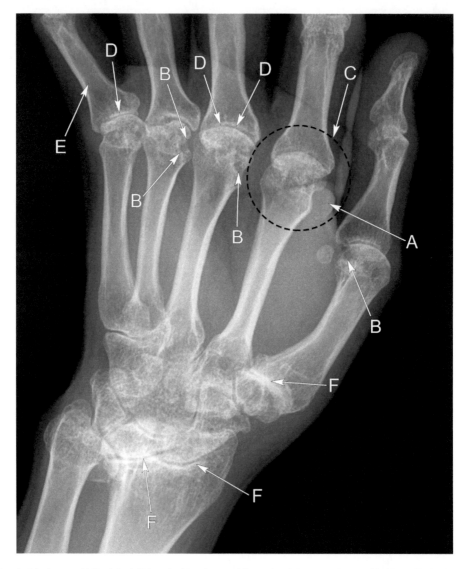

Fig. 8.8B Cropped XR of the left hand with advanced features of rheumatoid arthritis (RhA). Periarticular soft tissue swelling (A), marginal erosions (B), juxta-articular osteoporosis (C: ringed dotted line), joint space loss (D), ulnar subluxation (E), and secondary radiocarpal degenerative change (F).

2 What is the diagnosis?

The XR shows a bilateral, symmetrical, polyarthropathy in keeping with rheumatoid arthritis (RhA). The key radiological features include:

- Joint space narrowing.
- Marginal erosions.
- Juxta-articular osteoporosis.
- Periarticular soft tissue swelling.
- Ulnar subluxations.
- Secondary degenerative change at the wrists and base of thumbs.
- Proximal symmetrical distribution across the wrists and MCP joints.

RhA has a female predominance and tends to involve young and middle-aged individuals. It is characterised by joint pain and morning stiffness with overlying soft tissue swelling. Rheumatoid factor (RhF) is positive in the majority of patients (seropositive) but also present in about 6% of the normal population. HLA B27 is positive in <10% of patients with RhA.

3 What are the typical radiological features of this condition?

Periarticular soft tissue swelling, juxta-articular osteoporosis, marginal erosions, and uniform joint space narrowing are typical early features. A lack of reactive proliferative bone formation is typical.

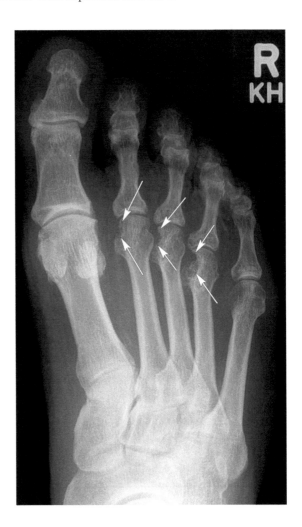

- In the hands and feet the distribution is proximal, involving the MCP joints before the PIP joints. The distal interphalangeal (DIP) joints are relatively spared (**Figure 8.8C**).
- These features are usually bilateral and symmetrical.
- Any joint can be affected. The appendicular skeleton is commonly involved, as are the distal clavicles (**Figure 8.8D**) and the atlantoaxial joint of the cervical spine.
- Features of RhA are included in *Tables 8.8A* and *8.8B*.

Fig. 8.8C Magnified XR of the right forefoot in the same patient as **8.8A** with marginal periarticular erosions at the 2nd–4th metatarsal heads (arrows).

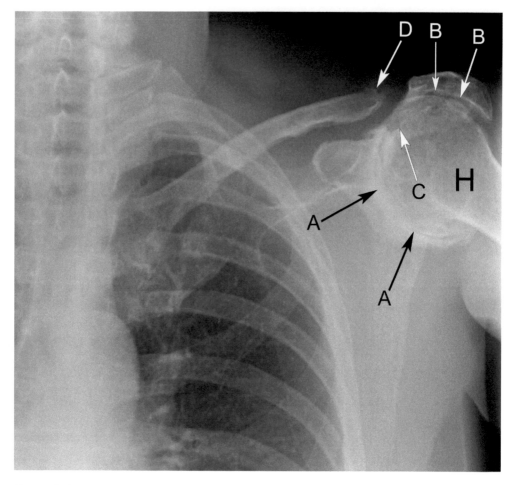

Fig. 8.8D Coned-in view of the left shoulder in a patient with RhA. The humerus (H) is 'high riding' with reduced glenohumeral (GH) joint space (A) and subacromial joint space (B). The latter is due to associated rotator cuff damage. There are marginal erosions of the humeral head (C) and distal end of the clavicle (D) with widening of the acromioclavicular joint space.

Table 8.8A Nonmusculoskeletal features of RhA

Pulmonary	Interstitial fibrosis (lower zone), rheumatoid nodules, pleural thickening, and pleural effusions
Cardiovascular	Accelerated coronary and cerebral artery atherosclerosis, pericarditis, and vasculitis
Cutaneous	Rheumatoid nodules in pressure areas such as elbows, occiput, and lumbosacral region in RhF-positive patients
Ocular	Uveitis, episcleritis, and keratoconjunctivitis sicca

Table 8.8B Clinical features of RhA

Mnemonic: RHEUMATISM	
R	RhF +ve in 80%/**R**adial deviation of wrist
H	**H**LA-DR1 and DR-4
E	**E**SR/**E**xtra-articular features
U	**U**lnar deviation of fingers
M	**M**orning stiffness/**M**CP + PIP joint swelling
A	**A**nkylosis/**A**tlanto–axial joint subluxation/**A**utoimmune/**A**NA +ve in 30%
T	**T**-cells (CD4)/**T**NF
I	**I**nflammatory synovial tissue (pannus)/**i**nterleukin-1
S	**S**wan-neck deformity, Boutonniere deformity, Z-deformity of thumb
M	**M**uscle wastage of small muscles of the hand

4 What are the diagnostic criteria?

The American College of Rheumatology revised criteria (1988) require four out of the following seven diagnostic criteria to be present for diagnosis of RhA:

- Morning stiffness lasting >1 hour.
- Soft tissue swelling of three or more joints observed by a physician.
- Soft tissue swelling of either the wrist, PIP or MCP joints on imaging.
- Symmetric swelling.
- Subcutaneous rheumatoid nodules.
- RhF (seropositive).
- Radiographic signs: erosions or periarticular osteopenia in the hand/wrist.

5 How would you manage this patient?

Treatment aims to improve symptoms and delay disease progression. Therapy is with a combination of corticosteroids, NSAIDs, disease modifying antirheumatic drugs (DMARDs) such as methotrexate, sulfasalazine, ciclosporin, and anti-tumour necrosis factor (TNF) agents. The anti-TNF treatments and variants of, which suppress the immune system, are known collectively as biological therapies.

LEARNING POINTS: RHEUMATOID ARTHRITIS

- Look for a bilateral, symmetrical and proximal polyarthropathy and periarticular erosions.
- Periarticular soft tissue swelling is an early sign.
- Rheumatoid factor is positive in the majority of cases.
- Early diagnosis and initiation of therapy is the key to altering the course of the disease.

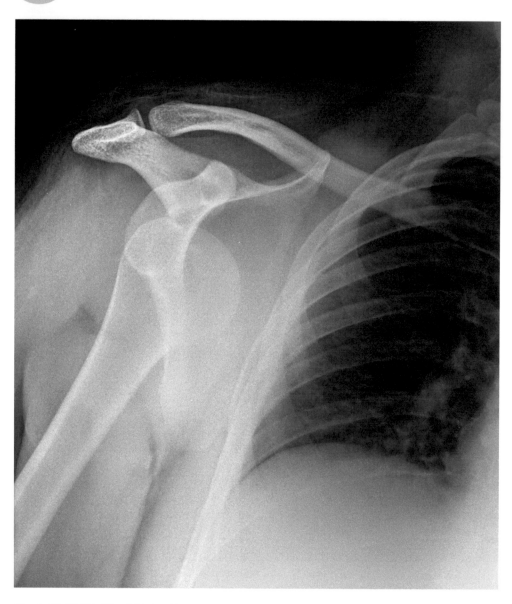

Fig. 8.9A AP XR of the right shoulder.

A 28-year-old female sustained a fall while playing volley-ball. She had extremely limited and painful movement in the right shoulder and was removed from the court. She attends the ED supporting her right arm with her other hand. You arrange an urgent XR (**Figures 8.9A** and **8.9B**).

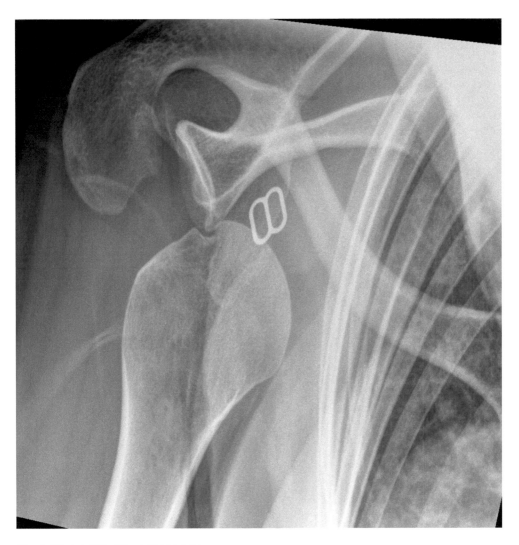

Fig. 8.9B Axial XR of the right shoulder.

CASE 8.9: QUESTIONS

1 What injury has this patient sustained?
2 How is this type of injury classified, and what other types are there?
3 How would you manage this patient?

CASE 8.9: ANSWERS

1 What injury has this patient sustained?

The XR shows an anterior dislocation of the right humeral head with an associated Hill–Sachs defect of the humeral head (**Figure 8.9C**). On the AP view the humeral head lies inferomedially in relation to the glenoid. An axial XR of the shoulder is obtained with the patient's upper arm elevated (may be difficult owing to pain) with the XR beam passing down in a head to foot direction (craniocaudal).

- Hill–Sachs lesions are compression fractures of the posterolateral humeral head, typically secondary to recurrent anterior shoulder dislocations as the humeral head comes to rest on the anteroinferior glenoid rim. If large, the wedge defect can also be seen on the post-relocation XR (**Figure 8.9D**).

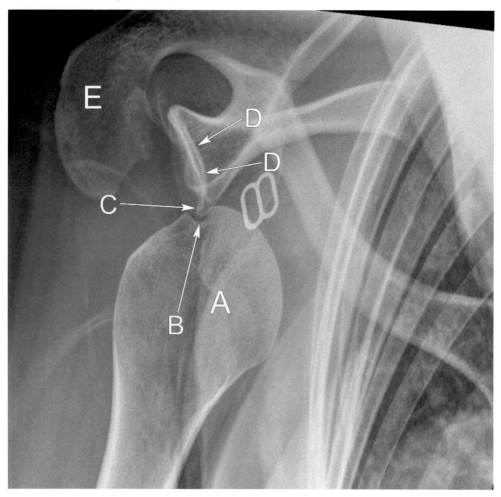

Fig. 8.9C Axial XR of the right shoulder showing anterior dislocation of the humeral head (A) with a Hill–Sachs defect (B) where the humeral head is perched on the anterior inferior glenoid rim (C). Glenoid (D), acromion (E). The humeral head lies anteriorly and has lost its normal glenoid articulation.

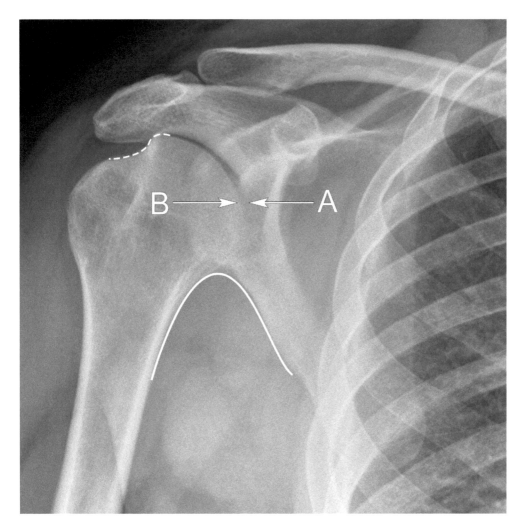

Fig. 8.9D AP XR of the right shoulder in a different patient following relocation of an anterior dislocation in the ED. A Hill–Sachs lesion (dotted line) is seen as a wedge defect in the humeral head. Normal glenoid (A) and humeral head (B) alignment is demonstrated by the tracing of a smooth continuous line along the scapulohumeral arch (solid line). This is also called the Bandi line.

- Bankart lesions are often seen in combination with Hill–Sachs lesions and are caused by humeral head impaction on the anteroinferior glenoid. They may constitute glenoid labral damage only ('soft Bankart') or an impaction fracture of the glenoid ('bony Bankart').

2 How is this type of injury classified, and what other types are there?

Shoulder dislocation may be anterior (most common), posterior (uncommon) or inferior (least common).

- Posterior dislocation makes up 2–4% of cases and is classically associated with a convulsive disorder, electrocution or high energy RTA, causing forced posterior displacement with the arm in abduction and internal rotation.

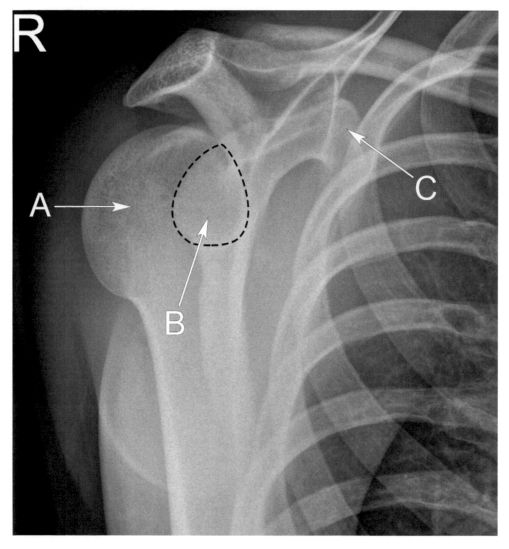

Fig. 8.9E Y-view (lateral) of the right shoulder showing a posterior dislocation. The central aspect of the humeral head (A) does not overlie the glenoid (B: outlined by dotted line) but is positioned posteriorly. The coracoid (C) is a useful anterior anatomical landmark.

- Posterior dislocation on frontal XR shows an internally rotated humeral head ('lightbulb sign'), loss of normal glenohumeral (GH) overlap with widening of the joint >6 mm, and disruption of the scapulohumeral arch. The axillary view is preferred as it directly shows displacement in the posterior direction (**Figures 8.9E** and **8.9F**).

3 How would you manage this patient?

Anterior dislocation is usually managed with closed reduction and a period of immobilisation to allow capsular healing. It is important that the patient undergoes a programme of physiotherapy to restore range of movement and muscle strength.

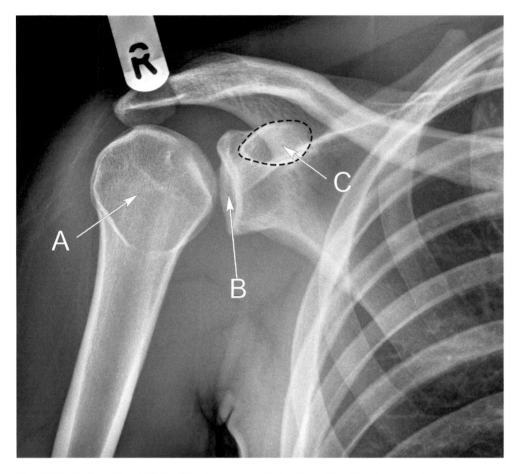

Fig. 8.9F AP view of the right shoulder showing a posterior dislocation. There is a rounded appearance of the humeral head ('light bulb sign') and absent GH overlap indicating widening of the GH joint. Humeral head (A), glenoid (B), and coracoid (C: dotted line).

SHOULDER RELOCATION PROCEDURE

- **W**ash hands, **I**ntroduce, ask the **P**atient's name and date of birth, **E**xplain the procedure and risks, and gain consent.
- *Review the* XRs (both views) before and after to determine pattern of dislocation/confirm relocation/exclude fractures (do not reduce if there is a fracture).
- *Examine* neurovascular status and document it. In particular axillary nerve sensation over the lateral deltoid.
- *Analgesia* and sedation with IV morphine, midazolam, and Entonox.
- *Technique* depends on pattern of dislocation:
  - Anterior: use Kocker's, Stimpson's or Modified Milch technique (look these up).
  - Posterior: pull arm gently forward and externally rotate.
- *Aftercare* with broad arm sling or polysling for 3 weeks and appointment at the fracture clinic.

LEARNING POINTS: SHOULDER DISLOCATION

- Always check the XR for associated fractures of the glenoid or humeral head.
- A Hill–Sachs lesion is a compression fracture of the posterolateral humeral head caused by impaction against the anterior glenoid rim.
- A bony-Bankart lesion is a fracture of the anteroinferior glenoid rim.
- Dislocations can usually be reduced in the ED with sufficient analgesia and sedation. Make sure to examine the neurovascular status of the arm before and after reduction, and document it in the notes.

Case 8.10

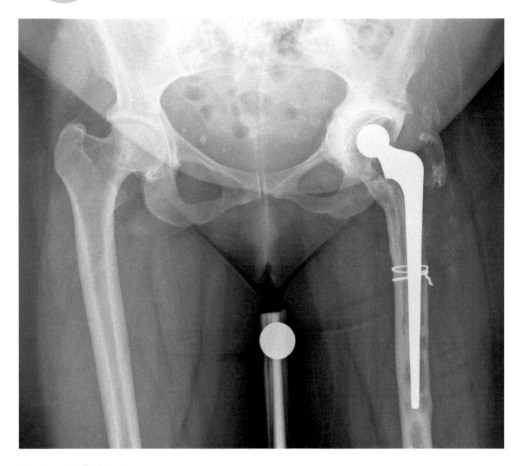

Fig. 8.10A XR of hips.

A 68-year-old female attends the orthopaedic clinic 4 years following revision of her left total hip replacement (THR), with worsening left groin and thigh pain. She is otherwise fit and well. On examination, there is a limited range of movement in the left hip owing to pain and there is some shortening of the left leg.

An XR of her pelvis and left hip is arranged (**Figure 8.10A**).

CASE 8.10: QUESTIONS

1 What does the XR show?
2 What is the cause of the pain?
3 What are the differential diagnoses?
4 What is stress shielding?
5 How should this patient be managed?

CASE 8.10: ANSWERS

1 What does the XR show?

The XR shows a left total hip arthroplasty (THA or THR [total hip replacement]). There is proximal osteolysis (bone resorption) of the calcar (ridge of dense bone in the posteromedial femoral neck that is important for mechanical support). There is also cortical thinning and bone loss within the nonweight-bearing greater trochanter and lateral femoral cortex in keeping with stress shielding (**Figure 8.10B**).

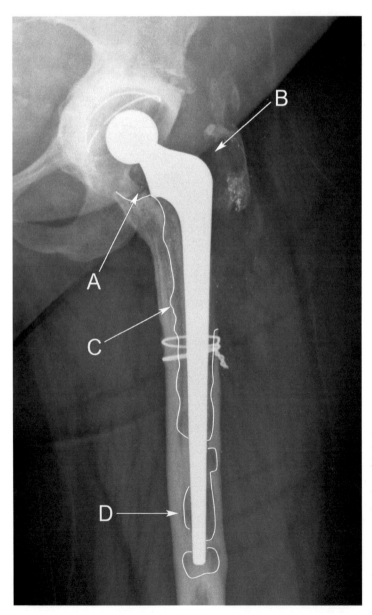

Fig. 8.10B Left THR with osteolysis of the calcar (A) and greater trochanter (B) owing to stress shielding. The calcar is a vertical plate of bone deep to the lesser trochanter. A large, concentric, linear, periprosthetic lucency (C) indicates loosening. Multifocal distal femoral lucencies with endosteal scalloping (D) suggest further foci of loosening secondary to particle disease.

A tension band wire has been used to stabilise the middle zones of the femoral prosthesis where there is a long, linear, concentric periprosthetic lucency measuring >2 mm depth. This is indicative of mechanical loosening.

Multiple discrete and well-defined lucencies surround the distal femoral prosthesis with smooth endosteal scalloping. This is the appearance of osteolysis caused by particle disease.

There are no signs of infection.

2 What is the cause of the pain?

The pain is caused by loosening of the femoral prosthesis. This is likely caused by a combination of mechanical loosening and particle disease. Importantly, there are no signs of infection.

- Particle disease is an aggressive granulomatous reaction that is caused by shedding of particles from the prosthesis, polyethylene cup, and/or cement. The submicron sized particles can migrate along the whole course of the prosthesis causing multiple foci of osteolysis and eventually prosthetic loosening.
- Clinical features: patients tend to be asymptomatic until there is substantial bone loss, then in severe pain. There may be limb shortening (as seen here) and limitation of movement.

3 What are the differential diagnoses?

Lucencies at the metal–cement or metal–bone interface >2 mm may indicate particle disease, loosening or infection, or all three.

- *Mechanical loosening* is the most common indication for revision surgery. It is characterised by a linear periprosthetic lucency, >2 mm depth. Component migration is a late but diagnostic sign.
- *Particle disease* usually produces multifocal lucencies with endosteal scalloping, which do not conform to the shape of the prosthesis. It tends to occur 1–5 years after surgery.
- *Infection* causes ill-defined, irregular, and eccentric bone resorption. There is also usually a periosteal reaction. It is important to check the inflammatory markers.

KEY POINTS: RISK OF INFECTION

- Infections <1 year after surgery are acquired during surgery. The risk of intraoperative infection is less than 1% owing to the use of antimicrobial prophylaxis and laminar airflow in the operating theatre.
- Infections later than this are acquired by haematogenous seeding from respiratory tract, dental, and urinary tract infections.

4 What is stress shielding?

Stress shielding is reduction in bone density, osteopenia, as a result of the removal of normal stress on the bone owing to a prosthesis. If bone loading decreases, the bone becomes less dense and weaker as there is no longer a stimulus to normal bone remodelling. First there is osteopenia, with thinning of the cortex, and then bone resorption. This is usually seen medially, deep to the lesser trochanter (at the calcar), where it can cause limb shortening. Stress shielding and calcar resorption are normal findings on follow-up and are not associated with loosening of the prosthesis.

5 How should this patient be managed?

Surgical revision is almost always necessary.

LEARNING POINTS: PROSTHETIC LOOSENING

- If you see a THA remember to check for signs of mechanical loosening, particle disease, and infection.
- A lucent zone >2 mm at the bone–prosthesis or bone–cement interface is indicative of loosening. A thinner zone of lucency is likely to be normal but take senior advice if you are unsure.
- Ask to see previous postoperative XRs for comparison.
- Other complications of THA include fracture and dislocation.

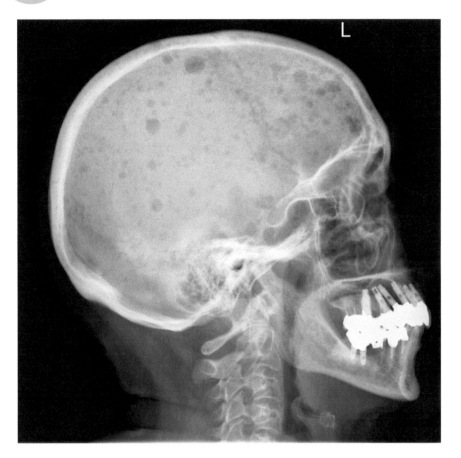

Fig. 8.11A Lateral skull XR.

A 72-year-old female has visited her GP several times in recent months complaining of tiredness and lower back pain, with an initial lumbar spine XR showing mild OA only. Her pain worsens and is not controlled by her prescribed analgesia (paracetamol and codeine). In addition to the back pain, she also now complains of head and arm pain.

On examination there is bony tenderness over the proximal left humerus. There is a palpable liver edge and the spleen also feels enlarged. Blood tests show:

Hb	86 g/L (125–165 g/L)
Total serum calcium	2.75 mmol/L (2.15–2.55 mmol/L)

There is also evidence of acute renal impairment. She is referred to a haematologist who requests an XR series (**Figure 8.11A**).

CASE 8.11: QUESTIONS

1 What is shown on the XR?
2 What is the most likely diagnosis?

3 Is any other imaging required?
4 How might this patient be managed?

CASE 8.11: ANSWERS

1 What is shown on the XR?

This is a selected image from a skeletal survey (a collection of XRs taken to demonstrate the whole skeleton). It is commonly performed in adults to investigate myeloma. Similar skeletal surveys are also used in children to look for fractures in cases of suspected nonaccidental injury (NAI).

The lateral skull XR shows multiple small lucencies, the so-called 'pepper pot' skull. This finding is most suggestive of myeloma. Bone metastases could give a similar appearance but are less likely given the patient's symptoms (**Figure 8.11B**). Hyperparathyroidism may also cause a 'pepper-pot skull'.

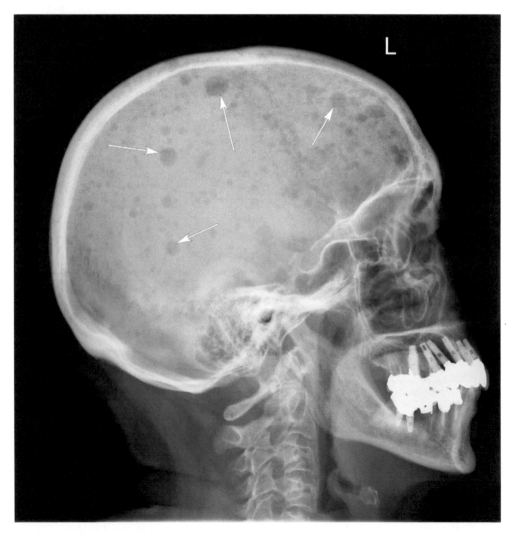

Fig. 8.11B Lateral skull XR with multiple small lucencies (arrows).

2 What is the most likely diagnosis?

The most likely underlying diagnosis is multiple myeloma.

- Multiple myeloma is a cancer of the plasma cells found in bone marrow. Plasma cell proliferation destroys the bone causing pain and releasing calcium.
- Bone destruction causes characteristic 'punched out' lytic lesions and increases the risk of pathological fracture.
- Erythropoiesis is hampered as bone marrow is replaced by plasma cells resulting in anaemia. Patients may present with marrow failure, also renal failure and hypercalcaemia.
- A plasmacytoma (not shown) is a larger lytic/expansile lesion associated with multiple myeloma usually found in the spine, pelvis or ribs.
- The diagnosis is made using a combination of biopsy (including bone marrow with >30% plasma cells), lytic bone lesions, and raised immunoglobulin levels (elevated M protein is the hallmark).
- XRs are frequently normal in myeloma: the commonest XR finding is actually osteopenia. Lytic bone lesions, when they occur, are usually pathognomonic. Bone scans are often negative and are of limited use in this condition.

3 Is any other imaging required?

No further XR imaging is required.

- Whole body MRI using diffusion-weighted techniques, however, is gaining popularity for the detection of bone lesions in multiple myeloma as it is more sensitive than XR. It is especially useful for assessment of the spine.

4 How might this patient be managed?

The patient should be managed by a haematologist specialising in myeloma.

- Multiple myeloma is an incurable disease with a variable prognosis depending on disease severity. The majority of patients have 'standard risk' disease with a median survival of approximately 10 years with modern treatment strategies.
- Treatment is complex and ranges from watchful waiting in early disease to chemotherapy or stem cell transplantation for eligible patients.

LEARNING POINTS: MULTIPLE MYELOMA

- Multiple myeloma is a haematological malignancy affecting the plasma cells.
- As plasma cells reside in the bone marrow, the disease may be diagnosed on XR or MRI.
- Bone lesions have a lucent, punched out appearance on XR.
- Whole body diffusion weighted MRI is gaining popularity for myeloma screening as it is more sensitive than XR for demonstrating bone disease.

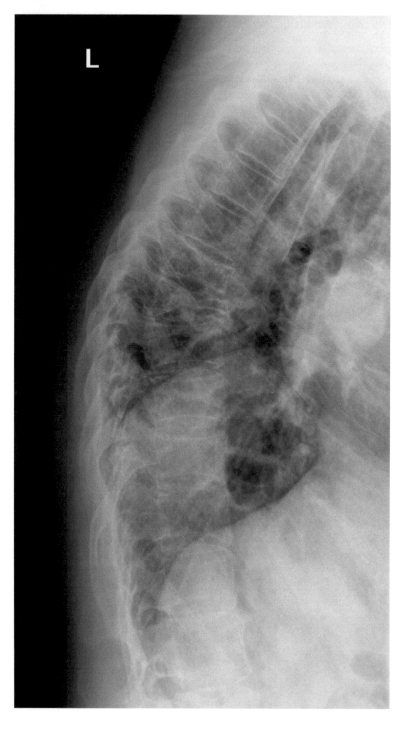

Fig. 8.12A
Lateral XR of the
thoracic spine.

A 68-year-old female presents to the orthopaedic clinic with a long history of back pain, exacerbated recently by lifting a heavy suitcase. Lying in the supine position relieves some of the discomfort but it is exacerbated by standing or walking. She reports having had a bone density scan carried out the previous week, with a T score of -2.9 (low). She denies any weight loss. She has a sedentary lifestyle, smokes 20 cigarettes per day, and drinks an excessive amount of alcohol.

On examination the thoracic spine is kyphotic and there is mid-thoracic tenderness on percussion. There is pain with forward and lateral flexion. The straight leg raise test is negative and neurological exam normal. Routine blood tests are unremarkable; in particular, serum calcium, phosphate, and ALP are normal.

An XR series of the thoracic spine is arranged. The lateral view is included (**Figure 8.12A**).

CASE 8.12: QUESTIONS

1 What are the XR findings?
2 What is the diagnosis?
3 What can you say about bone mineral density in this patient?
4 How would you manage this patient?

CASE 8.12: ANSWERS

1 What are the XR findings?

The XR shows severe compression fractures of the anterior aspects of the T7 and T8 vertebral bodies and a mild compression fracture of the central aspect of the T9 vertebral body. The posterior vertebral line is intact, as are the pedicles. There are no visible retropulsed fragments (**Figure 8.12B**).

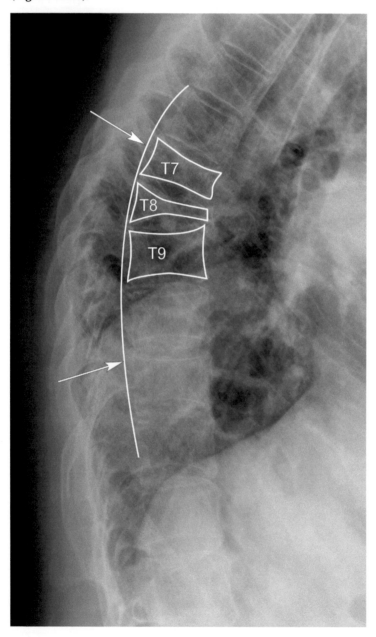

Fig. 8.12B Lateral XR of the thoracic spine showing severe anterior wedge compression of T7 and T8 vertebral bodies. Also mild biconcave compression fracture of T9. Intact posterior vertebral line (arrows). There is kyphotic deformity with reduced bone mineral density.

- Vertebral compression fractures (VCFs) are also called wedge fractures when either the anterior or posterior part of the vertebral body is compressed, and biconcave fractures where the central endplates are compressed.
- The most common causes of VCF:
  - Osteoporosis (also osteomalacia and hyperparathyroidism): consider a DEXA scan if not already done.
  - Trauma: consider a CT scan if not already done.
  - Metastasis/myeloma: consider MRI. Also a myeloma screen or CT body to look for a primary tumour.
- It is important to assess and comment on the neurological status of the patient as a retropulsed bony fracture fragment might narrow the spinal canal and cause cord/cauda equina compression. This may only be visible on CT. Look for posterior vertebral line alignment. Neurological symptoms would include:
  - Muscular weakness.
  - Abnormal sensation in the dermatomes below the vertebral level.
  - Increased tone in the lower limbs.
  - Increased reflexes in the lower limbs.
  - Cauda equina syndrome (paraparesis, urinary incontinence, saddle-like dermatome anaesthesia, and areflexia).
- If there are neurological signs, concerns over fracture stability or suspicion that the fracture may be pathological, a CT or MRI is indicated. MRI is particularly useful in distinguishing acute from chronic fractures, and tumour from infection.
- If there is concern over malignancy, FBC, ALP, LFTs, and CRP are indicated. If infection is suspected, FBC, inflammatory markers, and blood cultures should be obtained. For metabolic causes, serum calcium, albumin, PTH, phosphate, ALP, magnesium, creatinine, TFTs, and vitamin D should be tested.

2 What is the diagnosis?

Osteoporotic VCF.

- There are no features on the XRs to suggest pathology other than osteoporosis, although metastases and myeloma should be considered and excluded in the absence of trauma. It is important to note blood bone profile (calcium, phosphate, ALP) is normal, pointing to a nonmalignant aetiology.
- VCFs are often insidious and may produce only modest back pain early in the course of progressive disease. They are common and present in up to 14% of women over 60 years old. Modifiable risk factors are smoking, alcohol, insufficient physical activity, and oestrogen, calcium or vitamin D deficiency.
- VCFs can occur anywhere in the spine but are most common at the thoracolumbar junction. They are usually multiple and may be consecutive or at different levels. Therefore, ensure imaging of the whole spine.
- VCFs can be graded based on the degree of vertebral height loss:
  - Mild: 20–25%.
  - Moderate: 25–40%.
  - Severe: >40%.

TOP TIP

Remember! An osteoporotic spine is the most common XR abnormality in myeloma.

3 What can you say about bone mineral density in this patient?

There is increased radiolucency of the vertebral bodies with thinning of the cortices in keeping with low bone density. This is supported by the results of the preceding DEXA scan.

- DEXA scans assess bone mineral density in the femoral neck and lumbar spine. A T-score more than 2.5 standard deviations below the young adult female reference range (20–40 years) is diagnostic for osteoporosis (WHO guideline). A Z-score uses the same threshold but is matched for the patient's age and ethnicity, making it more accurate. This patient had a Z-score of -2.9 in the spine, which is diagnostic for osteoporosis.

DEXA SCAN REFERRAL CRITERIA

- All patients >50 years with a low trauma fracture.
- All patients on oral prednisolone >2.5 mg for >3 months.
- All >50 years with 1 risk factor for osteoporosis.
- All <50 years with 1 major risk factor for osteoporosis.

Major risk factors: malabsorption syndromes, rheumatic disorders, glucocorticoids, organ transplantation, chronic liver disease, thyrotoxicosis, primary hyperparathyroidism, prolonged immobilisation, alcohol excess, low BMI <20.

Minor risk factors: renal disease, diabetes, early menopause <45 years, anticonvulsants, antipsychotics.

---

4 How should this patient be managed?

VCFs are usually stable and are treated conservatively with analgesia and a short period of rest. Muscle relaxants, use of a back-brace, and physiotherapy may also help. Risk factor modification would include smoking and alcohol cessation, and an exercise programme with a home visit and fall prevention advice. Patients who do not respond to conservative treatment and continue to have severe pain may be candidates for percutaneous vertebroplasty. This involves injecting acrylic cement into the collapsed vertebra to stabilise and strengthen the vertebral body.

LEARNING POINTS: OSTEOPOROTIC SPINAL FRACTURES

- VCFs are usually due to osteoporosis but may also be due to trauma or metastatic infiltration.
- Request imaging (usually XR initially) of the whole spine, as fractures are often multiple.
- Always assess the posterior vertebral body line for alignment.
- Remember to check and comment on neurological status.

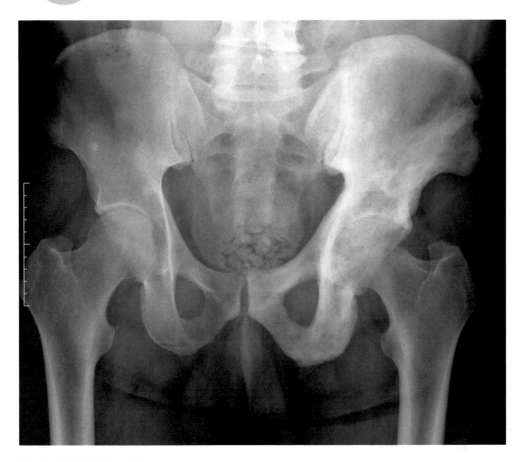

Fig. 8.13A XR of the pelvis.

A 67-year-old male visits his GP with a history of chronic pain in the left hip. On examination the GP elicits pain on external rotation of the hip and suspects OA.

An XR of the pelvis is performed (**Figure 8.13A**).

CASE 8.13: QUESTIONS

1 What are the XR findings?
2 What is the likely diagnosis?
3 Are there any risks associated with this disease?
4 Is any further imaging required?

CASE 8.13: ANSWERS

1 What are the XR findings?

There is cortical thickening, bone expansion, trabecular coarsening, and sclerosis of the left hemipelvis. This includes thickening of the iliopubic and ilioischial lines (**Figure 8.13B**).

The bone cortex is intact and there is no periosteal reaction or overlying soft tissue swelling to suggest an underlying aggressive process. There is no bone destruction. Note also the severe left hip OA.

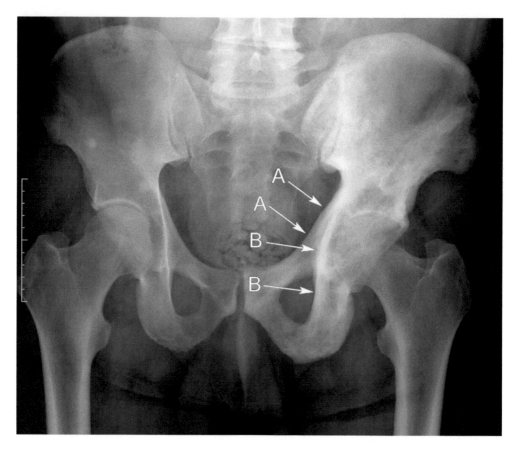

Fig. 8.13B AP XR of the pelvis. There is cortical thickening of the left hemipelvis with sclerosis and coarsening of the trabeculae. The iliopubic (A) and ilioischial (B) lines are also thickened. There is joint space narrowing and marginal osteophyte formation in the left hip joint, consistent with OA.

2 What is the likely diagnosis?

These are the characteristic appearances of Paget's disease of the bone, a common benign disorder, which results in disordered and excessive bone remodelling.

- Bone marrow is replaced by fibrous tissue with numerous vascular channels.
- It is rare under the age of 40 years and common over 80 years. The most common sites of involvement are the pelvis, spine, and skull.

- There are several stages of the disease ranging from initial active osteolysis (osteoclasts predominate), then a mixed phase, and then a chronic healing phase (osteoblasts predominate) with sclerosis.
- The inactive phase gives the classic XR appearance seen here, while the active phase produces a lytic appearance (**Figures 8.13C** and **8.13D**).
- Paget's disease usually affects more than one site (polyostotic) and is asymmetric in its distribution. In chronic Paget's disease the bones soften and long bones may bow (**Figure 8.13E**).
- There is often associated OA of the hips, with findings such as joint space narrowing and subchondral sclerosis.

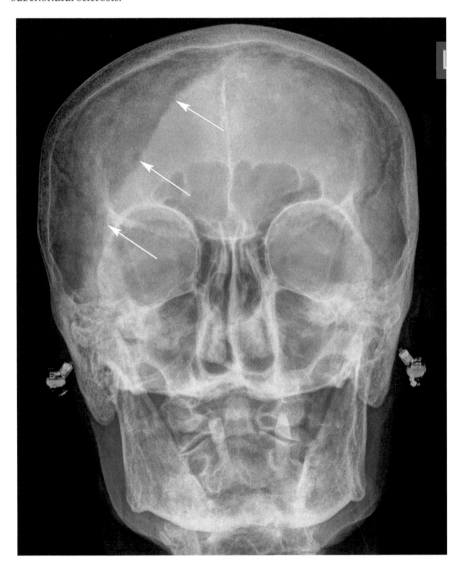

Fig. 8.13C AP skull XR showing geographic lysis (arrows) in the active phase of Paget's, also known as osteoporosis circumscripta.

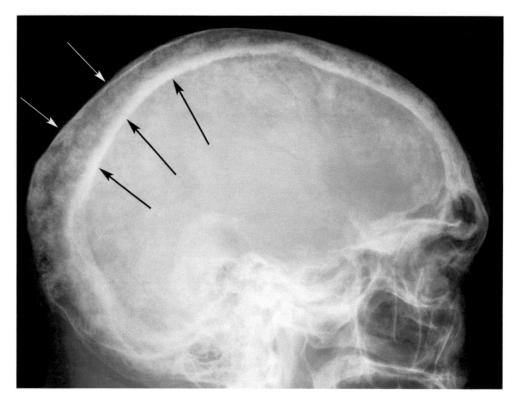

Fig. 8.13D Lateral skull XR in chronic Paget's disease with marked thickening of the calvarium.

3 Are there any risks associated with this disease?

The most serious complication is malignant transformation to osteosarcoma (rare).

- Concerning XR, features of malignancy would include cortical destruction, a 'moth-eaten' or 'permeative' pattern of lucency in the bone, periosteal reaction (fluffy edge to the bone cortex) or a soft tissue mass.
- Other potential complications of Paget's disease include insufficiency fractures (typically in a long bone) and nerve entrapment owing to bone softening and expansion (this might cause, for example, a radiculopathy or a cranial nerve palsy). Patients may be hypercalcaemic (rare, associated with immobilisation) and high output cardiac failure is described owing to new bone blood vessel formation.

4 Is any further imaging required?

Usually no further imaging is required. MRI may be used if there is ongoing concern regarding malignancy. A whole body isotope bone scan can be used to demonstrate the full extent of Paget's disease in the bone.

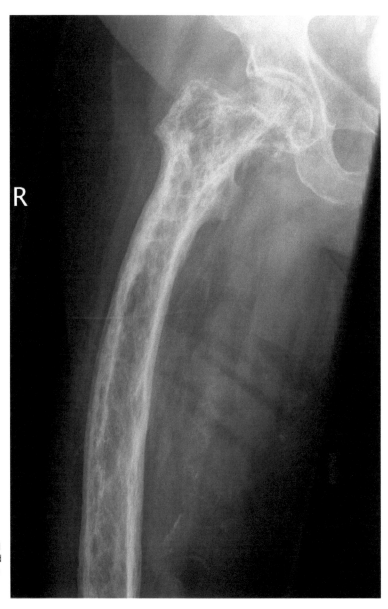

Fig. 8.13E AP view of the right femur in chronic Paget's, with trabecular coarsening, cortical thickening, and bowing of an expanded femur. No fractures are seen. Note: hip joint degenerative changes.

LEARNING POINTS: PAGET'S DISEASE

- Paget's disease is a benign disease of uncertain aetiology, more common in the elderly, involving abnormal bone remodelling.
- The pelvis or spine is affected in 75% of cases.
- There are different phases of the disease, which are reflected in the radiological appearance. Broadly speaking there is an active lytic phase followed by a chronic sclerotic phase.
- Complications include pathological fracture, nerve entrapment, and malignant conversion (rare).

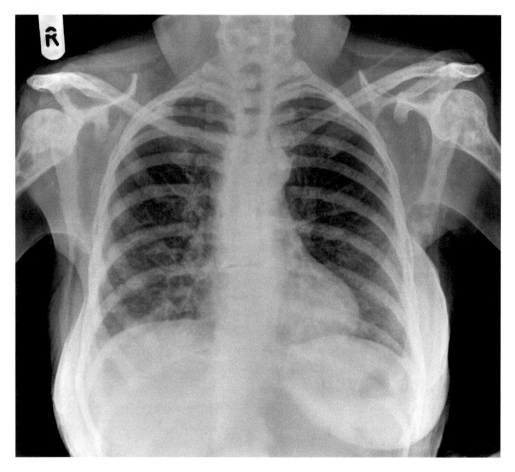

Fig. 8.14A CXR.

A 55-year-old female with a prior history of breast cancer treated with left wide local excision and axillary node clearance presents to her GP with several months of gradually worsening severe intractable pelvic, back, and chest wall pain. She delayed presentation having previously attributed the pain to a muscle strain. Today she presents with acute, severe worsening of pain in her right hip, which occurred while walking upstairs at home. A blood screen is taken, which shows a serum calcium of 3 mmol/L (2.15–2.55 mmol/L).

A CXR is arranged (**Figure 8.14A**), together with XRs of the pelvis and right hip (**Figure 8.14B**).

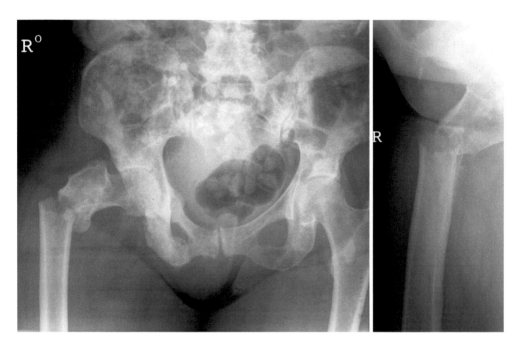

Fig. 8.14B AP XR of pelvis and lateral XR of the right hip.

CASE 8.14: QUESTIONS

1 Describe the XR appearances.
2 What is the diagnosis?
3 What other imaging tests would be justified?
4 How would you manage this patient?

CASE 8.14: ANSWERS

1 Describe the XR appearances.

The chest and pelvis XRs show multiple, sclerotic, osteoblastic bone lesions. These are best seen within the ribs and pubic rami. The bones appear generally dense and white (compare with other normal bones in this book). The lungs, hila, and pleural spaces are clear. There is also an angulated pathological subtrochanteric fracture of the right femoral neck, with healed right pubic rami fractures (**Figure 8.14C**). With the given history, these sclerotic lesions are likely to represent breast cancer metastases. Note: deformity of the left breast shadow on CXR owing to previous surgery.

- Sclerotic lesions are areas of increased bone density that result from overactivation of osteoblast cells. The differential diagnosis of multiple sclerotic lesions includes osteoblastic metastases, congenital bone islands, metabolic disorders, infection, and bone infarction.
- Multiple sclerotic or osteoblastic metastases can arise from a number of primary malignancies but are most commonly related to breast or prostate carcinoma. In breast cancer, lytic, sclerotic or mixed lesions may occur, and lesions may also become sclerotic as they heal post treatment.

Always suspect a pathological fracture, especially if the patient has a history of malignancy, when a fracture occurs that does not fit with the mechanism of injury. This area is covered in more detail elsewhere in the book.

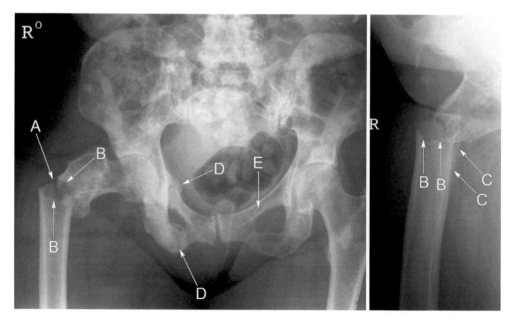

Fig. 8.14C The bone texture of the pelvis is generally abnormal. There is an angulated fracture of the subtrochanteric right femoral neck (A). On both AP and lateral views there is an area of ill-defined bone lysis (destruction) in the adjacent femur (B) with periosteal reaction seen (C). The XR findings and clinical history suggest fracture through an underlying lesion, which looks aggressive on radiology. With the patient history a lytic metastasis is most likely. There are old and healed pathological fractures of the right pubic rami (D). Compare the sclerotic density of the right pubic rami with normal bone density on the left side (E). Note the 'o' placed next to the R marker on the AP XR. Radiographers will place this if they suspect an abnormality/ fracture. This is a sign worth noting and discussing with the radiographer if necessary.

2 What is the diagnosis?

Metastatic breast cancer is the likely diagnosis, with associated pathological fracture of the right hip.

- Breast cancer is the most common site of origin of metastatic deposits in the female skeleton (comparable with prostate cancer in males). Bone is the most common site of recurrence of breast cancer.
- Breast cancer metastases most commonly affect the spine, ribs, pelvis, sternum, and proximal long bones.
- Systemic symptoms may occur, in particular those relating to hypercalcaemia such as bone pain, abdominal pain, renal or biliary stones, and depression (remember the mnemonic, 'stones, bones, groans and psychiatric overtones').

3 What other imaging tests would be justified?

This patient requires urgent orthopaedic referral for management and internal fixation of the right hip fracture, and discussion at the breast MDT meeting. She will need staging. This usually comprises CT chest/abdomen and pelvis, and a radionuclide bone scan. As always adopt an ABCDE approach initially, check bloods (exclude hypercalcaemia from widespread bone metastases, as in this patient) and manage the patient's pain.

- XR is the best first option usually for focal pain. Multiple, confluent, sclerotic, blastic bony lesions are typical of metastatic breast cancer. However, metastases may also present as purely lytic, aggressive, and destructive lesions. You may also see evidence of previous breast surgery on the CXR. It is important to identify both breast shadows in all female patients on CXR. XRs of the femoral necks are also sometimes performed in patients with bony metastatic disease to identify lesions at risk of fracture (these may undergo prophylactic nailing).
- Radionuclide bone scans are used to identify blastic lesions scattered throughout the skeleton, with these appearing as foci of increased radionuclide uptake (**Figure 8.14D**).
- CT is used to further stage the cancer, looking at the lungs, liver, and brain (brain only if symptomatic) particularly for soft tissue metastases, and also axillary and mediastinal nodes.
- MRI of the spine is used if there is clinical evidence to suggest nerve root or spinal cord compression (**Figure 8.14E**).
- PET/CT is useful in some cases for equivocal lesions.

4 How would you manage this patient?

Urgent orthopaedic, breast, and oncology team review with discussion at the breast cancer MDT meeting is required.

- Bone lesions of breast cancer may dramatically improve following bisphosphonate medications and chemotherapy or radiotherapy. Bisphosphonates reduce malignant bone pain and manage hypercalcaemia; they may also delay progressive bone disease. Urgent surgical decompression may be appropriate in some cases. Pre-emptive surgical fixation of the femoral necks should be considered if there are large lesions weakening the weight-bearing bone.

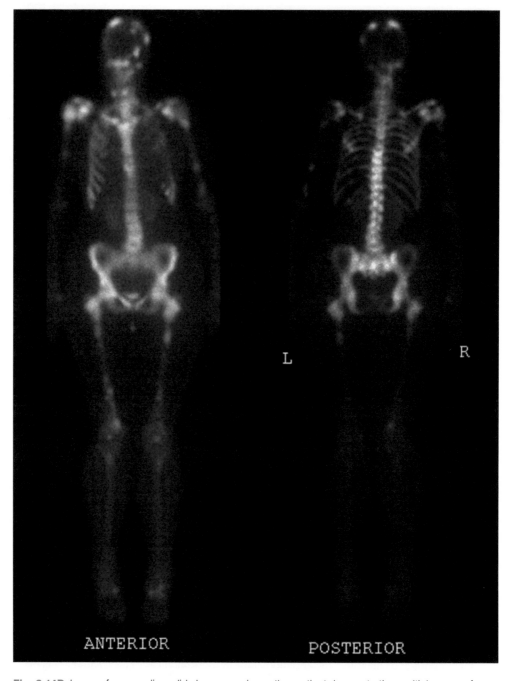

Fig. 8.14D Images from a radionuclide bone scan in another patient demonstrating multiple areas of metastatic increased uptake throughout the pelvis, femora, spine, ribs, and skull.

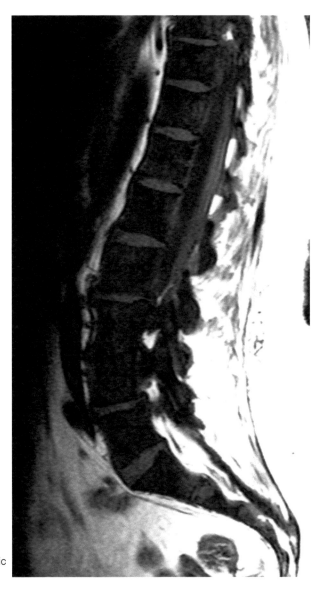

Fig. 8.14E Sagittal T1-weighted MR image of the lumbar spine. Note: the vertebrae are all markedly low signal – black – in keeping with sclerotic metastatic infiltration.

LEARNING POINTS: METASTATIC BREAST CANCER, SCLEROTIC BONE LESIONS

- When you see a woman aged over 40 years with a history of breast cancer and multiple bone lesions, think metastatic breast cancer.
- Potential complications include pain, pathological fracture, neural impingement, and symptoms relating to hypercalcaemia.
- A radionuclide bone scan, staging CT, and MRI spine may also be useful.
- In the exam (and real life!) remember to recommend urgent discussion at the relevant cancer MDT meeting.

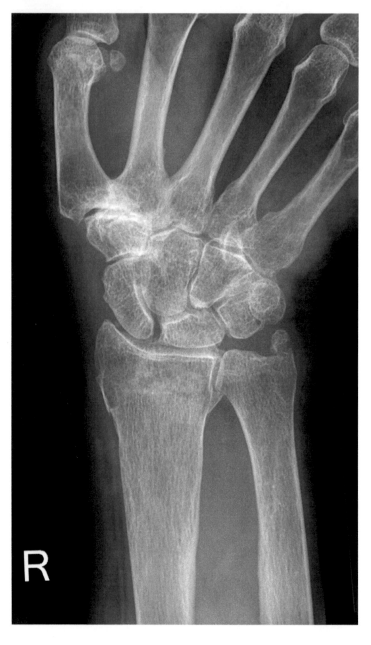

Fig. 8.15A AP XR of the right wrist.

A 68-year-old female presents to the ED having slipped on an icy pavement. She describes having fallen on her outstretched right hand with subsequent pain and swelling at the wrist.

On examination there is soft tissue swelling over the dorsum of the wrist with focal bony tenderness over the distal radius. Careful palpation of the carpal bones and proximal forearm and elbow reveal no further areas of tenderness. There are no signs of neurovascular compromise.

An XR of the wrist is arranged (**Figures 8.15A** and **8.15B**).

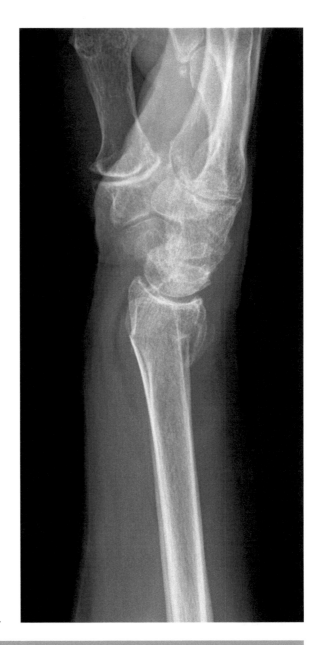

Fig. 8.15B Lateral XR of the right wrist.

CASE 8.15: QUESTIONS

1 Describe the XR findings.
2 What is the diagnosis?
3 What do you think of her bone mineral density?
4 What is happening at the base of the thumb?
5 How would you manage this patient?

CASE 8.15: ANSWERS

1 Describe the XR findings.

There is an extra-articular fracture of the distal radius with dorsal displacement and angulation. The medial fracture line passes proximal to the distal radial ulnar joint (DRUJ). There is also a minimally displaced avulsion fracture of the ulnar styloid tip (**Figures 8.15C** and **8.15D**).

- As with any fracture, it is worth commenting on degree of *displacement, angulation, impaction,* and *shortening.*

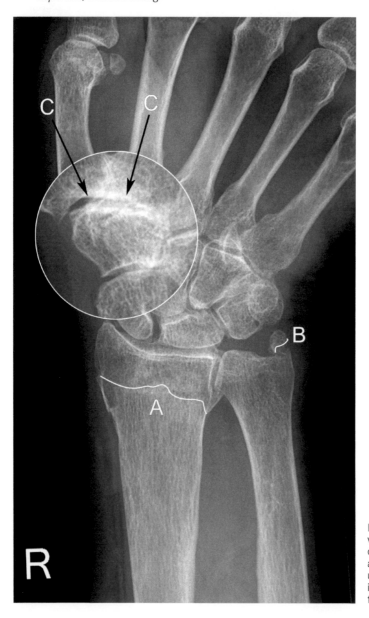

Fig. 8.15C AP XR of the wrist with a Colles fracture of the distal radius (line A) and additional fracture of the ulnar styloid tip (line B). OA is present at the base of the thumb (C).

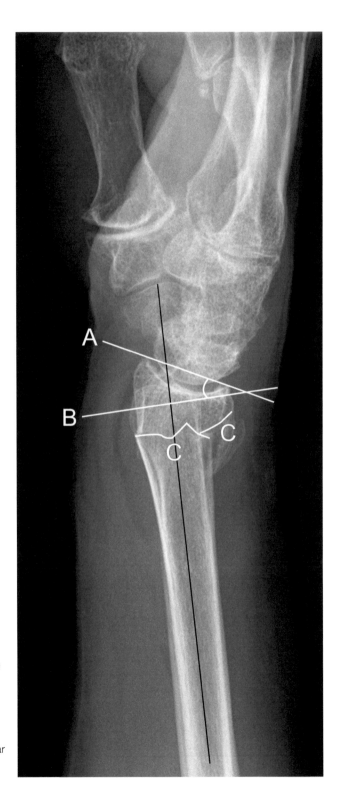

Fig. 8.15D Lateral XR of the wrist with a Colles fracture (C) showing dorsal angulation of the distal radial fracture fragment and some loss of palmar tilt. The palmar tilt angle is formed between a line drawn perpendicular to the long axis of the radius (B) and a second line drawn tangentially to the radial articular surface (A). In women the palmar tilt angle is about 12°; this will be reduced in compression fractures with dorsal displacement of the distal radial fragment. Loss of palmar tilt is also indicative of likely loss of function later on.

- Assessment of a wrist fracture must also include a description of the distal ulna and distal radioulnar joint (DRUJ). It is important to state whether or not there is articular communication of the fracture as this may indicate instability (high risk of secondary displacement). Subluxation or dislocation of the ulnar head as a result of avulsion of the base of the ulnar styloid, or tear of the TFCC or capsular ligaments will need reduction to avoid chronic instability. Avulsions of the tip of the ulnar styloid, as demonstrated in this case, however, are stable. Ulnar styloid fractures are present in up to 50% of cases.
- It is also important to scrutinise for evidence of intra-articular radiocarpal involvement as this may also indicate instability and lead to post-traumatic OA of the wrist. If you are unsure you could recommend a CT scan to look for intra-articular (radiocarpal or DRUJ) involvement and subluxation.
- Other signs of instability include radial shortening (where the distal radius is more proximal than the distal ulna), loss of radial height, and loss of radial inclination (**Figure 8.15E**).

Radial height: two lines are drawn perpendicular to the radial shaft, one along the articular surface and one along the radial styloid tip (T). The distance between them should measure >12 mm and is reduced to <9 mm in distal radial fractures.

Radial inclination: is the angle of the distal radial surface with respect to a line perpendicular to the shaft (A). A normal slope should be 15–25° and is also reduced when fractured.

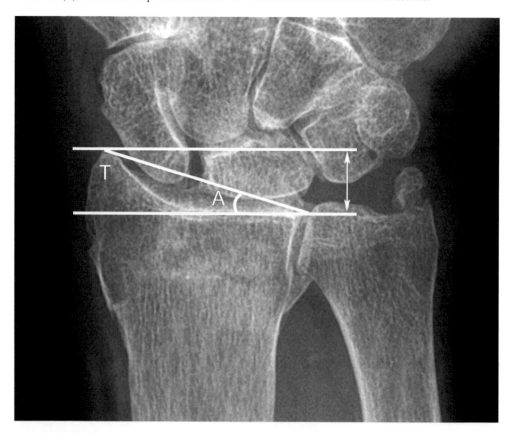

Fig. 8.15E AP XR of the wrist with annotations to illustrate radial height and radial inclination measurements.

2 What is the diagnosis?

These features are diagnostic of a Colles fracture.
  Classic features of a Colles fracture are:

- Transverse fracture of the distal metaphysis of the radius.
- Fracture is proximal to the DRUJ.
- Dorsal displacement and dorsal angulation ('dinner fork deformity').

A Smith's fracture is a reverse Colles; namely there is palmar angulation of the distal radial fracture fragment (caused by a fall on a flexed wrist).

3 What do you think of her bone mineral density?

The bone density appears normal.

- This is important to comment on, even if normal as in this case, as it demonstrates an understanding of the pathogenesis. Colles fracture usually occurs following a fall on an outstretched hand (FOOSH) in elderly postmenopausal women owing to decreased bone mineral density.
- A low energy fracture in the elderly may reflect previously undiagnosed osteoporosis or other metabolic bone disease. Take the opportunity to recommend a DEXA scan to assess bone fragility.

4 What is happening at the base of the thumb?

There is joint space loss and subchondral sclerosis at the thumb CMC joint, in keeping with OA. This is a common location for OA in the hand.

5 How would you manage this patient?

First check that the patient has been examined for:

- Acute carpal tunnel syndrome (weakness or altered sensation in the thumb or index finger).
- Vascular injury (rare).
- Concomitant injury to the ulnar side of the wrist, the elbow, and the carpal bones ('Always assess the joints above and below the known injury'.)

The fracture can then be managed in the ED with closed reduction and cast immobilisation using a 'backslab'. Analgesia and sedation will be required.
  If there are signs of instability (fractures that are displaced, comminuted, or articular), specialist orthopaedic opinion is required with a view to open reduction and internal fixation (ORIF) surgery.

LEARNING POINTS: COLLES FRACTURES

- Colles fractures are extra-articular fractures of the distal radius with dorsal angulation.
- Check for fracture extension into the radiocarpal joint and/or distal radioulnar joints as these will effect stability.
- Check for an ulnar styloid fracture.
- Always comment on bone mineral density.
- Remember to also assess the elbow and the carpal bones for injury.

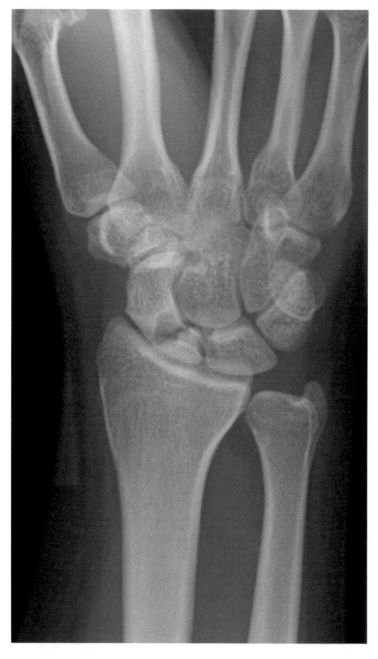

Fig. 8.16A AP view of the wrist.

A 45-year-old female attends the ED having had a FOOSH that day. She has pain and swelling of the right wrist, which was exacerbated when she attempted to grip the steering wheel of her car.

Examination confirms marked swelling of the radial aspect of the right wrist. The patient complains of pain on deep palpation of the anatomical snuff-box.

XRs of the wrist are requested (**Figures 8.16A** and **8.16B**).

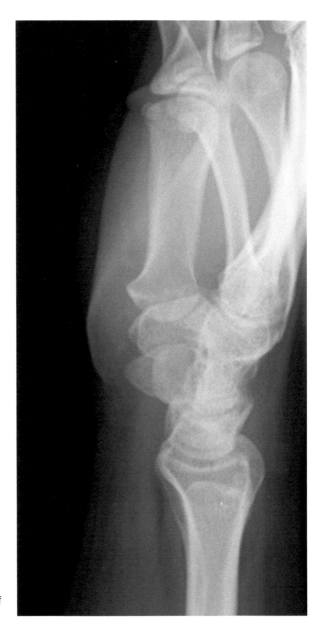

Fig. 8.16B Lateral view of the wrist.

CASE 8.16: QUESTIONS

1 What abnormality is demonstrated?
2 How should this patient be managed?
3 What complications may arise from this injury?
4 Is any further imaging required?
5 Can you identify the carpal bones?

CASE 8.16: ANSWERS

1 What abnormality is demonstrated?

There is a displaced fracture of the waist of the scaphoid bone. The other carpal bones are intact and normally aligned (**Figure 8.16C**).

- Usually when a scaphoid fracture is suspected a dedicated 'scaphoid series' is performed: this comprises AP, lateral, pronated oblique, and supinated oblique views.
- Up to 25% of scaphoid fractures are occult on initial XR. Therefore, if no fracture is seen the patient should still be managed as if a fracture is present and an MRI arranged.

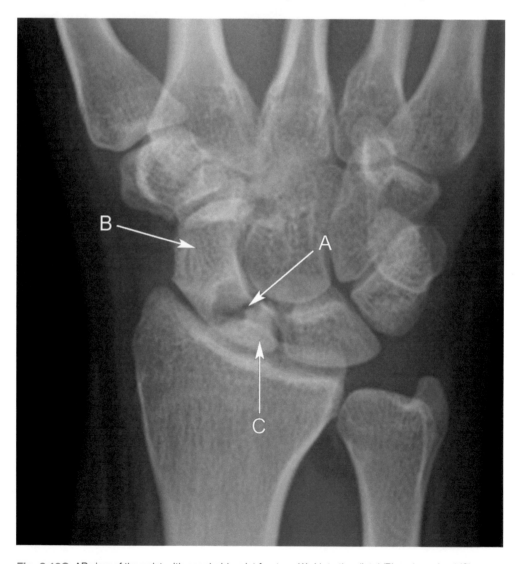

Fig. 8.16C AP view of the wrist with scaphoid waist fracture (A). Note the distal (B) and proximal (C) fracture fragments.

- Transverse fractures through the waist (middle one-third) of the scaphoid are most common, and result from compression of the scaphoid against the distal radius (such as occurs with FOOSH).
- A minority of patients with a scaphoid fracture have either a dislocation or fracture elsewhere. **Figures 8.16D** and **8.16E** show a scaphoid waist fracture with lunate dislocation. This is a rare but serious injury requiring surgical management (trans-scaphoid perilunate dislocation).

2 How should this patient be managed?

The patient should be given adequate analgesia, the wrist immobilised, and an appointment made for review in the fracture clinic.

- The thumb and wrist is immobilised with a below-elbow cast.
- The patient may be reviewed in clinic 2 weeks later with repeat XR. If the fracture is confirmed the cast is reapplied for a further 6–8 weeks. A further XR is taken to check for bone union.

3 What complications may arise from this injury?

Avascular necrosis, nonunion, and osteoarthritis are potential complications of scaphoid fracture.

- The blood supply to the scaphoid enters the bone at the distal one-third. Displaced fractures of the scaphoid waist risk interrupting the blood supply to the proximal fragment and may result in avascular necrosis. The proximal fragment may appear sclerotic on follow-up XR. This is managed surgically with a bone graft.
- Nonunion is the failure of a fracture to heal. OA, pain, and limitation of movement may result.

4 Is any further imaging required?

Further imaging is used in equivocal fractures, to demonstrate avascular necrosis not demonstrated on XR, or to plan for surgery.

- MRI is the most sensitive tool for diagnosing scaphoid fractures and complications and is increasingly being used in place of XR.
- Bone fractures appear as a low signal (dark) line on T1 imaging.
- A bone affected by avascular necrosis will appear as diffuse low T1 signal (dark) owing to replacement of the normal fatty bone marrow.

5 Can you identify the carpal bones?

For nomenclature of the carpal bones see **Figure 8.16D**.

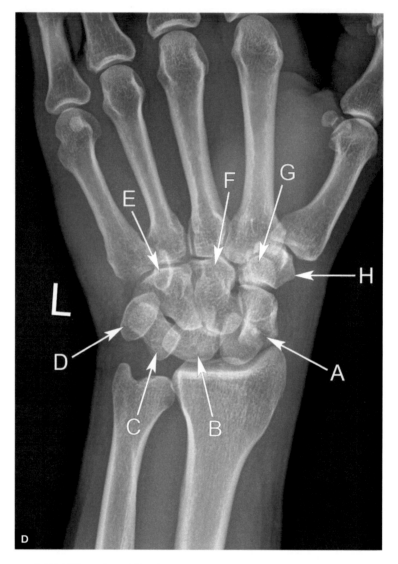

Figs. 8.16D, E AP (**8.16D**) and lateral (**8.16E**) XRs of the wrist in another patient showing a displaced fracture of the scaphoid (A) with palmar rotation of the proximal fragment and lunate and dorsal migration of the capitate. On the lateral view the capitate can be seen to have slipped posteriorly (F) and the lunate has tipped forwards (B). This is a serious injury and requires urgent surgical management. This is a trans-scaphoid perilunate dislocation – on the lateral view the carpus can be seen to have dislocated posteriorly in relation to the lunate/radius. The lunate has slipped/rotated a little and looks triangular on the AP view. *Carpal bones:* scaphoid (+ fracture) (A), lunate (B), triquetral (C), pisiform (D), hamate (+ hook) (E), capitate (F), trapezoid (G), trapezium (base of the thumb) (H).

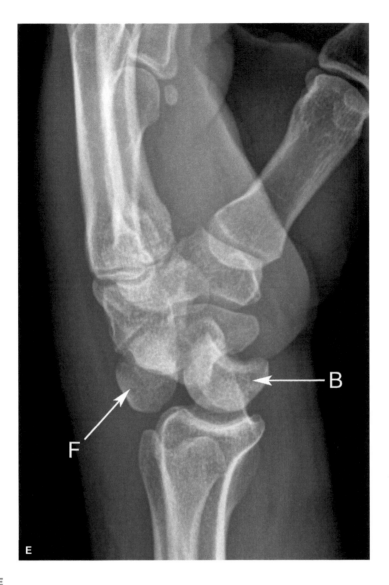

Fig. 8.16E

LEARNING POINTS: SCAPHOID FRACTURE

- Scaphoid fracture is a common injury resulting from a FOOSH – it is frequently occult on the standard XR series.
- Scaphoid fracture should be suspected where there is an appropriate clinical history and anatomical snuffbox tenderness.
- If there is adequate clinical suspicion but a normal XR, the patient may either proceed to MRI or be managed as a fracture, reviewed in fracture clinic in 2 weeks, and a repeat XR taken.
- Avascular necrosis and nonunion are recognised complications of scaphoid fractures that require operative management.

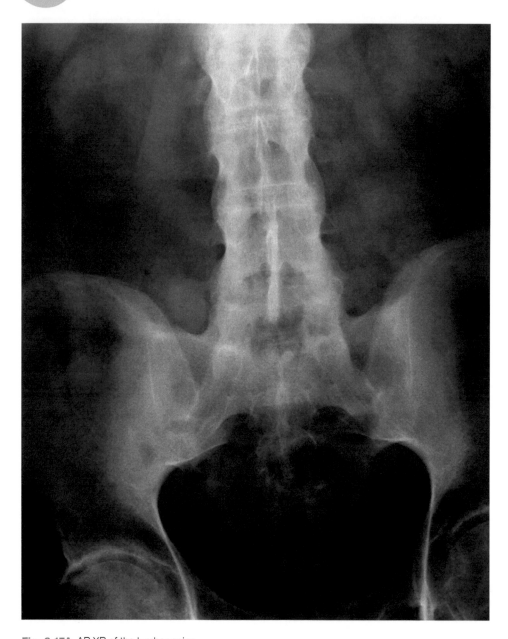

Fig. 8.17A AP XR of the lumbar spine.

A 65-year-old male with a long history of back pain and stiffness comes to see his GP with worsening lower back pain, which came on as the patient attempted to stand up.

Examination reveals some generalised tenderness over the lumbar spine but neurological examination is normal. The patient is referred for XR of the lumbar spine (**Figures 8.17A** and **8.17B**).

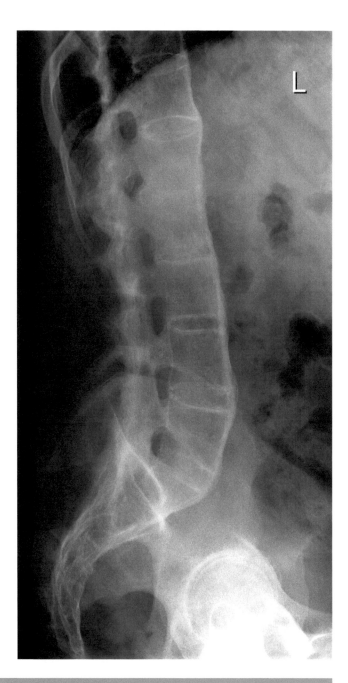

Fig. 8.17B Lateral XR of the lumbar spine.

CASE 8.17: QUESTIONS

1 What are the key XR findings?
2 What is the underlying diagnosis?
3 What other imaging may be helpful?
4 What are the complications of this condition?

CASE 8.17: ANSWERS

1 What are the key XR findings?

The sacroiliac joints are not clearly visible (**Figures 8.17C** and **8.17D**), with a thin sclerotic line only present. The joints have fused.

Abnormalities are also seen in the lumbar spine:

- Vertebral body squaring.
- Diffuse interspinous ligament calcification, 'dagger spine'.
- Diffuse syndesmophyte ankyloses, 'bamboo spine'.
- Diffuse ossification of spinal ligaments.

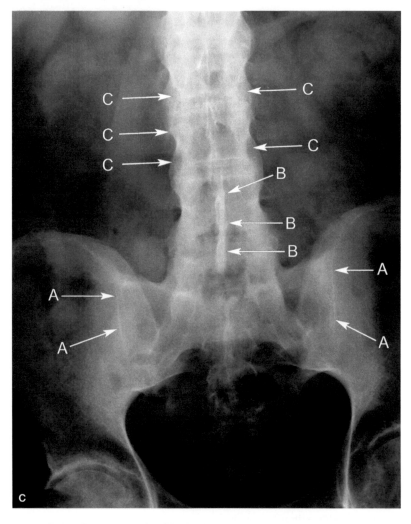

Figs. 8.17C, D AP (**8.17C**) and lateral (**8.17D**) XRs of the lumbar spine demonstrating sclerosis and fusion of the sacroiliac joints (A). There is interspinous ligamentous calcification (arrows B) 'dagger spine' and also flowing syndesmophyte calcification and ankylosis seen on both views (arrows C, 'bamboo spine'). No fractures are visible.

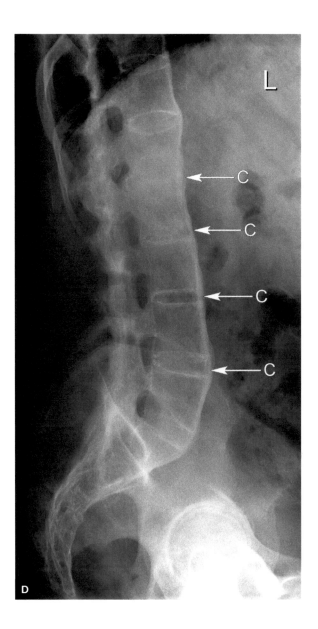

Fig. 8.17D

2 What is the underlying diagnosis?

The diagnosis is ankylosing spondylitis. The fused sacroiliac joints indicate endstage disease. Earlier in the disease process the joints may widen secondary to active inflammation but will then become progressively more erosive and sclerotic.

Ankylosing spondylitis is a seronegative spondyloarthropathy with a male predilection (male:female = 3:1), which usually manifests in the third decade; 90% of Caucasian patients are HLA-B27 positive. The disease commonly involves the spine and sacroiliac joints but may also affect other small and large joints. Sacroiliitis, symmetrical and bilateral, is the commonest first manifestation. Early spondylitis in the spine is associated with small erosions at the corners of vertebral bodies, with sclerosis as they heal (Romanus lesions). Progressive erosion leads to sclerosis, fusion, and ankylosis.

3 What other imaging may be helpful?

MRI is the technique of choice for demonstrating the early changes of sacroiliitis (**Figure 8.17E**). CT is useful in the assessment of spinal fractures to which these patients are prone. Bone scintigraphy has a role in equivocal cases.

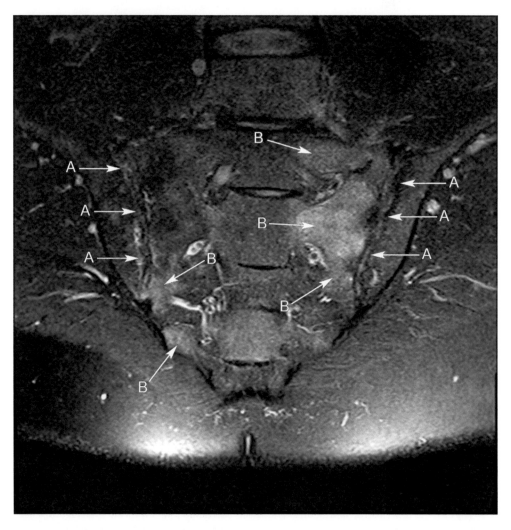

Fig. 8.17E MRI of the sacrum in another patient with early stage ankylosing spondylitis. This is a STIR sequence (short tau inversion recovery): do not worry overly about the physics or nature of the sequence, it is designed to highlight fluid/oedema and is very useful in assessing early joint inflammatory changes. This image is in the coronal plane and shows the sacroiliac joints (A). The joints have rather irregular margins and there is significant adjacent high signal (white) oedema change adjacent to the joints, indicative of active inflammation (B).

4 What are the complications of this condition?

Ankylosing spondylitis is associated with a number of potentially serious complications.

- The diffusely ossified spine is brittle and highly susceptible to pathological fracture. Fractures are often highly unstable and can occur with only minimal trauma. Cervical spine fractures are particularly hazardous and can cause cord compression/transection.
- Other associations include:
  - Anterior uveitis.
  - Inflammatory bowel disease.
  - Interstitial lung fibrosis (1% of patients, predilection for upper lobes).
  - Aortic valve disease and aortitis.
  - Amyloidosis.

LEARNING POINTS: ANKYLOSING SPONDYLITIS

- Ankylosing spondylitis is a cause of low back pain, which can radiate to the lower limbs or groin.
- The condition is more common in males and is associated with HLA-B27 positivity.
- MRI is the imaging technique of choice, it is nonionising, and can detect early stage sacroiliitis,
- The ankylosed spine is brittle and prone to unstable, pathological fracture.

Neurology cases

9

VINCENT HELYAR AND EDWARD SELLON

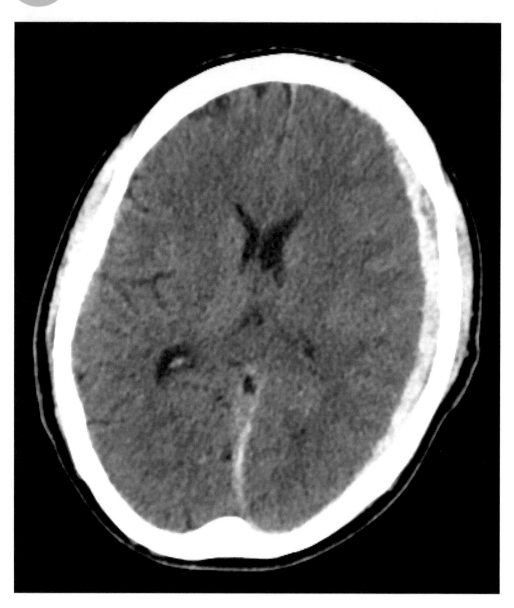

Fig. 9.1A Unenhanced (noncontrast) axial CT image of the brain at the level of the frontal horns of the lateral ventricles.

A 76-year-old male presents to the ED with new-onset slurred speech and right-sided facial and limb weakness. He lives on his own in a warden-controlled flat and has had a series of falls, according to his daughter.

On examination, there is no sign of a head injury and the patient is alert, although mildly disorientated. There is, however, a clear motor weakness on the right side of the body affecting the face, arm, and leg. There is also expressive dysphasia. Routine blood tests are unremarkable. A CT scan of the head is arranged (**Figure 9.1A**).

CASE 9.1: QUESTIONS

1 What are your provisional differential diagnoses given the history and examination findings?
2 What findings are shown in **Figure 9.1A**?
3 How should this patient be managed?

CASE 9.1: ANSWERS

1 What are your provisional differential diagnoses given the history and examination findings?

The main differential diagnoses to consider are transient ischaemic attack/stroke and intracranial haemorrhage. The focal neurological signs are nonspecific.

- In order to determine the diagnosis and to rule out haemorrhage, a CT scan of the head is required. The presence of focal neurology indicates this scan should be performed urgently.
- The CT scan will be initially performed without IV contrast ('unenhanced') to allow detection of acute haemorrhage, which may be obscured by contrast.

2 What findings are shown in Figure 9.1A?

CT shows a shallow, hyperdense extra-axial (i.e. not within neuroaxis or brain parenchyma) collection overlying the left cerebral hemisphere (**Figure 9.1B**). The appearance is typical for a

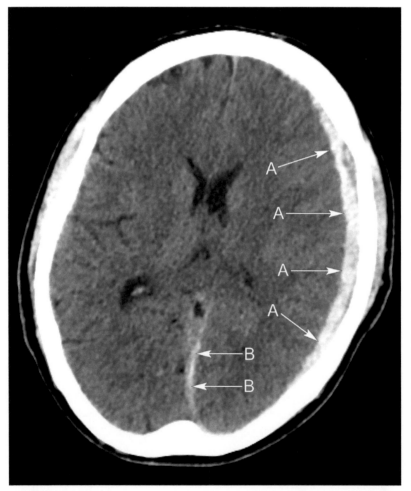

Fig. 9.1B
Unenhanced axial CT of the brain demonstrating a thin hyperdense collection overlying the left cerebral hemisphere (A) and extending along the posterior falx cerebri (B) in keeping with subdural haematoma. There is also some mass effect, with midline and ventricular shift to the right. Note also the sulcal effacement of the left cerebral hemisphere, and the normal right sulci.

subdural collection. Note: it has a concave inner margin, not biconvex as is seen in extradural haematoma, it overlies most of one hemisphere, is not contained by the sutures of the cranium, and pushes away the brain parenchyma in an undulating fashion.

- Acute intracranial blood appears white, hyperdense on CT. As blood matures it becomes isodense to brain by 7–10 days, and by about 1 month blood methaemoglobin converts to haemosiderin and appears dark and hypodense when compared with the brain. The appearances may be confusing as rebleeds are common in subdural haematoma and acute blood can mix with older blood products (**Figure 9.1C**).
- Subdural haematoma is common and often caused by laceration of the superficial bridging cortical veins. The risk of haemorrhage is increased in those with reduced brain volume (e.g. old age, chronic alcohol abuse, dementia) owing to stretching of the bridging veins.
- Subdural haematoma may be spontaneous; however, it is often precipitated by trauma or anticoagulation.

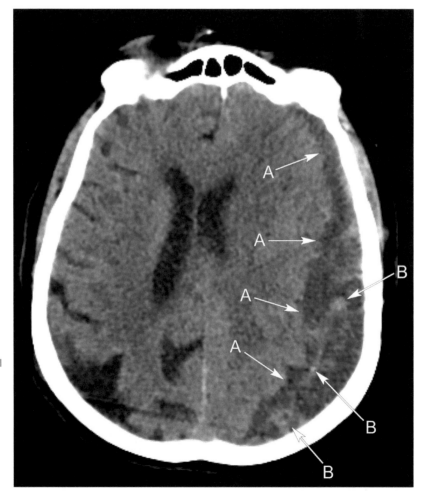

Fig. 9.1C Unenhanced axial CT in another patient showing maturation of a subdural haematoma (A). This left subdural haematoma is also associated with mass effect but note the mixed density; it is mature, hypodense but contains internal high density rebleeds (B).

3 How should this patient be managed?

These findings require urgent action. You should seek senior advice and speak to a neurosurgeon for their opinion.

- The mortality of subdural haematoma in this age group is about 65%.
- The morbidity is also high with many patients being unable to return to their previous level of function, especially if the haematoma was severe enough to warrant surgery.
- Craniotomy may be considered where the depth of acute blood measures >5 mm or where there is significant mass effect.

LEARNING POINTS: SUBDURAL HAEMATOMA

- Subdural haematoma may follow minor head trauma and is more common in the elderly or those with a history of alcohol abuse.
- The presence of mass effect and midline shift may require urgent neurosurgical intervention.
- Rebleed is common with subdural haematoma. Acute and chronic blood products give a mixed density appearance (i.e. areas of high density acute blood with low density old blood).

Case 9.2

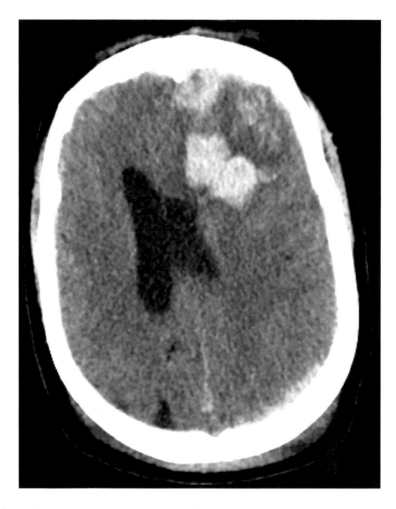

Fig. 9.2A Axial unenhanced CT of the brain at the level of the bodies of the lateral ventricles.

A 22-year-old male is brought unconscious to the ED by ambulance in the early hours of a Sunday morning. The patient smells strongly of alcohol and was found by passers-by at the bottom of a flight of stairs. No further history is available.

Initial examination reveals a Glasgow Coma Scale (GCS) of 8 (E2 V2 M4) (E = eye opening; V = verbal response; M = motor response) and signs of an injury to the back of the head. While the anaesthetic registrar intubates the patient you expose the patient to complete your examination. You palpate the occiput and find a large swelling, which feels 'boggy.' The patient is referred for CT (**Figure 9.2A**), intubated, and his cervical spine immobilised prior to imaging.

CASE 9.2: QUESTIONS

1 What is your provisional clinical diagnosis? What additional imaging should you request?
2 What is shown in **Figure 9.2A**?

3 What is the pathophysiology for this abnormality?
4 What will you do next?

CASE 9.2: ANSWERS

1 What is your provisional clinical diagnosis? What additional imaging should you request?

The history is of a head injury in a young, intoxicated patient with resulting severe impairment of consciousness. Your first thought should be that of an intracranial haemorrhage.

- The boggy swelling overlying the occiput most likely represents a haematoma. A depressed skull fracture could also feel boggy.
- An emergency CT scan of the brain and cervical spine are required; these should be reported urgently.

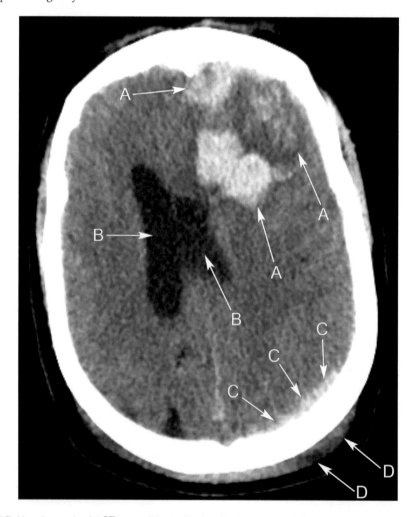

Fig. 9.2B Unenhanced axial CT scan of the brain showing hyperdense left frontal lobe parenchymal haemorrhage (A) with associated oedema and mass effect. The bodies of the lateral ventricles are distorted and displaced to the right (B). There is some compression of the body of the left lateral ventricle and dilatation of the body of the right lateral ventricle. Shallow left posterior subdural haematoma (C) and overlying soft-tissue swelling (D) are also demonstrated.

- Imaging of the cervical spine is mandated owing to the impaired consciousness and mechanism of injury. Further CT imaging of the rest of the body would be advised if the patient had fallen from a significant height (e.g. >5 steps).

2 What is shown in Figure 9.2A?

Figures 9.2A and **9.2B** show extensive hyperdense material in the left frontal lobe representing acute intra-axial (i.e. parenchymal) haemorrhage.

- There is adjacent oedema and significant mass effect, which causes partial effacement of the anterior horn of the left lateral ventricle.
- There is also hyperdense material posteriorly, which overlies the left occipital lobe, consistent with an acute subdural haematoma.
- There is superficial soft-tissue swelling overlying the left occipital bone, which is the swelling felt when palpated (**Figure 9.2C**).

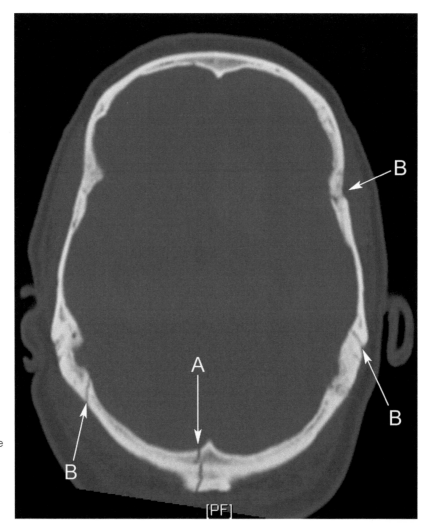

Fig. 9.2C Unenhanced axial CT scan of the brain slightly inferior to that in **9.2B** displayed on a bone window setting. Note the occipital bone fracture (A). Normal sutures (B) should not to be confused with fractures.

3 What is the pathophysiology for this abnormality?

The pattern of injury is the result of trauma to the back of the head. This is demonstrated by the site of the fracture and soft-tissue swelling.

- The pattern of parenchymal injuries is known as 'coup' (same side of the brain as the trauma) and 'contrecoup' (on the opposite side of the brain to the trauma).
- Coup injury is caused by the direct effect of the trauma, while contrecoup is usually the result of brain shaking.
- Parenchymal haemorrhage arising from trauma typically occurs where the brain is thrown against bone, most commonly seen in the inferior frontal and temporal lobes.

4 What will you do next?

The patient should be discussed urgently with the neurosurgical team with a view to transfer to a neurosurgical unit for further management. This may involve surgical decompression of the haematoma and also shunting of the lateral ventricles.

LEARNING POINTS: INTRACEREBRAL HAEMATOMA

- When you spot an intracranial haemorrhage, comment on any mass effect and search for an underlying fracture, or possible lesion if no history of trauma.
- The most common sites of intra-axial haemorrhage following head injury are the inferior frontal lobes and inferior temporal lobes.
- The site of the haematoma may be on the same (coup) or opposite (contrecoup) side to the site of trauma.

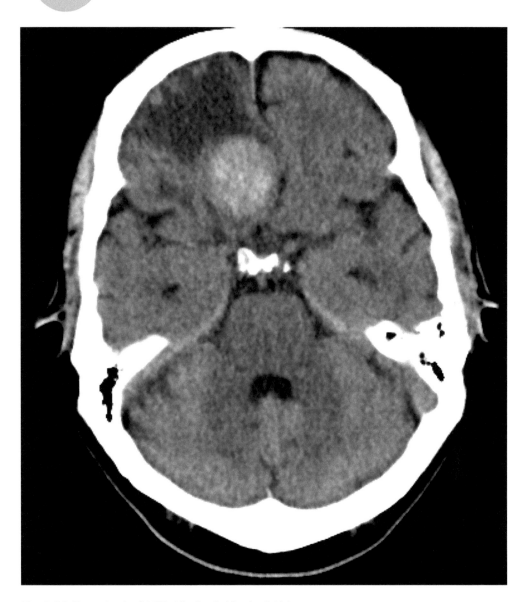

Fig. 9.3A Precontrast axial CT at the level of the frontal lobes.

A 56-year-old female visits her GP with a long history of headache and visual disturbance. More recently her son has noticed some short-term loss of memory and erratic behaviour. The patient is concerned that she might have dementia.

Your examination reveals near blindness in the right eye and diffuse weakness on the left side of the body. There is evidence of both anterograde and retrograde amnesia.

Routine blood tests are unremarkable. The patient is referred for urgent CT of the brain (**Figures 9.3A–9.3C**).

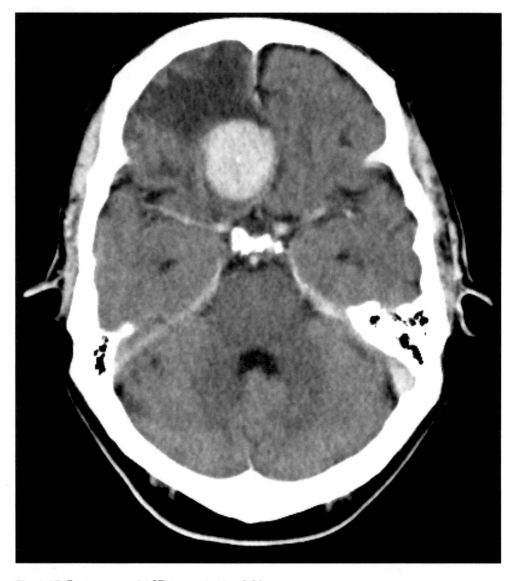

Fig. 9.3B Postcontrast axial CT at same level as **9.3A**.

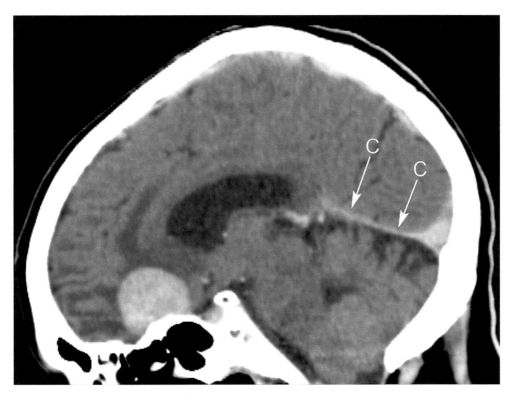

Fig. 9.3C Precontrast midline brain sagittal CT reconstruction.

CASE 9.3: QUESTIONS

1 What differential diagnoses would you consider from the history and examination?
2 What other imaging tests are indicated?
3 How would you describe the abnormality shown in **Figures 9.3A–9.3C**? What is the normal structure 'C'?
4 Do you think this pathology has developed slowly or quickly?
5 How should this patient be managed?

CASE 9.3: ANSWERS

1 What differential diagnoses would you consider from the history and examination?

The main concerns are those of a brain tumour (primary or secondary), while dementia, stroke, and chronic subdural haematoma are also possibilities.

- The presence of focal neurology makes dementia less likely.
- The insidious onset of symptoms makes a stroke less likely.

2 What other imaging tests are indicated?

A CT scan of the brain is usually requested in the first instance, especially if stroke or bleed are in the differential diagnosis. If tumour is suspected CT should be performed before and after an IV infusion of contrast. A precontrast scan is required to assess for the presence an infarct or, if a

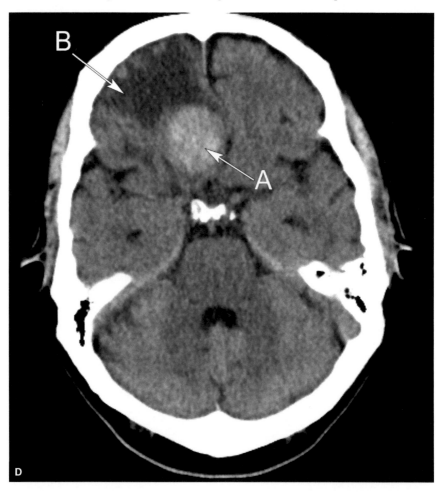

Figs. 9.3D, E Precontrast (**9.3D**) and postcontrast (**9.3E**) CT scans of the brain. There is a large and rounded lesion in the frontal region to the right of the midline (A); on the sagittal image this is seen to arise from the floor of the anterior cranial fossa (**Figure 9.3C**). Precontrast this lesion is mildly hyperdense – note the adjacent low density tumoural type oedema (B) – and the lesion enhances avidly and homogeneously postcontrast.

lesion is present, to assess lesional haemorrhage/calcification and to compare with the postcontrast images to see if there is lesional enhancement.

A contrast-enhanced MRI scan may also be requested (usually following specialist neurology review). This would be a useful investigation if the CT scan is normal (as it is more sensitive for hyperacute strokes and small mass lesions than CT) or to further characterise a lesion if the CT scan is positive. If CT and MRI demonstrate possible intracranial malignancy, then further imaging via CT chest/abdomen and pelvis may be undertaken to look for a possible primary tumour.

3 How would you describe the abnormality shown in Figures 9.3A–C? What is the normal structure 'C'?

There is a large, circumscribed mass lesion in the right frontal region with surrounding perilesional oedema (**Figures 9.3D** and **9.3E**). There is shift of midline structures to the left but no significant effacement of the CSF spaces on the left. The mass shows homogeneous enhancement after IV contrast (it appears more dense in **Figure 9.3E** than **9.3D**).

- The lesion arises from the floor of the anterior cranial fossa. The lesion is therefore likely to be extra-axial (i.e. not arising from the brain parenchyma itself).

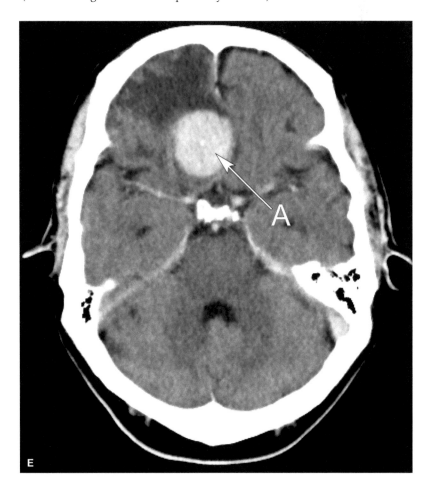

Fig. 9.3E

- Structure 'C' (**Figure 9.3C**) is the straight sinus overlying the tentorium cerebelli, below which lies the cerebellum. Anything above the tentorium cerebelli is described as being 'supratentorial' in location.

4 Do you think this pathology has developed slowly or quickly?

The extent of oedema (relatively small amount) in relation to the size of the lesion may suggest that this is a low-grade tumour (i.e. slow growing). The patient history supports this.

- Homogeneous contrast enhancement is also more often a feature of slow growing lesions. Fast growing lesions tend to outstrip neovascularisation, so parts of the tumour become ischaemic and then necrotic. This produces a heterogeneous pattern of enhancement postcontrast.
- Areas of necrosis are low density (dark) on CT.
- Overall, the appearance of this lesion is typical for a meningioma.

   Meningiomas are the second most common primary brain tumour after glioma. They are more common in women aged 50–60 years.

- 95% of meningiomas are low-grade (benign) tumours and 90% are supratentorial.
- They may cause thickening of the adjacent bone (hyperostosis) and a dural tail of enhancement is a typical feature.

5 How should this patient be managed?

The patient should be referred urgently to a specialist neurosurgical centre for discussion at a neuro-oncology MDT meeting.

- The MDT meeting would include a neuroradiologist, a neurosurgeon, a neurooncologist, a neuropathologist, and specialist nurses.
- The purpose of the MDT meeting is to agree a management plan. This might include conservative measures (e.g. follow-up imaging) or active treatment (e.g. surgery to remove the tumour) depending on the age, condition, and wishes of the patient.

LEARNING POINTS: BRAIN TUMOUR, MENINGIOMA

- Postcontrast CT scans of the brain are useful to diagnose brain tumours and brain abscesses. A precontrast scan is also performed for comparison and to exclude stroke or acute blood.
- Low-grade tumours tend to have a more homogeneous enhancement pattern while high-grade tumours enhance heterogeneously.
- A meningioma is a relatively common, low-grade, extra-axial tumour associated with hyperostosis and a dural tail of enhancement.

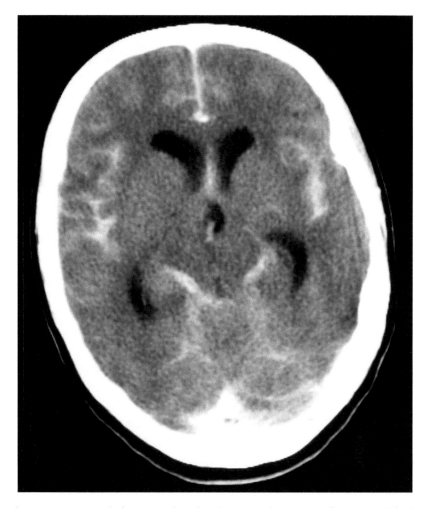

Fig. 9.4A
Unenhanced
CT brain at
the level of the
basal cisterns
and frontal
horns of the
lateral ventricles
performed
at the time of
presentation to
hospital.

A 45-year-old male arrives in an ambulance intubated to the ED with a history (from his wife) of prior sudden-onset 'thunderclap' headache. This had been followed by several episodes of vomiting, a seizure, and loss of consciousness. A collateral history reveals that the patient receives haemodialysis three times a week owing to end stage renal failure caused by 'kidney cysts'. There is also a history of hypertension.

On examination you find brisk reflexes and severe impairment of consciousness with GCS 6 (E2 V2 M2). Baseline observations are stable and he is apyrexial. There is neck rigidity and up-going plantar reflexes. You request a CT scan of the brain (**Figure 9.4A**).

CASE 9.4: QUESTIONS

1 What does the clinical scenario suggest?
2 What is the diagnosis as shown in
   Figure 9.4A?
3 What further investigations might you
   consider?
4 How should this patient be managed?

CASE 9.4: ANSWERS

1 What does the clinical scenario suggest?

Sudden onset of severe headache is suggestive of a subarachnoid haemorrhage in this patient. This provisional diagnosis is supported by subsequent events (collapse, vomiting, and seizures), which suggest raised intracranial pressure (ICP).

- 'Kidney cysts' are also a clue – these are clearly severe as the patient is on dialysis and likely represent polycystic kidney disease (PKD), which is associated with intracerebral 'berry' aneurysms in up to 7% of cases.
- 85% of saccular aneurysms occur in the anterior circulation. Saccular aneurysms (berry aneurysms) are the most common type of cerebral aneurysm and appear as a round outpouching of the vessel.
- Only 50% of patients with an aneurysmal subarachnoid haemorrhage are alive at 6 months.

2 What is the diagnosis as shown in Figure 9.4A?

CT shows an extensive subarachnoid haemorrhage (hyperdense fresh blood) lying within the basal cisterns and the sulcal spaces of both hemispheres (**Figure 9.4B**).

- Also, the CT section shows dilatation of the temporal horns of the lateral ventricles indicative of early hydrocephalus. Hydrocephalus in this instance is most likely caused by obstruction of CSF flow by blood products.
- Smaller subarachnoid bleeds may be occult on CT (10%). Such cases should be considered for lumbar puncture and CSF examination for xanthochromia where appropriate, assuming no clinical evidence of raised ICP, which may be underestimated on CT.

3 What further investigations might you consider?

Further imaging is required to look for the underlying cause of haemorrhage. The history of PKD suggests that the likely cause here is an underlying intracranial aneurysm.

- A CT angiogram of the intracerebral vessels should be considered in order to demonstrate the location of the aneurysm.
- MR angiography is also used in some cases.
- Further investigations should be performed in a centre that offers interventional neuroradiology and neurosurgery, as part of the work-up prior to potential endovascular coiling or surgical clipping.

   Figure 9.5C shows an MR image of a cerebral aneurysm in another patient.

4 How should this patient be managed?

You should expect to receive an urgent verbal and then written report from the radiologist. Urgent transfer to a neurosurgical centre is required.

- The patient is at risk of brain stem herniation (so called 'coning') due to cerebral oedema and obstructive hydrocephalus. Hydrocephalus may be managed by placement of an intraventricular shunt.

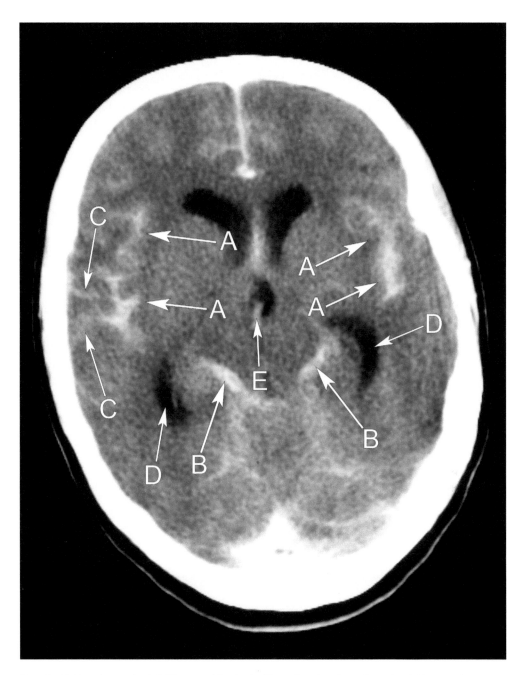

Fig. 9.4B Unenhanced axial CT scan of the brain. There is extensive subarachnoid haemorrhage with blood seen in the basal cisterns (B), Sylvian fissures (A), and within the sulci (C). Note: there is also dilatation of the temporal horns of the lateral ventricles indicative of early hydrocephalus (D). The third ventricle also appears dilated (usually slit-like) and contains a small focus of intraventricular haemorrhage (E).

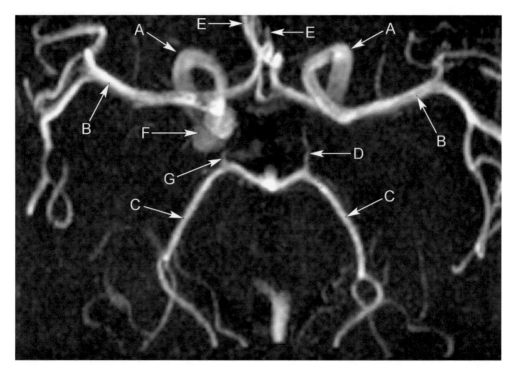

Fig. 9.4C Axial MR angiogram image of the circle of Willis in another patient. Internal carotid (A), middle cerebral (B), and posterior cerebral (C) arteries are shown, together with the left posterior communicating artery (D) and anterior cerebral arteries (E). Note: aneurysm (F) arising from the right posterior communicating artery (G).

- The risk of rebleed is nearly 20% in the first 14 days post haemorrhage and carries a high mortality (80%). The risk of rebleeding is reduced by medical measures and by aneurysm coiling or clipping.
- Aneurysm coiling is often preferred to open surgery. It is a procedure performed by interventional neuroradiologists with access to the arterial vasculature via the common femoral artery.
- 25% of those surviving a subarachnoid haemorrhage have a permanent neurological deficit.

LEARNING POINTS: SUBARACHNOID HAEMORRHAGE

- Subarachnoid haemorrhage is characterised by haemorrhage in the subarachnoid space (sulci and CSF spaces).
- Small subarachnoid haemorrhages may be occult on CT. Check the posterior aspects of the lateral ventricles for a small dense fluid level.
- Subarachnoid haemorrhage carries a high mortality and morbidity with a minority of patients able to return to their previous level of functioning.

Case 9.5

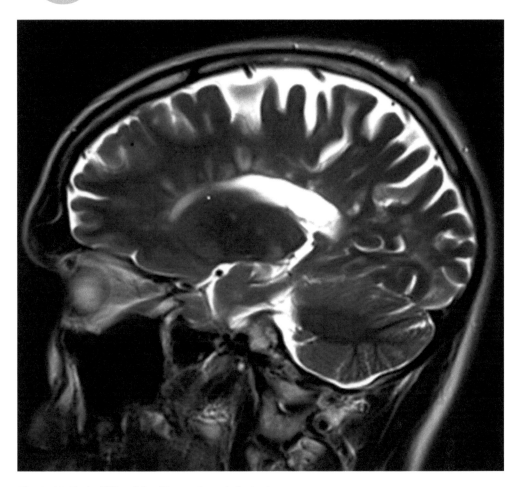

Fig. 9.5A Sagittal T2-weighted image through the brain.

A 29-year-old female is referred to the neurology clinic complaining of several weeks of muscle cramps and episodes of urinary incontinence. Your history reveals that the patient has also been feeling more tired than usual recently. You notice that the patient suffered an episode of optic neuritis 18 months ago but was lost to follow-up.

A neurological examination reveals mild loss of power in the lower limbs, more pronounced on the left. There is increased tone on the left and plantars are up-going bilaterally. The reflexes are brisk. The retinas have a slightly pale appearance on ophthalmoscopy but are otherwise unremarkable. Routine bloods performed by the GP are normal.

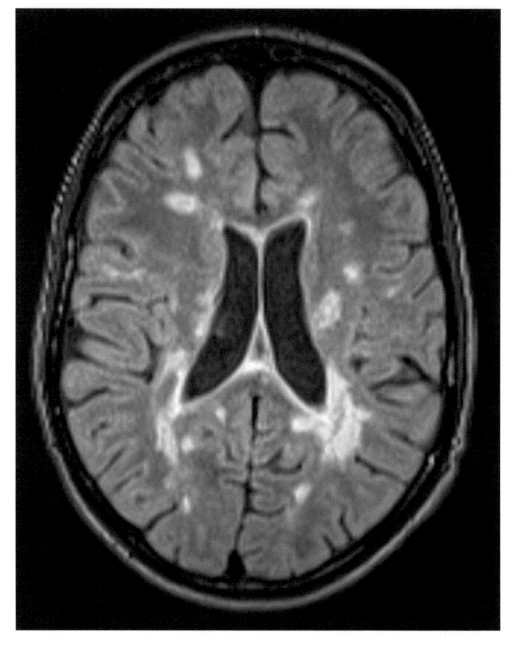

Fig. 9.5B Axial FLAIR sequence through the brain at the level of the bodies of the lateral ventricles.

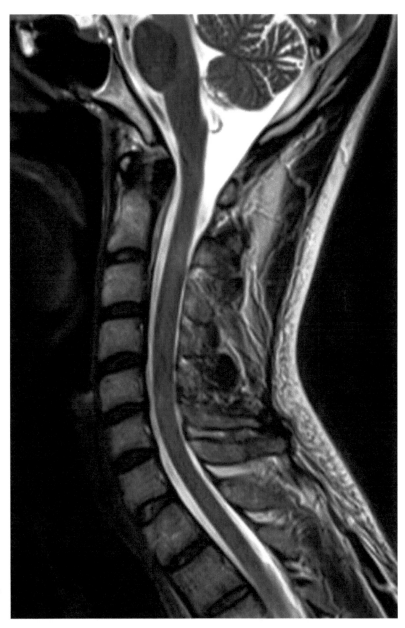

Fig. 9.5C Sagittal T2-weighted image of the cervical spine.

CASE 9.5: QUESTIONS

1 What is your working diagnosis? What other investigations would you consider?
2 What do the MR images demonstrate (**Figures 9.5A–9.5C**)?
3 Where are the abnormalities in **Figures 9.5A** and **9.5B** located? How would you describe these?
4 What additional abnormality is demonstrated in **Figure 9.5C**?
5 What is the likely course of this disease?

CASE 9.5: ANSWERS

1 What is your working diagnosis? What other investigations would you consider?

The clinical presentation is typical for demyelination as occurring in multiple sclerosis (MS), an immune-mediated inflammatory disease that attacks myelinated axons in the CNS. Characteristically the disease produces symptomatic episodes that occur months or years apart and in varying anatomical locations. MRI is the imaging technique of choice for diagnosing demyelinating lesions in the brain and spine, and for monitoring response to treatment.

A variety of other tests will be performed including visual evolved potentials and CSF examination on lumbar puncture for oligoclonal bands of IgG production. The diagnosis ultimately is made clinically.

2 What do the MR images demonstrate (Figures 9.5A–9.5C)?

The MR images demonstrate multiple high signal lesions in the supratentorial white matter in a periventricular distribution with further high signal lesions seen in the cervical cord (**Figures 9.5D** and **9.5E**). These appearances are typical for plaques of demyelination.

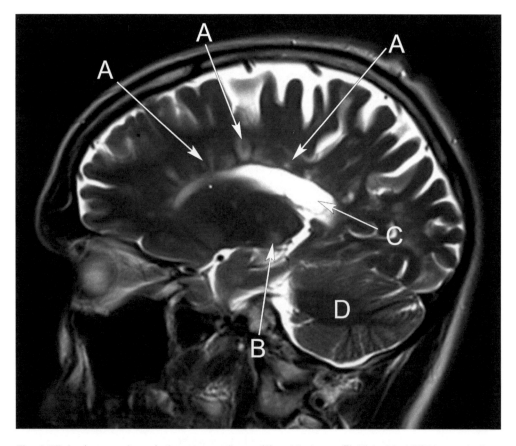

Fig. 9.5D Lesions are shown in the corpus callosum (A) and thalamus (B). High signal CSF is seen in the lateral ventricle (C) and around the cerebellum (D).

3 Where are the abnormalities in Figures 9.5A and 9.5B located? How would you describe these?

The intracranial lesions labelled in this patient (**Figure 9.5D**) are found in a classic location for MS on the underneath of the corpus callosum, known as the 'callosal septal interface.'

- Typical for MS, there are multiple high T2 signal white matter lesions in a periventricular distribution.
- The lesions are predominantly round, oval or flame shaped.

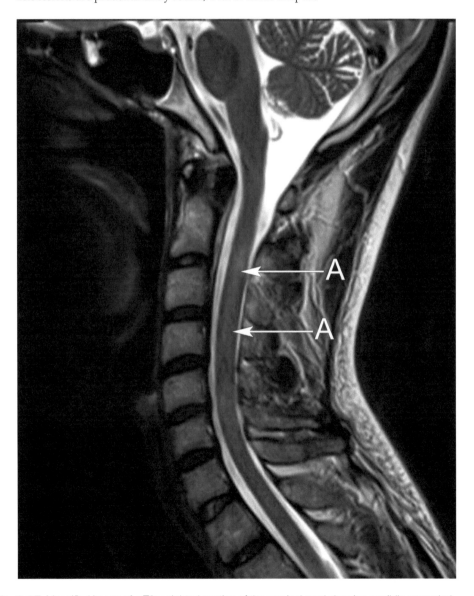

Fig. 9.5E Magnified image of a T2-weighted section of the cervical cord showing a mildly expanded cervical cord and a high signal focus of demyelination in the cord (A). Note: CSF around the cord appears high signal, white on T2 weighting.

- The arrangement of multiple lesions along the underside of the corpus callosum is a classic feature of MS known as 'Dawson's fingers'.
- The lesions represent foci of demyelination (destruction of the myelin sheath), known as plaques. Foci of active inflammation may enhance after contrast administration.
- Aggressive MS, known as tumefactive MS, can resemble a primary brain tumour.

4 What additional abnormality is demonstrated in Figure 9.5C?

Figures 9.5C and **9.5E** show focal high signal on T2 weighting located in the cervical cord, consistent with a plaque of demyelination. The cervical cord is mildly expanded at this level owing to oedema.

5 What is the likely course of this disease?

Modern diagnostic criteria for MS require the following:

- Objective evidence of two separate CNS lesions compatible with MS and separated by both space and time.
- Other causes for CNS lesions to have been excluded.

A unilateral and painful optic neuritis is a common first presentation, as in this patient.

MS is of unknown aetiology, more common in women with increasing prevalence. It is thought to be autoimmune with immune system malfunction destroying myelin.

The most common subtype of the disease is known as relapsing remitting MS, which accounts for about 85% of cases.

- Treatment is aimed both at the underlying autoimmune disease involving the myelin sheaths and at symptom control.
- Life expectancy is not shortened significantly by most forms of MS. However, rare fulminant subtypes can be rapidly fatal.

LEARNING POINTS: MULTIPLE SCLEROSIS

- MS is a diagnosis made by combining clinical findings, imaging, and other tests (e.g. CSF analysis, evoked potentials).
- MRI is also used for monitoring the disease and assessing response to treatment.
- The periventricular white matter is affected most commonly by MS plaques: the characteristic MRI appearance is known as Dawson's fingers.

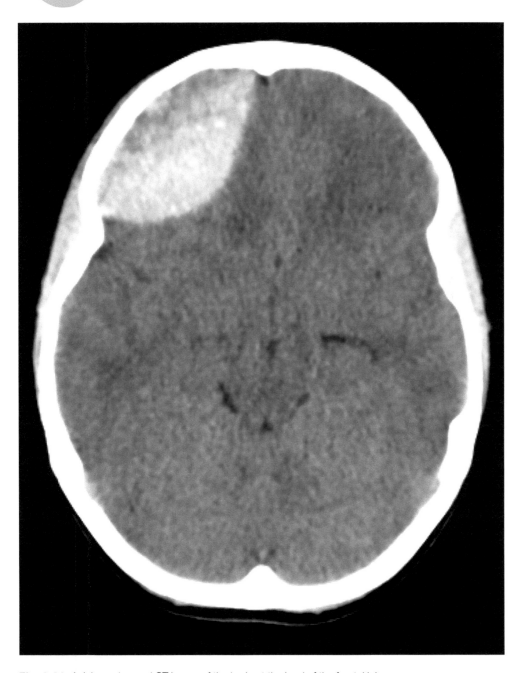

Fig. 9.6A Axial unenhanced CT image of the brain at the level of the frontal lobes.

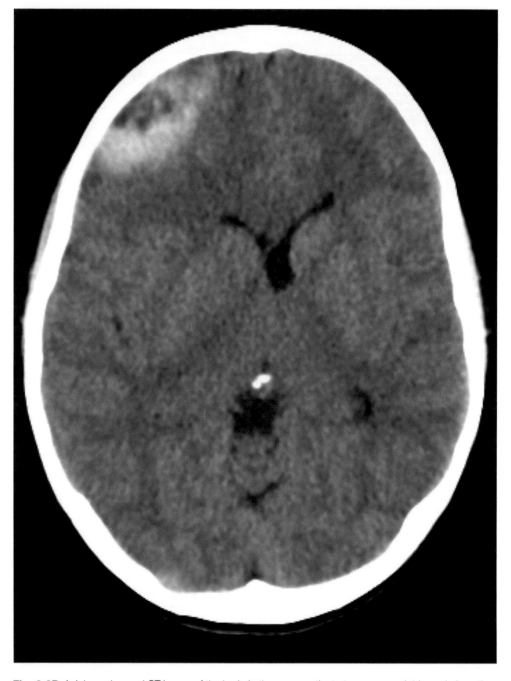

Fig. 9.6B Axial unenhanced CT image of the brain in the same patient at a more cranial (superior) section (at the level of the frontal horns of the lateral ventricles).

A 26-year-old female is brought to the ED by helicopter following a head injury sustained by a fall from a bicycle after a low speed collision with a car. Bystanders saw the patient fall on to the right side of her head. She lost consciousness and a helicopter was dispatched owing to the remote location.

The patient was awake by the time the helicopter arrived 20 minutes later, although slightly disorientated (GCS 13). Initial assessment showed no cervical spine tenderness or focal neurology and a small laceration to the right frontal region.

As the patient was being immobilised for transfer to the local trauma unit she became unresponsive. Eye opening and limb flexion could be elicited only with a painful stimulus (GCS now 7). She was intubated and transferred to hospital for further management. Urgent cranial CT is undertaken (**Figures 9.6A** and **9.6B**).

CASE 9.6: QUESTIONS

1 Assuming the patient is currently stable, what additional imaging would you consider? What is your working diagnosis?
2 What key imaging findings are demonstrated in **Figure 9.6A**?
3 What important additional finding is illustrated in **Figure 9.6B**?
4 How should this patient be managed?

CASE 9.6: ANSWERS

1 Assuming the patient is currently stable, what additional imaging would you consider? What is your working diagnosis?

The patient should undergo additional CT imaging at the same sitting as CT head. In the context of major trauma, this would involve CT of the cervical spine and also the chest, abdomen, and pelvis owing to the mechanism of injury (so-called 'traumagram').

- The principal concerns are those of intracranial haemorrhage and possible cervical spine fracture.
- The lucid interval, which preceded significant drop in consciousness, is particularly suggestive of an extradural haematoma.

2 What key imaging findings are demonstrated in Figure 9.6A?

CT shows a lenticular, biconvex-shaped hyperdense extra-axial (i.e. outside in the brain parenchyma) collection overlying the right frontal lobe (**Figure 9.6C**). The appearance is in keeping with an acute extradural haematoma.

The hyperdense (hyperattenuating) nature of the haemorrhage means it is acute. As blood products age they become less dense on CT and eventually become the same density as water or CSF when chronic (weeks old). See *Table 9.6*.

- There is 'mass-effect' and sulcal effacement (the sulci are compressed and no longer visualised) and the temporal horn of the right lateral ventricle is also effaced.
- 85% of extradural haematomas are associated with a fracture. Temporal bone fractures classically tear the middle meningeal artery and cause arterial pressure haemorrhage between the dura mater and the periosteum.

3 What important additional finding is illustrated in Figure 9.6B?

Figure 9.6B shows the 'mass effect' from the right frontal haematoma with a clear midline shift. There is displacement of the anterior horns of the lateral ventricles to the left and the frontal horn of the right lateral ventricle is partly effaced (**Figure 9.6D**).

- The haematoma displaces the entire right cerebral hemisphere. The cranium is essentially a closed box (see the Monro–Kellie hypothesis), and the extra volume caused by the haematoma inevitably effaces the CSF spaces (sulci, ventricles) and displaces structures, initially across the midline (subfalcine herniation).
- As intracranial pressure increases further, the brain is pushed inferiorly through the tentorium cerebelli (tentorial herniation). The uncus may also be displaced inferiorly (uncal herniation).
- Uncal herniation is typically a preterminal event as vital brainstem function is compromised.

4 How should this patient be managed?

These findings are a neurosurgical emergency. The reporting radiologist should telephone a report to the requesting clinician and advise that an urgent neurosurgical opinion be sought.

- This patient is already intubated. All patients with head injury will need urgent ABCDE assessment, IV access, bloods and monitoring, and urgent discussion with seniors.

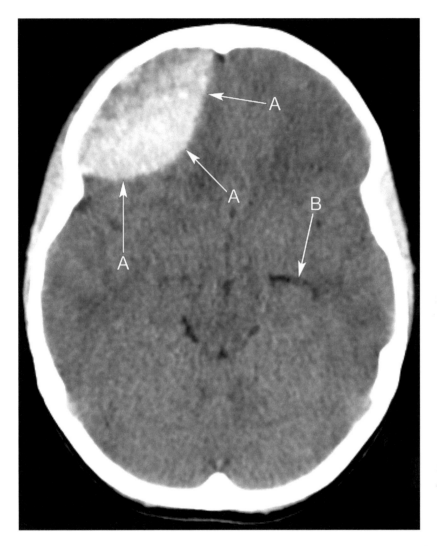

Fig. 9.6C Axial CT image of the brain without contrast showing a large right frontal (biconvex) lenticular-shaped, acute extra-axial haemorrhage (A). There is mass effect with effacement of the temporal horn of the right lateral ventricle. Note the mildly dilated temporal horn of the left lateral ventricle (B); the right temporal horn is effaced.

Table 9.6 Hounsfield units (HU) – CT density

The inventor of CT, Sir Godfrey Hounsfield, gave his name to the CT unit of measurement of tissue radiodensity

- The more a tissue attenuates the CT XR beam, the more dense and whiter it appears on CT (e.g. bone, typically 700–3000 HU)
- The more easily the CT XR beam passes through tissue, the less dense and darker the tissue appears (e.g. lung, typically –500 HU)
- The HU scale is centred on water, defined as 0 HU

Acute intracranial blood is hyperdense (i.e. more dense than water) and ranges from 40 to 80 HU

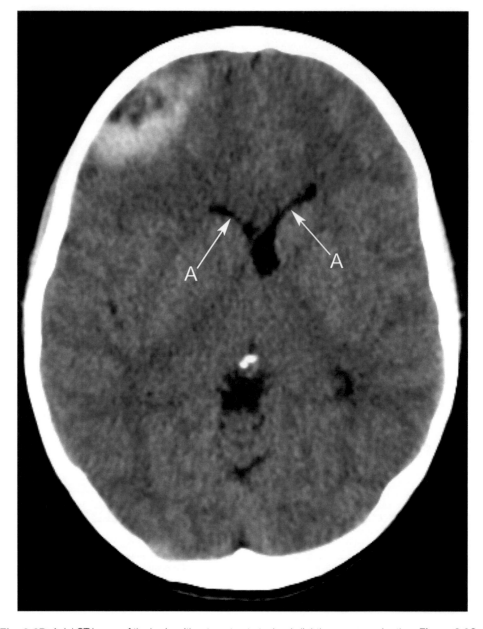

Fig. 9.6D Axial CT image of the brain without contrast at a level slightly more superior than **Figure 9.6C**. There is mass effect from the right frontal haematoma causing midline shift of the anterior horns of the lateral ventricles to the left (A).

If a CT scan is indicated then there needs to be discussion with radiology and then the radiographers in CT. It is essential that patients who go to CT are haemodynamically stable and can maintain their airway – if the airway is, or may be, compromised, then urgent anaesthetic involvement is needed.

- The patient must be transferred urgently to a neurosurgical centre for further management (e.g. Burr hole to relieve intracranial pressure).

LEARNING POINTS: EXTRADURAL HAEMATOMA

- Extradural haematoma is life threatening and requires urgent neurosurgical intervention.
- It is typically a complication of a skull fracture and is characterised clinically by a lucid interval before loss of consciousness.
- Acute blood is hyperdense or hyperattenuating on unenhanced CT: as a haematoma ages it becomes less dense.
- Midline shift of ≥3 mm on CT is significant.

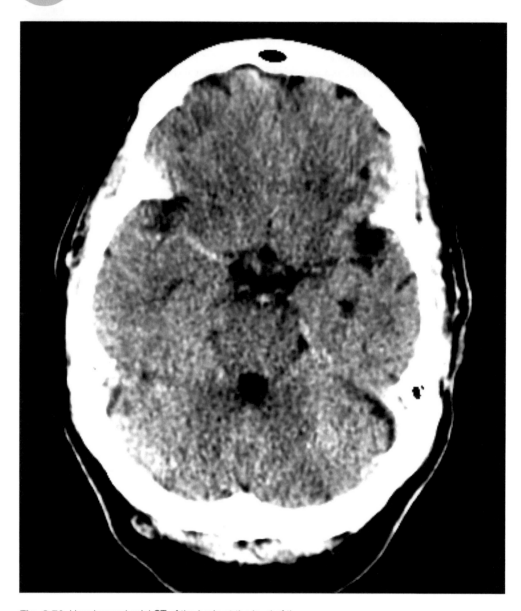

Fig. 9.7A Unenhanced axial CT of the brain at the level of the pons.

A 67-year-old male presents to the ED with a history of sudden-onset left-sided weakness 3 hours previously and altered sensation to the left side of his face. He gives a longstanding history of hypertension and type 2 diabetes, and a 30 pack-year history of smoking.

On examination, there is a dense left hemiparesis and facial droop, also paraesthesia, particularly on the left side of the face. The plantar reflex is up-going on the left. His BP is 180/110 mmHg, pulse 100 bpm and regular, and he is apyrexial. Urgent cranial CT is arranged (**Figures 9.7A** and **9.7B**).

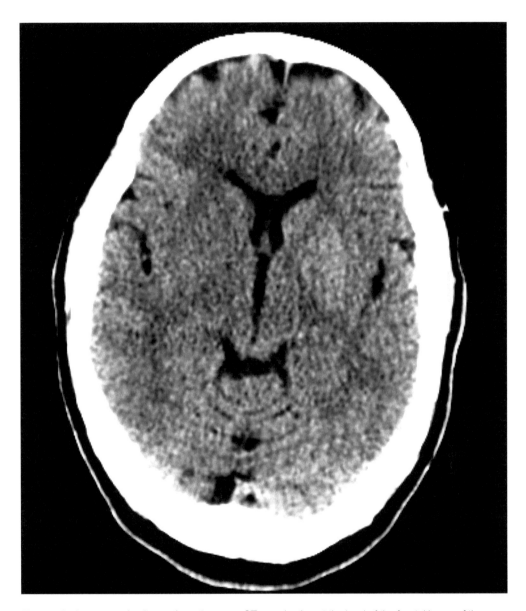

Fig. 9.7B Accompanying image from the same CT examination at the level of the frontal horns of the lateral ventricles.

CASE 9.7: QUESTIONS

1 What is your provisional diagnosis?
2 How will you manage this patient?
3 What findings are demonstrated in **Figures 9.7A** and **9.7B**?
4 What are the treatment options?

CASE 9.7: ANSWERS

1 What is your provisional diagnosis?

The symptoms and examination findings are suggestive of an ischaemic stroke (or transient ischaemic attack: TIA). Hypertension, smoking, and type 2 diabetes are all risk factors. The differential diagnosis is intracerebral haematoma, although this is less likely given the lack of predisposing factors such as recent head injury or anticoagulant therapy.

2 How will you manage this patient?

The patient should be referred urgently to the stroke team. Providing there are no contraindications, the patient may be treated with IV thrombolysis. The stroke team will request an urgent unenhanced CT scan of the brain.

- The purpose of the CT scan is principally to exclude intracerebral haematoma (or haemorrhagic stroke) or a focal intracranial mass lesion. If there is no evidence of haemorrhage or other contraindication, the patient may be eligible for thrombolysis.

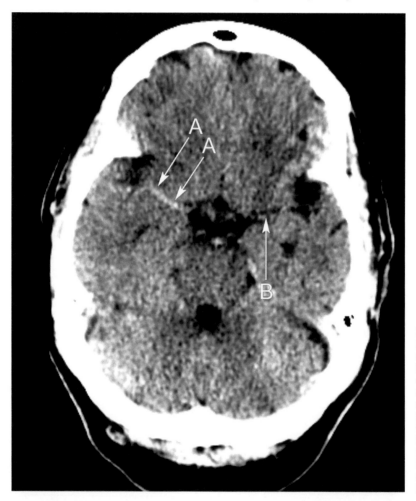

Fig. 9.7C Axial unenhanced CT showing increased density of the right middle cerebral artery (MCA) (arrows A), highly suggestive for acute thrombosis. Note the normal appearing left MCA (B).

- The initial CT scan may show no signs of ischaemic stroke; indeed at 3–4 hours after a stroke 40% of patients have a normal CT scan. A normal scan, therefore, should not deter thrombolysis.

3 What findings are demonstrated in Figures 9.7A and 9.7B?

The CT scans show a hyperdense right middle cerebral artery (MCA). The hyperdensity is caused by occlusive thrombus within the artery and is an early sign of ischaemic stroke (**Figure 9.7C**).

- The MCA is involved in 75% of infarcts, mostly due to atheroma rupture at or near the bifurcation of the common carotid artery.

The second CT image (**Figure 9.7B**) does not show a definite focal lesion at this stage in MCA distribution.

The infarcted brain parenchyma gradually reduces in density on CT over time owing to cell death and liquefaction. **Figure 9.7D** shows the same patient 3 days after the infarction. The low density corresponds to part of the vascular territory supplied by the MCA.

- Eventually (months after infarction), the infarcted brain tissue is absorbed by macrophages and the affected area adopts a density similar to water or CSF. The loss of brain volume may cause dilatation of an adjacent ventricle, known as *ex-vacuo* dilatation.

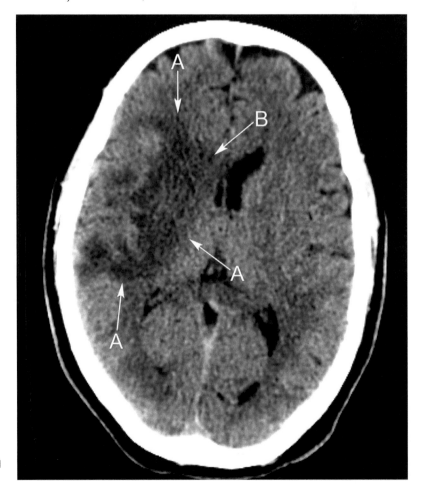

Fig. 9.7D Follow-up CT performed 3 days later showing diffuse low density (A) in keeping with acute right MCA infarction with mass effect and effacement of the frontal horn of the right lateral ventricle (B).

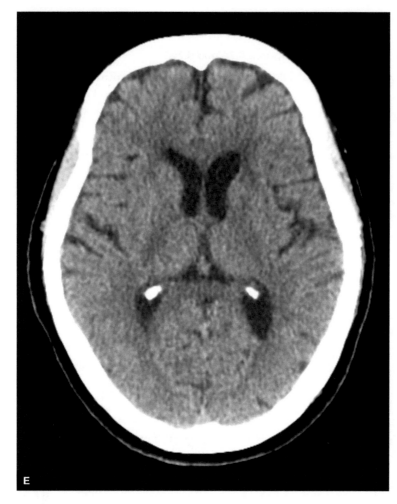

Figs. 9.7E, F Axial CT (**9.7E**) in another patient at the level of the lateral ventricles/basal ganglia in a patient with acute left-sided weakness: no definite lesion is seen on CT. The patient proceeded urgently to MRI. A DW image (**9.7F**) at the same level as the CT confirms an area of high signal, restricted diffusion, consistent with an acute infarct in the right basal ganglia (A).

E

- MRI has superior sensitivity to CT for diagnosing hyperacute stroke and can add value in this setting. Diffusion-weighted imaging (DWI) is the most sensitive and can be positive within minutes of an infarct occurring (**Figures 9.7E** and **9.7F**). Infarcted tissue with restricted diffusion appears as high signal on DWI and normalises after about 4 days.

4 What are the treatment options?

Suspected strokes are best managed at hospitals with a hyperacute stroke service.

- IV thrombolysis (recombinant tissue plasminogen activator, r-TPA) is currently licensed for patients with symptom onset of <4.5 hours, having been reviewed by a stroke specialist.
- After 4.5 hours, thrombolysis is associated with an increased mortality.
- CT or MR cerebral angiography can also be performed in hospitals with an interventional neuroradiology service with a view to clot retrieval if clinically appropriate.
- Following confirmation of a stroke and initial management, the patient should be transferred to a specialist stroke unit for further assessment and rehabilitation.

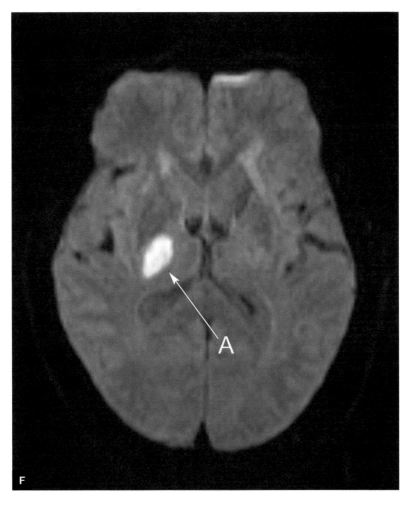

Fig. 9.7F

- If there is further deterioration in neurological status a follow-up CT scan can be performed to look for haemorrhage, either as a complication of thrombolysis or from haemorrhagic conversion of an ischaemic stroke.

LEARNING POINTS: STROKE

- Patients with suspected acute stroke must be referred urgently to the stroke team for consideration of thrombolysis.
- CT is performed in the acute setting to exclude haemorrhage (an absolute contraindication to thrombolysis) but is often normal early on.
- Diffusion-weighted MRI is the most sensitive imaging modality for hyperacute stroke. MRI is not widely available for hyperacute stroke assessment and some stroke patients find it difficult to tolerate.
- Review the CT for an area of low density (this may be very subtle) corresponding to a vascular territory. Additional signs include mass effect or a hyperdense MCA.

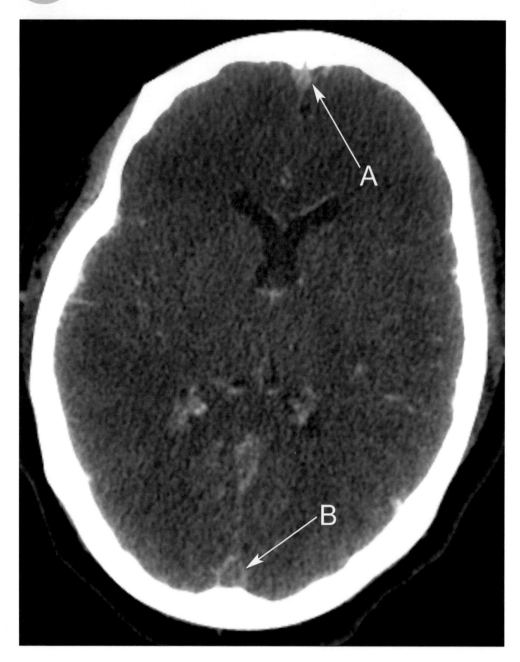

Fig. 9.8A

A 19-year-old female presents to the ED with a 2-day history of constant severe headache, nausea, and several episodes of vomiting. The patient also complains of unsteadiness on her feet and double vision. She has tried paracetamol to no avail. The patient is overweight (BMI 30) although otherwise fit and well. She takes no medication other than the oral contraceptive pill.

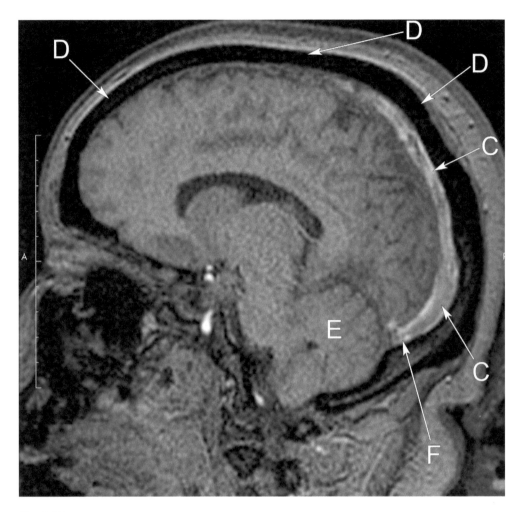

Fig. 9.8B

Observations are stable and the patient is apyrexial. Neurological examination shows a palsy of the left VI cranial nerve and cerebellar signs (Rhomberg test is positive). Ophthalmoscopy shows early papilloedema. There is a mild impairment of consciousness with GCS 14 (E4 V4 M6).

CASE 9.8: QUESTIONS

1 What is your working differential diagnosis? What imaging would you consider in this situation?
2 What imaging has been performed in **Figures 9.8A** and **9.8B**?
3 What normal structure is labelled 'A' and what abnormality is shown by 'B' (**Figure 9.8A**)?
4 How would you describe the abnormality labelled 'C'? What normal structures are shown by arrows D, E, and F (**Figure 9.8B**)?

CASE 9.8: ANSWERS

1 What is your working differential diagnosis? What imaging would you consider in this situation?

The symptoms and signs are nonspecific. Differential diagnoses to be considered include meningoencephalitis, an intracranial mass, and venous sinus thrombosis.

- A CT scan of the brain pre and post-IV contrast is the most useful initial investigation in the acute setting. It is more readily accessible than MRI and a normal CT scan would rapidly and effectively exclude an intracranial mass.
- A CT venogram (postcontrast) can be performed easily at the same sitting if venous sinus thrombosis is suspected. MRI and MR venography are also highly accurate for diagnosing tumours and sinus thrombosis but are more time consuming and less well tolerated.

2 What imaging has been performed in Figures 9.8A and 9.8B?

Figure 9.8A is an axial CT slice of the brain from a postcontrast venogram examination. **Figure 9.8B** is a selected sagittal image from a postcontrast MR venogram.

- CT is often performed first as it is readily accessible and helps to exclude other differential diagnoses. CT can also be performed rapidly and may be easier for an ill patient to tolerate.
- Hyperdense dural sinuses on an unenhanced CT scan of the brain can suggest a dural venous sinus thrombosis. Other features to support the diagnosis include cerebral oedema or venous infarctions (these do not correspond to a vascular territory). A postcontrast study will confirm a sinus filling defect/thrombus.
- There is little difference in diagnostic performance between a CT venogram and an MR venogram for the investigation of sinus thrombosis, with sensitivities of approximately 95% with each.
- MR venogram may, however, have added value where there are equivocal findings on CT or in looking for subtle complications of a sinus thrombosis (i.e. venous infarction).

3 What normal structure is labelled 'A' and what abnormality is shown by 'B' (Figure 9.8A)?

Arrow A points to the anterior portion of the superior sagittal sinus. It is filled with contrast as expected on this CT venogram and appears normal. Arrow B points to the posterior portion of the superior sagittal sinus. There is no contrast filling the sinus (the 'empty delta sign') because it is obstructed by thrombus. The diagnosis is, therefore, venous sinus thrombosis: this appears as low density material within the sinus. A thin layer of contrast can be seen to outline the low density, dark, thrombus.

- Venous sinus thrombosis is a poorly understood condition associated with risk factors including the oral contraceptive pill, pregnancy, prothrombotic states, and malignancy. The presentation often is nonspecific.
- Sinus thrombosis may lead to venous hypertension, cerebral oedema, and venous infarction.

4 How would you describe the abnormality labelled 'C'? What normal structures are shown by arrows D, E, and F (Figure 9.8B)?

The image demonstrates extensive low signal filling defect (C) within the superior sagittal sinus posteriorly in keeping with thrombus. The filling defect extends posteriorly to the confluence of sinuses (at the level of the tentorium cerebelli). Label D points to the normal bony cranium, which has low signal. E is the cerebellum and F is the sinus confluence.

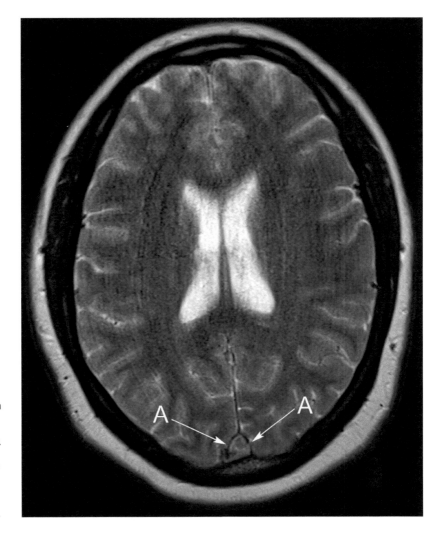

Fig. 9.8C
Axial
T2-weighted
MR image
showing a
mixed signal
filling defect in
the superior
sagittal sinus
(A) posteriorly.
On this
sequence the
sinus should
appear black
owing to
flowing blood.

Figure 9.8C is a single axial slice of a T2-weighted MR image in this same patient. A filling defect is again demonstrated, in keeping with thrombus.

- The signal characteristics of thrombus change over time on T1 and T2-weighted imaging so that it is possible to age thrombus. You do not need to know details of this for finals.

LEARNING POINTS: SAGITTAL SINUS THROMBOSIS

- The presentation of dural venous sinus thrombosis is nonspecific and the differential is broad.
- There are numerous risk factors, more commonly the oral contraceptive pill, pregnancy, prothrombotic states, and malignancy.
- A CT venogram and/or MR venogram are most useful for diagnosis. Which investigation is performed will depend on availability, contraindications to iodinated CT contrast, pregnancy (ionising radiation in CT), and patient cooperation.
- Management is with systemic anticoagulation with LMWH or warfarin.

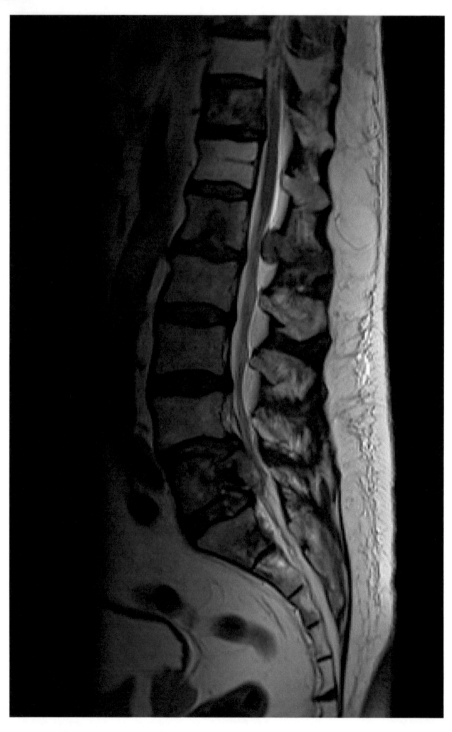

Fig. 9.9A Sagittal T2-weighted MR image of the lumbar spine.

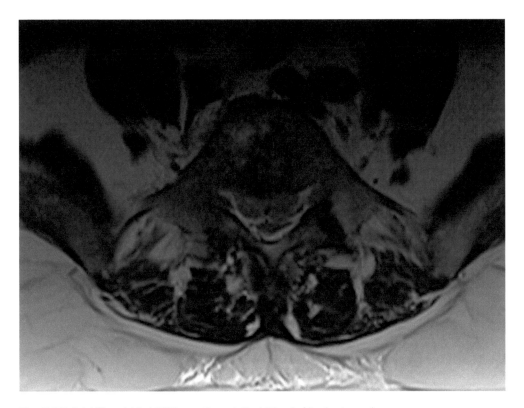

Fig. 9.9B Axial T1-weighted MR image through the L5 level of the lumbar spine.

A 72-year-old female is referred to the oncology team having presented to the ED with a 24-hour history of increasing lower back pain on a background of chronic back pain. There is no history of trauma. The patient denies any urinary or faecal incontinence. There is a past medical history of breast cancer, and this was treated with a mastectomy, radiotherapy, and chemotherapy 3 years ago.

On examination, there is 4/5 power in the lower limbs and reflexes cannot be elicited. There is loss of perianal sensation but anal tone is maintained. There is diffuse tenderness on palpation of the lumbar spine, most severe at L5.

CASE 9.9: QUESTIONS

1 What is your provisional diagnosis?
2 What priority would you give to this patient's problem and what investigations are indicated?
3 What do the images show (**Figures 9.9A** and **9.9B**)?
4 How should the patient be treated?

CASE 9.9: ANSWERS

1 What is your provisional diagnosis?

The history of chronic lower back pain with acute deterioration in pain and associated lower limb neurology in the last 24 hours with focal neurology is indicative of cauda equina compression syndrome. Cauda equina syndrome is said to be 'complete' once there is urinary dysfunction.

- Common causes for this presentation include disc prolapse or vertebral collapse causing nerve root compression. Pathological vertebral collapse is to be excluded given the history of breast cancer.
- The patient's presentation is likely to represent a recurrence of breast cancer.
- There are recognised 'red-flag' symptoms that should alert the clinician to a possible serious underlying cause for low back pain and these include:
  - Unrelenting pain, worse at night.
  - Pain in patients <18 years, >50 years of age.
  - Previous history of cancer.
  - Associated systemic symptoms/signs, e.g. weight loss, fever, malaise.
  - Radiation of pain.
  - Change in perianal sensation, incontinence.

2 What priority would you give to this patient's problem and what investigations are indicated?

Cauda equina syndrome is a radiological and surgical emergency (*Table 9.9*):

- This patient requires urgent MRI of the spine in the first instance – liaise with seniors and then radiology to arrange the scan. This must be done as soon as possible after diagnosis. Once suspected cord compression is suspected clinically, MRI must not wait until the next day or after the weekend – if local MRI facilities do not exist out of hours then the patient should be transferred urgently to a neurosurgical unit for imaging.
- Emergency surgical decompression is generally the preferred approach to decompressing the lumbosacral nerve roots in patients with no history of cancer and needs to be performed, if appropriate, urgently after the diagnosis is made. In patients with known cancer and likely metastatic compression, it may be more appropriate to arrange urgent radiotherapy to the affected area having started the patient on high-dose steroids to reduce swelling.
- The urgency of surgery is greatest with incomplete cauda equina syndrome, and neurological/urological outcomes are best when there is no progression to complete cauda equina.
- Remember also to check bloods, address patient pain, check urine output if urinary catheterisation is needed, and exclude hypercalcaemia in likely malignancy.

Table 9.9 Cauda equina syndrome

- The cauda equina refers to the nerve roots originating from the conus (the cord termination)
- These lumbosacral roots provide sensory innervation to the saddle area, motor innervation to the lower limbs, and voluntary control of the anal and urinary sphincters
- The most common cause of cauda equina syndrome is a disc herniation at L4–5 or L5–S1

3 What do the images show (Figures 9.9A and 9.9B)?

They are MR images of the spine and confirm bony metastases and malignant compression of the cauda equina at L5 (**Figures 9.9C** and **9.9D**).

- A typical MRI of the spine for suspected cauda equina syndrome includes sagittal and axial T1-weighted imaging (to assess the bone marrow), sagittal and axial T2-weighted imaging (for assessment of the cord), and postcontrast or STIR imaging if there is suspicion of infection (spondylodiscitis).

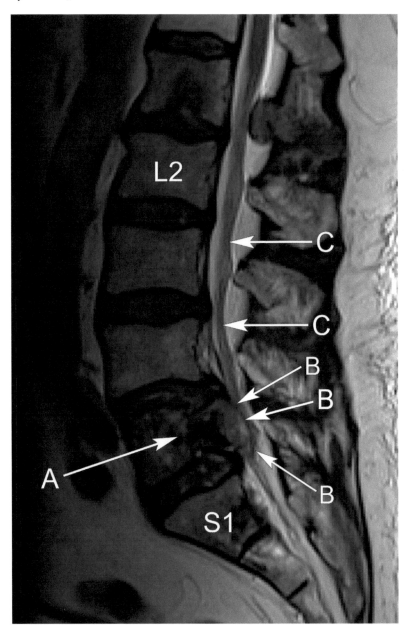

Fig. 9.9C Sagittal T2-weighted MR image of the lumbar spine. A low signal (dark) lesion consistent with vertebral metastasis is seen at the L5 vertebral level (A). The tumour extends posterior to L5 causing significant canal compression and cauda equina compromise (B). The L2 vertebra and S1 segment are labelled. The cauda equina nerve roots are shown (C) within a CSF filled thecal sac.

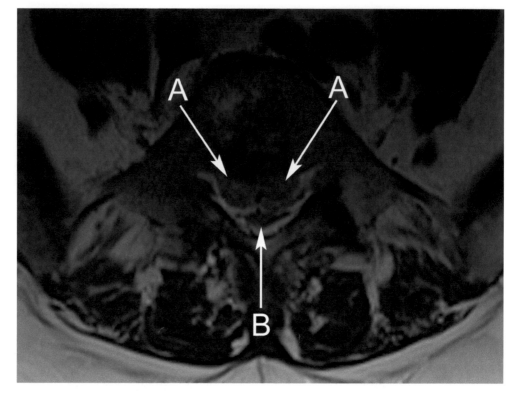

Fig. 9.9D Axial T1-weighted MR image at L5 level. Note the tumour extending from the posterior vertebra (A) and compressed thecal sac (B).

4 How should the patient be treated?

This patient requires urgent MDT discussion between radiology, oncology, and neurosurgery. She should be started on high-dose dexamethasone by mouth to reduce oedema and then be considered for further treatment, most likely spinal radiotherapy in view of her previous history: neurosurgical decompression is less likely in this case. The patient also needs urgent restaging (CT chest, abdomen, pelvis, and radionuclide bone scan) of her breast cancer prior to consideration of any further treatment (chemotherapy).

LEARNING POINTS: MALIGNANT SPINAL CORD/CAUDA EQUINA COMPRESSION

- Think of bone metastases in patients over 40 years with bone pain, especially if there is a given past history of malignancy.
- Cauda equina syndrome (and cord compression) is a diagnostic and surgical emergency. The evidence regarding optimal time for surgical decompression is mixed; however, most surgeons intervene within 24–48 hours.
- Patients with incomplete cauda equina syndrome are the highest priority for intervention.
- Cauda equina syndrome is uncommon and mostly caused by disc prolapse.

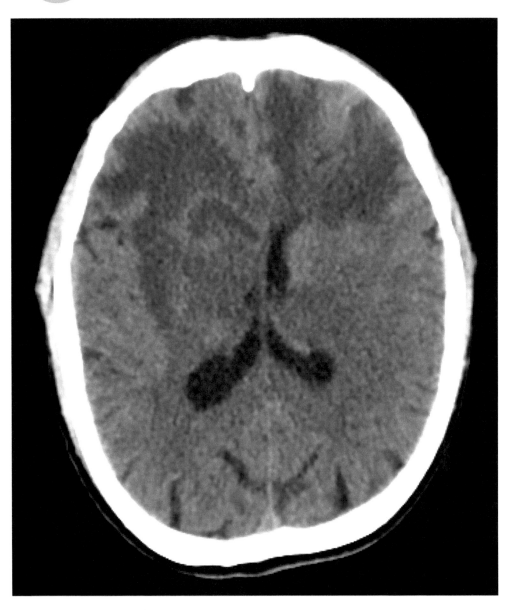

Fig. 9.10A

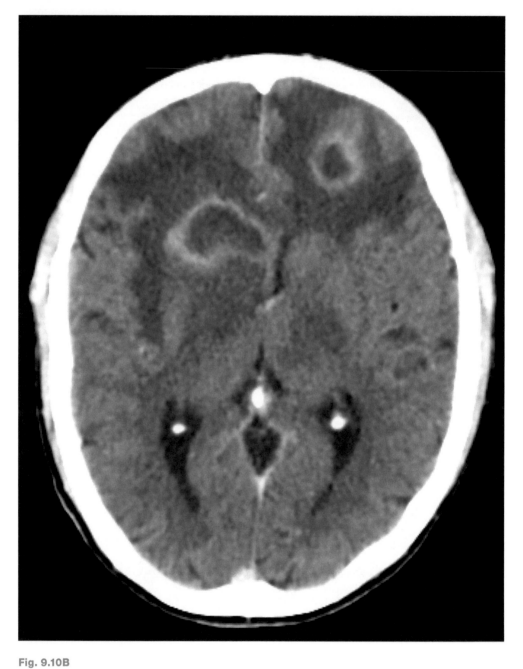

Fig. 9.10B

A 45-year-old male lorry driver attends the ED with his wife. Although the patient is slightly drowsy, you are able to take a brief history. He describes several weeks of feeling unwell with a productive cough and worsening headache. More recently he has felt tired and irritable. There is a 30 pack-year history of smoking.

On clinical examination his abdomen is soft and nontender. On auscultation of the chest there are crackles at the right base. There is a mild impairment of consciousness with GCS 13 (E3 V5 M5). There is reduced power in all limbs (slightly worse on the left) and hyperreflexia.

His BP is 150/90 mmHg, HR 115 bpm, and respiratory rate 22 bpm. Oxygen saturation is 92% on room air and he is pyrexial at 37.9°C. Routine bloods show:

Elevated serum glucose	18 mmol/L (normal fasting level 3.9–5.5 mmol/L)
WCC	22×10^9/L $(4–11 \times 10^9$/L)
CRP	220 mg/L (<5 mg/L)

Urine dipstick is positive for glucose only. You request a CXR, which reports 'Focal airspace opacification in the right lower lobe in keeping with infection.'

CASE 9.10: QUESTIONS

1 Does this patient require any immediate further imaging?
2 What studies are shown in **Figures 9.10A** and **9.10B** and what do they show?
3 What further steps should you take in this patient's management?

CASE 9.10: ANSWERS

1 Does this patient require any immediate further imaging?

You have already established a probable diagnosis of pneumonia. A follow-up CXR at 6 weeks after treatment is advisable to ensure that the consolidation has resolved and that there is no underlying malignancy.

Pneumonia alone, however, does not account for the patient's neurological symptoms and collapse. Urgent cross-sectional imaging of the brain is required. CT is usually used in the acute situation, as it is quick to undertake and is sensitive for stroke and blood and tumour. IV contrast is used following the initial precontrast scan in certain situations, for example suspected tumour or mass lesion or venous sinus thrombosis.

- The differential for the neurological symptoms include tumour (primary or secondary), infection, and stroke (ischaemic or haemorrhagic).

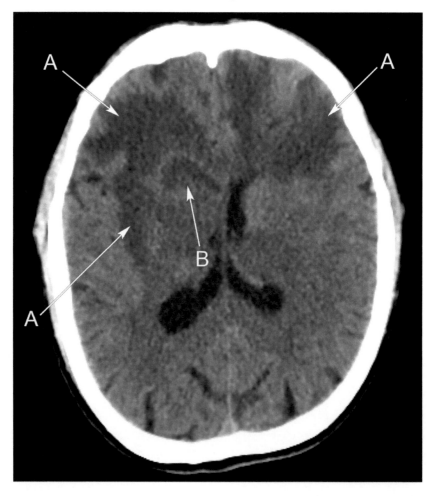

Fig. 9.10C Precontrast axial CT section of the brain at the level of the bodies of the lateral ventricles showing extensive oedema (A) and an ill-defined periventricular lesion (B).

- Given the impaired consciousness, an anaesthetic assessment prior to CT would be appropriate. Remember in the exam to mention urgent discussion with seniors and radiology. If the patient has altered conscious level or if his airway is at risk then he will need intubating prior to CT.
- Given that the patient is septic and an undiagnosed diabetic, acute kidney injury should also be excluded. If the estimated glomerular filtration rate (eGFR) is <30 mL/min there is increased risk of contrast-induced nephropathy (the patient may require prehydration).

2 What studies are shown in Figures 9.10A and 9.10B and what do they show?

They are CT images of the brain and are repeated here as **Figures 9.10C** and **9.10D**. **Figure 9.10C** is a precontrast axial CT image of the brain. After reviewing the images, the on-call radiology registrar asked the radiographers to repeat the scan after IV contrast administration (**Figure 9.10D**). Pre-IV contrast there are large areas of low density in the right frontal and parietal lobes and left frontal lobe. The appearance is in keeping with vasogenic oedema, and the distribution and appearance is not typical for stroke (*Table 9.10*).

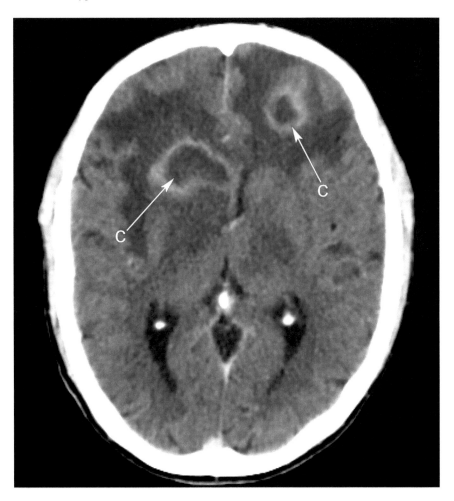

Fig. 9.10D Postcontrast scan performed at almost the same level as in Figure 9.10C showing ring-enhancing lesions (C) and associated vasogenic oedema.

Table 9.10 CT findings

Cytotoxic oedema

Appears following ischaemic infarction. It is an area of low density involving the white matter and the
   cortex where extracellular water passes into cells with swelling and no disruption of the blood/brain
   barrier

Vasogenic oedema

Associated with brain tumours and abscesses. Mainly involves the white matter and associated with
   disruption of the blood/brain barrier. Irregular low density change extends towards the cortex with
   finger-like projections

Following IV contrast, ring-enhancing lesions are clearly seen within the oedema. There is
mass effect with effacement of cerebral sulci and distortion/compression of the frontal horns of
the lateral ventricles.

- This appearance could represent either multiple malignant tumours (metastases) or
  intracerebral abscesses. The history of chest sepsis, however, favours abscesses. It is
  characteristic of brain abscesses to have a thinned enhancing rim on their medial side
  (owing to the relatively avascular white matter medially). Eventually the abscess may
  rupture into the ventricle and cause ventriculitis.
- The presence of a smooth, thin enhancing rim and central low density (necrosis) is typical
  for the 'early capsule' abscess phase. This occurs about 1–2 weeks after onset.
- Most abscesses in the CNS arise owing to bacteraemia typically arising from lung or cardiac
  infection. Immunocompromise, congenital heart disease, skull fractures, and neurosurgery
  are key risk factors.
- MRI can be helpful in some cases to potentially differentiate abscess from tumour using
  DWI techniques.

3 What further steps should you take in this patient's management?

This is a neurosurgical emergency. The reporting radiologist should telephone a report to the
requesting clinician and advise a neurosurgical opinion.

- Further urgent actions would include prompt broad-spectrum antibiotics following blood
  cultures, fluid resuscitation, prophylactic anticonvulsants, and possible surgical excision/
  drainage. Lumbar puncture would be contraindicated in a case such as this owing to risk
  of coning caused by raised intracranial pressure. He will also need careful observation and
  anaesthetic review if his airway is at risk.
- The patient should be transferred to a neurosurgical unit where he will be managed by a
  MDT, including neurosurgery, neurology, microbiology, and neuroradiology.

LEARNING POINTS: CEREBRAL ABSCESS

- A brain abscess is a neurosurgical emergency.
- The appearance of a brain abscess is nonspecific on CT without corroborative clinical findings.
  It is important, therefore, that you provide the radiologist with accurate clinical information.
- Most brain abscesses arise due to sepsis elsewhere in the body and are more likely in the
  presence of immunocompromise, congenital heart disease, skull fracture or recent neurosurgery.
- Rarely, brain abscesses arise owing to direct spread from an infected facial sinus.

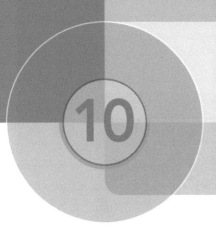

Paediatric cases

UDAY MANDALIA AND LUCY SHIMWELL

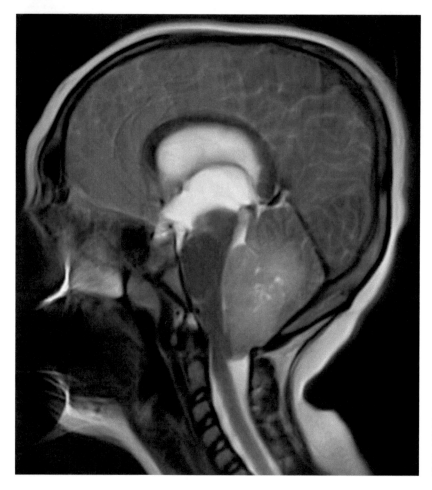

Fig. 10.1A
Sagittal
T2-weighted
MR image of
the brain.

A 6-year-old male presents with a 2-week history of nausea, headache, and double vision. His mother has also noticed that he has become increasingly clumsy and his speech has become slurred.

On examination the child appears lethargic. He is mildly hypertensive with a systolic blood pressure of 115 mmHg (90–110 mmHg). He has papilloedema and signs of cerebellar dysfunction with ataxia and poor balance.

He is seen by the paediatricians and an urgent MRI of the brain is requested (**Figures 10.1A** and **10.1B**).

CASE 10.1: QUESTIONS

1 What are the abnormal findings?
2 What is the likely diagnosis?
3 What is the investigation of choice for children who present in this way?
4 How should this patient be managed?

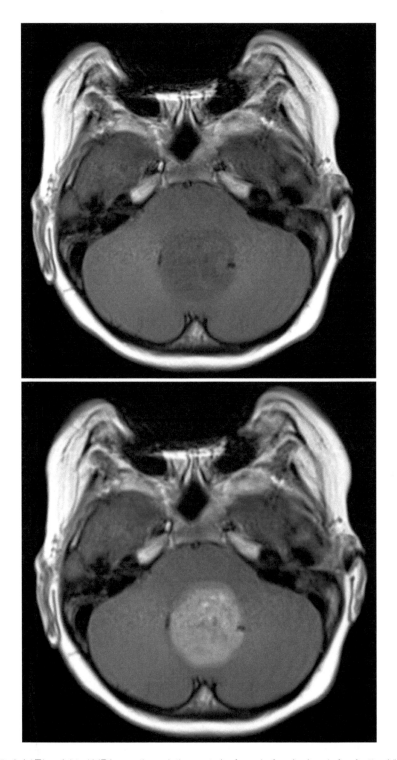

Fig. 10.1B Axial T1-weighted MR image through the posterior fossa before (top) and after (bottom) IV contrast.

CASE 10.1: ANSWERS

1 What are the abnormal findings?

There is a large midline mass in the posterior fossa, centred within the 4th ventricle (**Figures 10.1C** and **10.1D**). The lesion is obstructing the flow of CSF and is causing obstructive hydrocephalus with distension of the third ventricle.

The child presents with red flag features of raised intracranial pressure (ICP). Signs of raised ICP include headaches, which are worse on lying down or in the morning, vomiting, papilloedema, seizures, speech disturbance, and visual disturbance. Cranial nerve palsies are also common in posterior fossa tumours owing to compression or infiltration of the brain stem.

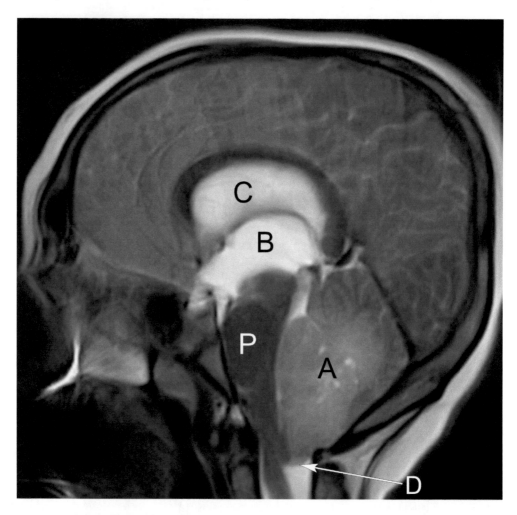

Fig. 10.1C Sagittal T2-weighted MR image showing a large mass (A) compressing the 4th ventricle with consequent distension of the 3rd (B) and lateral (C) ventricles. There is also mass effect on the pons (P) anteriorly and crowding of the foramen magnum (D) inferiorly owing to inferior extension of the mass. Note the impingement on the spinal cord/medulla.

2 What is the likely diagnosis?

This lesion is likely to represent a medulloblastoma. This is the commonest posterior fossa tumour of childhood and accounts for 15–20% of all paediatric brain tumours. These tumours commonly arise from the roof of the 4th ventricle and are made of densely packed cells with a high nuclear to cytoplasmic ratio giving them a characteristically dense appearance on CT (**Figure 10.1E**). On MRI they are typically heterogeneous but bright on T2 and enhance avidly with contrast.

Other posterior fossa tumours of childhood include brainstem gliomas, ependymomas, cerebellar astrocytomas, and atypical teratoid rhabdoid tumours.

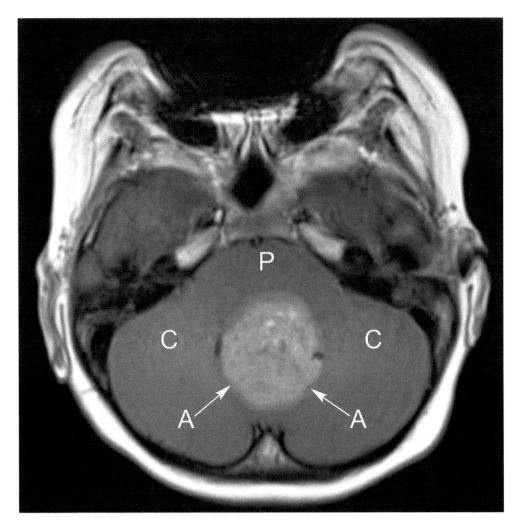

Fig. 10.1D Axial T1 with contrast MR image showing a large mass (A) filling the 4th ventricle. The pons (P) is compressed anteriorly and the cerebellar hemispheres (C) are compressed laterally. Note: the mass is low signal precontrast (see Figure 10.1B, top) and enhances in this figure (the degree of enhancement can be variable).

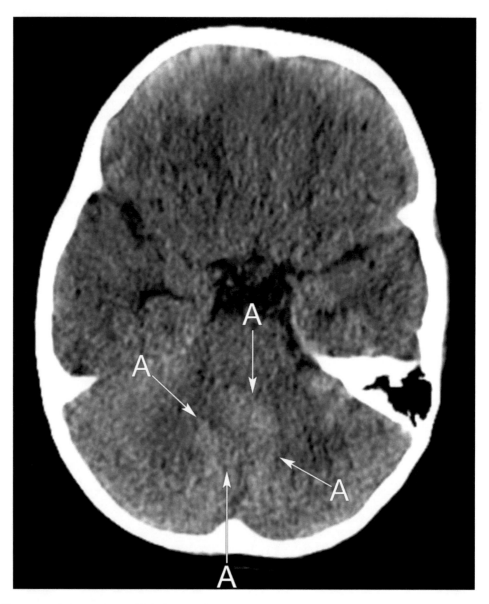

Fig. 10.1E Axial unenhanced CT of a posterior fossa medulloblastoma (A) in another child with a characteristically dense appearance.

3 What is the investigation of choice for children who present in this way?

In a child with suspected brain tumour an MRI scan with contrast would be the initial imaging investigation of choice, as this will best demonstrate the surrounding anatomy and origin of the tumour. A CT scan may help in the first instance if MRI is not available or the child is unable to lie sufficiently still. MRI can be performed on young/uncooperative children using general anaesthesia. MRI brain is combined with MRI spine also in suspected malignant tumours to check for 'drop' spinal metastases from the cranial primary.

4 How should this patient be managed?

The child needs to be managed initially using an ABCDE approach. It is important to assess the child's neurological status including GCS and cranial nerve assessment. The child should also be examined for evidence of raised ICP.

Urgent discussion with paediatricians and neurosurgeons is needed.

If there are signs of raised ICP then neuroprotective measures should be undertaken. These include:

- Nursing the child with the head up to increase cerebral venous drainage.
- Administration of hypertonic solutions, such as mannitol, and also steroids to reduce cerebral oedema.

Once the child is stabilised they will require emergency neurosurgical intervention in order to decompress the ventricles and relieve the hydrocephalus. This is usually achieved by inserting a ventricular shunt. Further definitive treatment in a specialist paediatric neuro-oncology centre is recommended to optimise the patient's care. Treatment will be with a combination of neoadjuvant chemoradiotherapy and surgery. Prognosis will depend on the amount of tumour left after resection and the presence of any metastases.

LEARNING POINTS: PAEDIATRIC BRAIN TUMOURS

- Red flag signs of raised ICP include decreased conscious level, seizures, change in behaviour, persistent and progressive headaches, vomiting, papilloedema, speech and visual disturbance, and cranial nerve palsies.
- Posterior fossa tumours can obstruct the 4th ventricle and the flow of CSF into the subarachnoid space leading to obstructive hydrocephalus.
- Differential diagnoses for a posterior fossa brain tumour in children include medulloblastoma, astrocytoma, ependymoma, and atypical teratoid/rhabdoid tumour.
- Immediate management of raised ICP may include intubation and ventilation if the child is comatosed, urgent neuroimaging, administration of hypertonic solutions and steroids, and transfer to a neurosurgical unit.

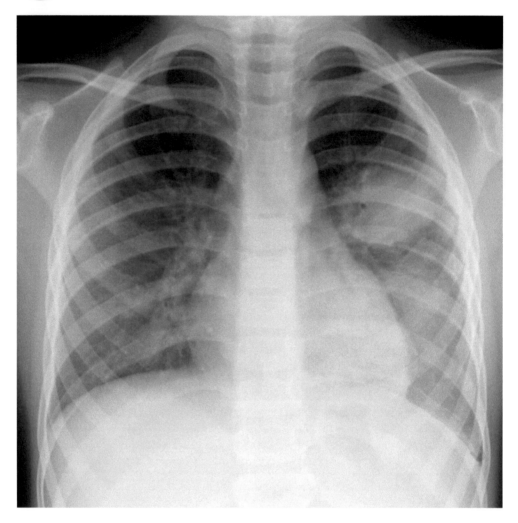

Fig. 10.2A Erect AP CXR.

A 7-year-old male presents to his GP with fever, cough, pleuritic chest pain, and lethargy following a upper respiratory tract infection. He has a fever of 39°C. He has some dullness to percussion and decreased breath sounds on the left.

The GP requests a CXR (**Figure 10.2A**), suspecting a chest infection, and commences antibiotic treatment empirically.

The reporting radiologist is concerned by the XR findings and recommends a repeat XR in 6 weeks after treatment (**Figure 10.2B**).

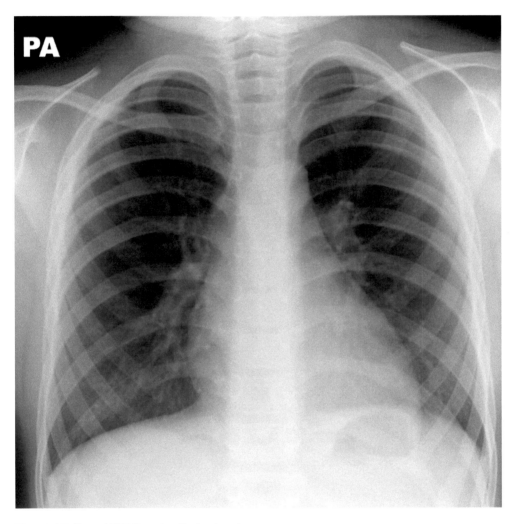

Fig. 10.2B Repeat CXR 6 weeks after treatment.

CASE 10.2: QUESTIONS

1 What do the CXRs show and what is the diagnosis?
2 Why was the radiologist concerned?
3 What are the common XR appearances of lower respiratory tract infections in children?
4 What normal structure is often mistaken for a mediastinal tumour in children?

CASE 10.2: ANSWERS

1 What do the CXRs show and what is the diagnosis?

The initial XR shows an ill-defined opacity in the left mid-zone with additional left lower zone opacity (**Figure 10.2C**). The opacity is rounded with poorly defined margins. There is no cavitation or calcification. On the subsequent CXR the abnormality has completely resolved. The clinical features and rapid resolution with antibiotics are consistent with a diagnosis of pneumonia. This XR pattern in children is known as a round pneumonia.

Round pneumonia is a pattern of infection typically seen in children under the age of 8 years. It is thought to occur because children have underdeveloped collateral air circulation through the channels of Lambert and the pores of Kohn, which limits the spread of infection and allows the formation of a contained rounded area of pneumonia.

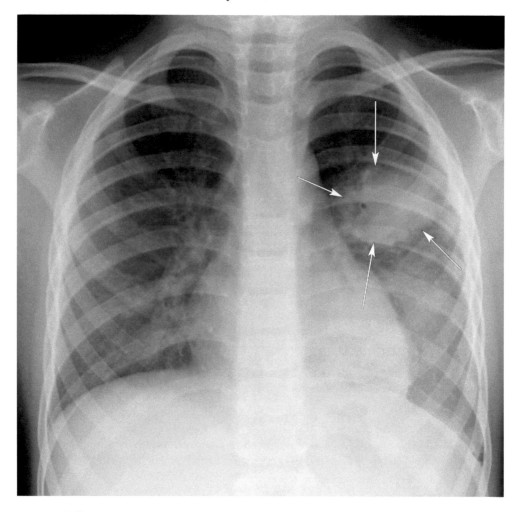

Fig. 10.2C The rounded opacity in the left mid-zone (arrows) can be seen. There is further additional opacity in the left lower zone extending behind the left heart. Note: the left heart border (LHB) is clearly seen so this additional density must lie within the left lower lobe posterior to the heart: silhouette sign.

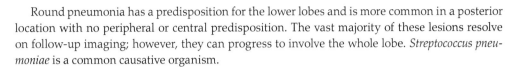

Round pneumonia has a predisposition for the lower lobes and is more common in a posterior location with no peripheral or central predisposition. The vast majority of these lesions resolve on follow-up imaging; however, they can progress to involve the whole lobe. *Streptococcus pneumoniae* is a common causative organism.

2 Why was the radiologist concerned?

Not uncommonly pneumonic consolidation, which assumes this spherical shape, can be mistaken for a pulmonary neoplasm and is known as a pseudotumour of the lung. If there is concern regarding a mass on the CXR then a follow-up XR several weeks after completion of antibiotic treatment will help to resolve any diagnostic dilemma, as infection will show resolution.

If the opacity is persistent or if there is suspicion of a lung tumour then a CT scan should be performed after paediatric review. A differential diagnosis for paediatric CXR masses is included in *Table 10.2*.

Table 10.2 Solitary pulmonary masses on a paediatric CXR

Pseudotumours	Round pneumonia
	Encysted pleural effusion
	Mucous plug
Non-neoplastic lesions	Pulmonary sequestration
	Congenital pulmonary airway malformation
	Intrapulmonary bronchogenic cyst
	Granuloma
	Inflammatory pseudotumour
	Pulmonary arteriovenous malformation
Neoplastic lesions	Solitary metastasis (usually Wilm's tumours and sarcomas)
	Bronchial carcinoid/adenoma
	Pleuropulmonary blastoma
	Hamartoma
	Thoracic neuroblastoma

3 What are the common XR appearances of lower respiratory tract infections in children?

The radiographic appearances of pneumonia vary according to the age of the patient and the pathogen. Several factors contribute to the differences in infection patterns seen in infants and adults:

- The peripheral airways are smaller and have less conductance.
- The collateral pathways of circulation are less well developed.
- There are more mucous glands.
- The airways are more collapsible.

These factors make the smaller airways more susceptible to narrowing, and this predisposes to air trapping and hyperexpansion or segmental collapse. The XR may demonstrate asymmetrical appearances. Thickening of the bronchial wall is a further feature seen in paediatric lower respiratory infections. These changes are secondary to oedema and inflammation in the bronchial walls.

The majority of pneumonias in children are viral and these radiographic changes are mostly associated with viral infections (**Figure 10.2D**). The classic lobar changes associated with bacterial infection are less common.

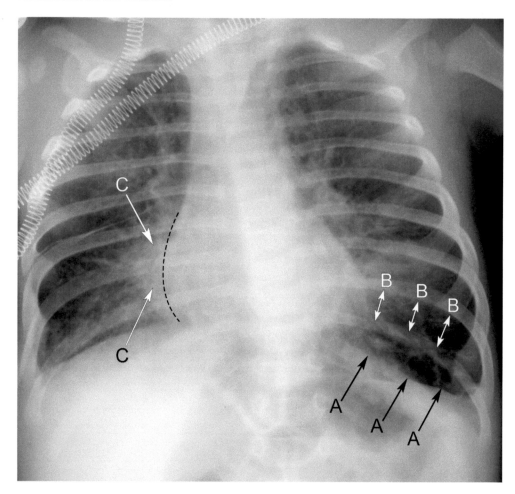

Fig. 10.2D CXR of a 1-year-old infant with a viral bronchopneumonia. The lung appearances are asymmetrical. There is hyperexpansion in the left lower zone with flattened left hemidiaphragm (A) and splaying of the ribs (arrows B). On the right there is an area of opacification (C) adjacent to and obscuring the RHB (border is seen as a dotted line) consistent with collapse and consolidation in the middle lobe (silhouette sign – opacified lung obliterates the normal air/soft tissue interface of aerated lung and right heart). Further consolidation is seen in the left mid and lower zone.

4 What normal structure is often mistaken for a mediastinal tumour in children?

The mediastinum in infants can appear abnormally wide owing to the variable appearances of the thymus, which can be misinterpreted as pathology particularly in those who do not look at paediatric CXRs routinely. The normal thymus can have a variable size and shape particularly in infants. It can extend up to the right or left chest wall, inferiorly to the cardiophrenic angles, and superiorly into the neck. Larger thymuses tend to be commoner in boys.

After the age of 5 years, the thymus becomes less visible on XR with a relative decrease in size and it should not be visible during the second decade. In infants it is often visible as a triangular extension, usually on the right, known as the 'sail sign' (**Figure 10.2E**).

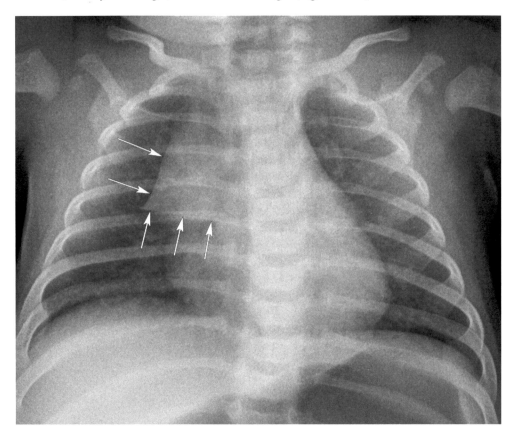

Fig. 10.2E The normal thymus in an infant. The gland extends lateral to the right mediastinal border forming a sail sign (arrows), not to be confused with a mediastinal mass.

LEARNING POINTS: PAEDIATRIC PNEUMONIA

- Several factors contribute to the differences in infection patterns seen in infants and adults owing to smaller and more collapsible airways as well as underdeveloped collateral pathways.
- Round pneumonia is an unusual appearance of pneumonia in children, which can be misinterpreted as a tumour. Radiographic follow-up to normality post-treatment is essential.
- Most paediatric pneumonias are viral and manifest with air trapping, atelectasis, and bronchial wall thickening.
- The thymus is prominent in infants and manifests as a widened mediastinum. It becomes less visible after the age of 5 years. The sail sign is a common appearance of a normal thymus.

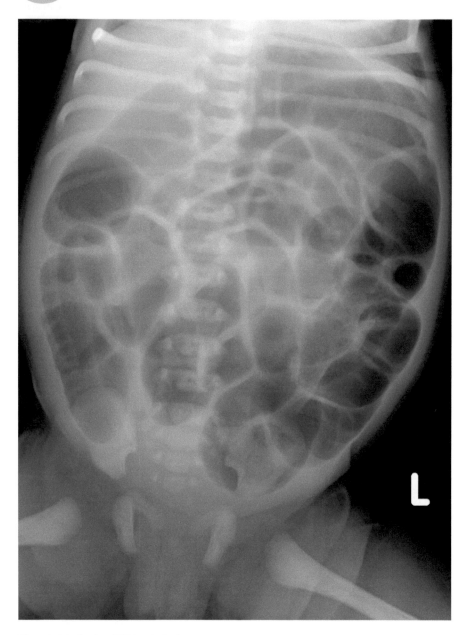

Fig. 10.3A Supine AXR in a baby boy.

A newborn male on the postnatal ward has a distended abdomen and has not passed meconium in the first 24 hours of life. He is breastfeeding well and not vomiting. On examination the abdomen is tense and distended but not peritonitic. You request an AXR (**Figure 10.3A**).

The baby is transferred to the neonatal unit for closer monitoring. In view of the AXR appearances, a contrast enema is performed using a water-soluble contrast agent, (**Figure 10.3B**).

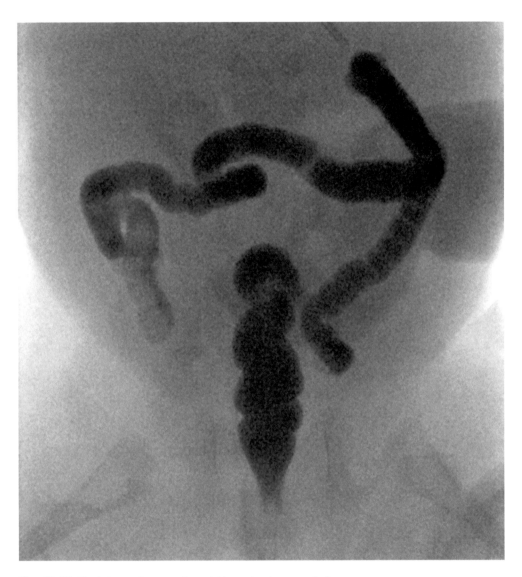

Fig. 10.3B Single image from a water-soluble contrast enema study.

CASE 10.3: QUESTIONS

1 What does the AXR show?
2 What does the contrast enema show and what is the most likely diagnosis?
3 What are the complications of this condition?
4 What are the other features of this condition?

CASE 10.3: ANSWERS

1 What does the AXR show?

Multiple dilated loops of bowel are visible (**Figure 10.3C**). It is not possible to differentiate large and small bowel on a neonatal AXR as both are of a similar calibre and the haustral folds of the colon have not yet fully developed. As a rule of thumb, however, bowel that is wider than the width of a lumbar vertebral body is considered dilated. The clinical and radiological features in this baby are consistent with bowel obstruction.

The causes of neonatal bowel obstruction can be divided into high or low level obstruction (*Table 10.3A*). The bowel gas pattern on this AXR demonstrates multiple loops and the pattern is consistent with a distal 'low level' obstruction. High obstructions tend to present with vomiting whereas low obstructions tend to present with the delayed passage of meconium.

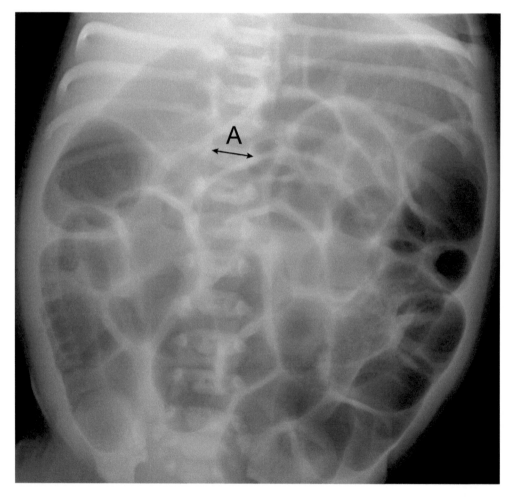

Fig. 10.3C AXR with multiple dilated loops of bowel wider than a vertebral body (arrows, A), in keeping with bowel obstruction.

Table 10.3A Causes of high and low level bowel obstruction in neonates

High obstruction	Low obstruction
Pyloric stenosis	Meconium ileus
Duodenal web	Ileal atresia
Duodenal atresia	Incarcerated inguinal hernia
Malrotation/volvulus	Small left colon
Annular pancreas	Hirschsprung's disease
Jejunal atresia	Anorectal malformations/imperforate anus

2 What does the contrast enema show and what is the most likely diagnosis?

A small atretic colon. Contrast refluxes into the terminal ileum where it outlines several pellets of meconium (**Figure 10.3D**).

The findings are consistent with meconium ileus. Up to 90% of patients with meconium ileus have cystic fibrosis (CF) and 10–20% of patients with CF will present in this manner.

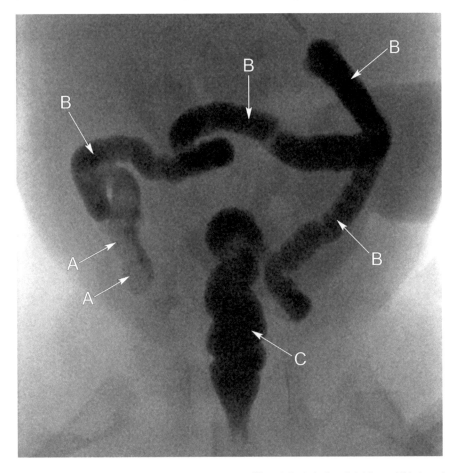

Fig. 10.3D Water-soluble contrast enema demonstrates filling defects in the distal ileum (A) in keeping with meconium ileus. The colon (B) and rectum (C) are empty and atretic with a microcolon appearance.

CF is caused (in most cases) by a mutation in the CF transmembrane conductance regulator (*CFTR*) gene on chromosome 7. This leads to faulty chloride transport across epithelial membranes. This increases the viscosity of meconium, which becomes thick and inspissated in the terminal ileum. The meconium can then impact and cause obstruction. The commonest CF mutation is screened for by heel prick blood test in the neonatal period.

3 What are the complications of this condition?

Complications of meconium ileus include ileal atresia, perforation, and volvulus.

Infants should be managed with an ABCDE approach. IV fluid resuscitation will be necessary as the child is kept nil-by mouth. The contrast enema has therapeutic as well as diagnostic value as the hyperosmolar contrast draws fluid into the bowel lumen and acts as a lubricant, easing the passage of meconium. If conservative measures fail, surgery is then considered.

4 What are the other features of this condition?

Other features of CF are included in *Table 10.3B*. **Figure 10.3E** is a CXR demonstrating thoracic complications of CF.

Table 10.3B Manifestations of CF

Thoracic	Peribronchial thickening
	Bronchial dilatation (bronchiectasis)
	Mucus plugging
	Air trapping, which can lead to a pneumothorax
	Cystic changes
	Pulmonary hypertension
	Hilar lymphadenopathy
GI	Meconium ileus
	Distal intestinal obstruction (equivalent of meconium ileus but in older children)
	Rectal prolapse
Hepatobiliary/ pancreatic	Fatty infiltration in the pancreas
	Chronic pancreatitis
	Hepatomegaly
	Gallstones
	Liver cirrhosis
Skeletal	Delayed skeletal maturation
	Clubbing and hypertrophic cardiomyopathy
Head and neck	Chronic sinusitis
	Nasal polyps

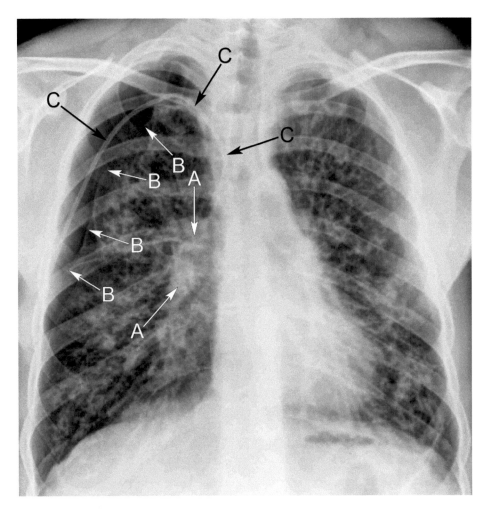

Fig. 10.3E CXR of a teenager with CF. The lungs are mildly hyperinflated. There are changes consistent with bronchiectasis with dilated thick-walled bronchi present. The right hilum appears bulky and dense consistent with lymphadenopathy (A). Note the patient has developed a right pneumothorax (lung edge – B). There is a right-sided central line used to administer long-term IV antibiotics (C). In the exam it is important to ascertain if the central line has just been inserted (so pneumothorax may be a complication of insertion) or if the pneumothorax is a complication of the disease.

LEARNING POINTS: CYSTIC FIBROSIS/MECONIUM ILEUS

- CF is an autosomal recessive genetic disease that affects the exocrine function of the lungs, liver, pancreas, and small bowel.
- 10–20% of patients present with meconium ileus.
- Meconium ileus causes 'low level' bowel obstruction in neonates and causes a 'microcolon' appearance on contrast enema.
- Treatment of CF usually involves long-term antibiotics, steroids, and supplements of vitamins and pancreatic enzymes. Physiotherapy and lung transplantation may also be required.

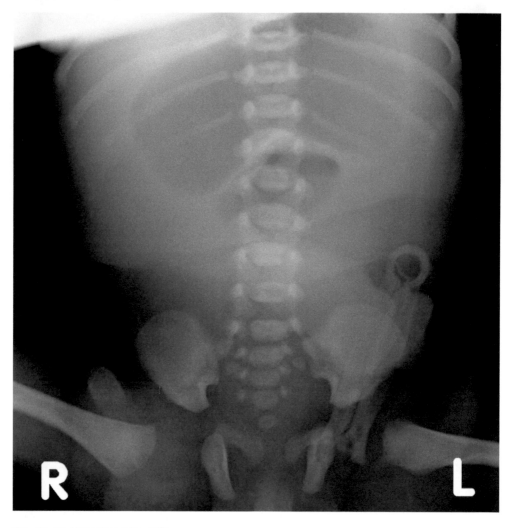

Fig. 10.4A Neonatal supine AXR.

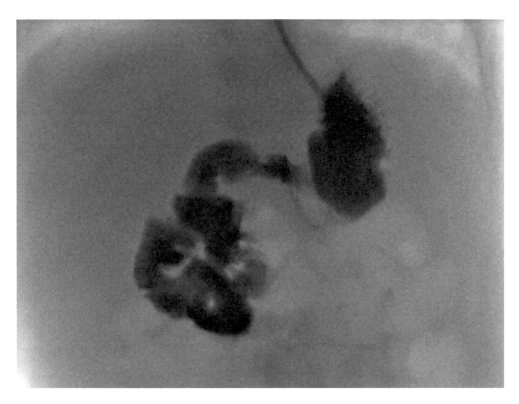

Fig. 10.4B Single image from an upper GI tract contrast study.

A 6-week-old neonate presents to the ED with bilious vomiting. On examination the child is in shock and the abdomen is tender and distended. The baby is stabilised and a NG tube inserted. An AXR is performed (**Figure 10.4A**) after which the patient is urgently transferred to a paediatric surgical unit.

On arrival at the specialist surgical unit, an upper GI (UGI) contrast study is arranged (**Figure 10.4B**).

CASE 10.4: QUESTIONS

1 What do the AXR and the UGI contrast study show and what is the likely diagnosis?
2 What is the pathophysiology of this condition?
3 What are the complications of this condition?
4 What are the differential diagnoses?

CASE 10.4: ANSWERS

1 What do the AXR and the UGI contrast study show and what is the likely diagnosis?

A distended gas-filled stomach and duodenum are seen with a virtually gasless abdomen distally (**Figure 10.4C**). This 'double bubble' appearance is suggestive of a high gastrointestinal obstruction at the level of the duodenum.

The UGI contrast study shows contrast in the stomach, duodenum, and proximal jejunum. The purpose of this study is to locate the position of the duodenojejunal (DJ) flexure. In this study a bolus of the radiopaque contrast agent is injected into the NG tube and followed from the stomach to the duodenum. Normally the course of the duodenum forms a 'C'-shaped loop as it leaves the stomach, such that the DJ flexure is sited in the LUQ of the abdomen to the left of the midline. However, in this case the DJ flexure and proximal small bowel are positioned inferiorly and to the right of the proximal duodenum (**Figure 10.4D**). The findings are consistent with malrotation.

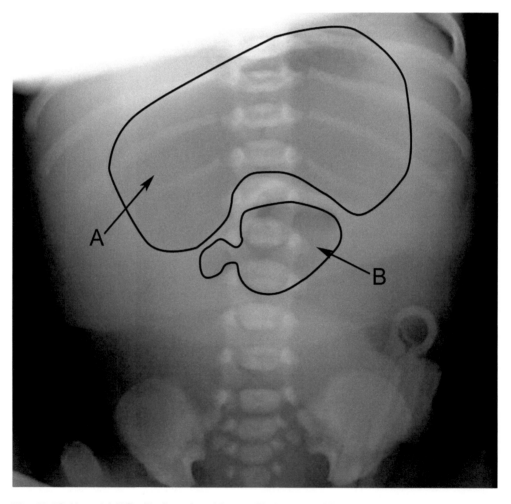

Fig. 10.4C Neonatal AXR with distension of the gas-filled stomach (A) and duodenum (B) with absent distal bowel gas.

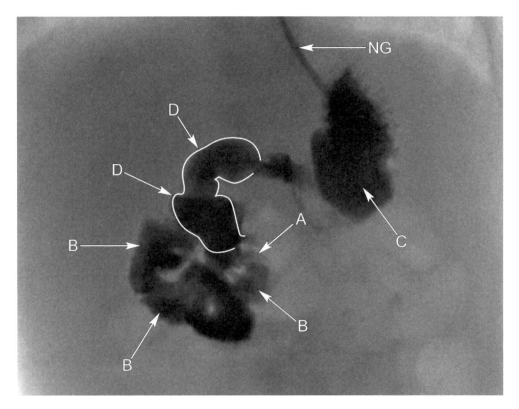

Fig. 10.4D Single image from an upper GI tract contrast study showing the DJ flexure (A) to the right of the midline. The proximal jejunal loops (B) are also located on the right side. Note the NG tube within the stomach (C) and the contour of the duodenum (D). The stomach is now collapsed as it has been drained with the NG tube. There is narrowing of the bowel lumen at the level of the abnormally orientated DJ flexure (A).

2 What is the pathophysiology of this condition?

During the 6th week of embryonic development the bowel undergoes a process of elongation, which leads to a physiological herniation of bowel into the umbilical cord. As the bowel returns back into the abdominal cavity it undergoes a rotation of approximately 270° anticlockwise. If the intestines fail to rotate then the DJ flexure comes to lie on the right of the midline and the caecum floats freely in the upper abdomen. This is known as malrotation.

The bowel becomes fixed in this abnormal position by peritoneal bands called Ladds bands. These stretch from the caecum to the duodenum and attach to the anterior and posterior abdominal walls.

3 What are the complications of this condition?

Because the DJ and ileocaecal junctions are not in their normal positions (malrotated), the base of the small bowel mesentery, which extends between these two points, is narrow. This predisposes to twisting of the bowel known as midgut volvulus. The bowel twists around the mesenteric vessels, which can lead to fatal midgut strangulation; hence the need for emergency treatment if a diagnosis of malrotation is being considered.

4 What are the differential diagnoses?

Malrotation complicated by midgut volvulus is considered a 'high' obstruction as the obstruction is proximal to the jejunum (*Table 10.4*). These cases often present with vomiting. 'Low' obstructions usually present with delayed passage of meconium.

Table 10.4 Causes of high intestinal obstruction in infants

Malrotation

Duodenal atresia/stenosis, jejunal atresia

Duodenal web

Annular pancreas

Pyloric stenosis – nonbilious vomiting

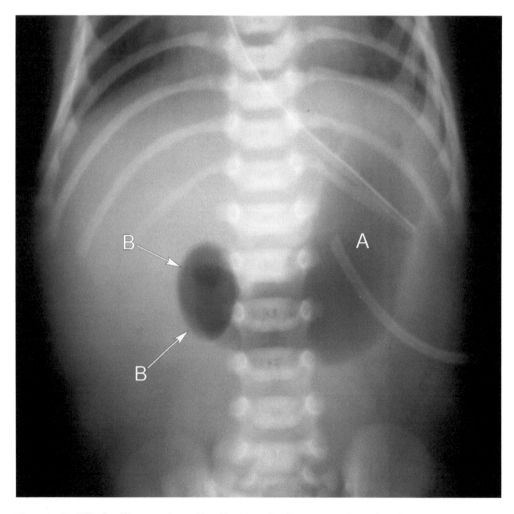

Fig. 10.4E AXR of a different patient with a 'double bubble' caused by distension of the stomach (A) and proximal duodenum (B). There is absence of distal bowel gas in keeping with complete duodenal obstruction. This child had duodenal atresia, which has a 30% association with Down's syndrome.

If the volvulus is partial, there may be no evidence of duodenal obstruction and the AXR may be normal. However, if the obstruction is complete the stomach and duodenum will distend with gas. The appearances can mimic other forms of high obstruction such as duodenal atresia where there is often complete duodenal obstruction with absence of distal gas (**Figure 10.4E**). The distended stomach and duodenum produce what is known as the 'double bubble' sign.

Pyloric stenosis is a common case in finals and you must know the details of this condition. Following AXR, US is used to diagnose these cases with the hypertrophied pylorus having a characteristic sonographic appearance. You are unlikely, however, to be shown this type of US image in finals.

LEARNING POINTS: MALROTATION

- Bowel obstruction in babies can be divided into 'high' and 'low' GI obstruction.
- Causes of a high obstruction include malrotation, duodenal atresia, duodenal web, annular pancreas, pyloric stenosis, and jejunal atresia.
- Malrotation is a congenital abnormality of intestines leading to abnormal fixation of the bowel within the abdomen. This can lead to twisting of the bowel known as midgut volvulus, a potentially life-threatening complication.
- Malrotation can often present with bilious vomiting. The diagnosis is made by a UGI contrast study.
- Treatment of malrotation includes stabilisation and resuscitation of the sick child followed by emergency surgery.

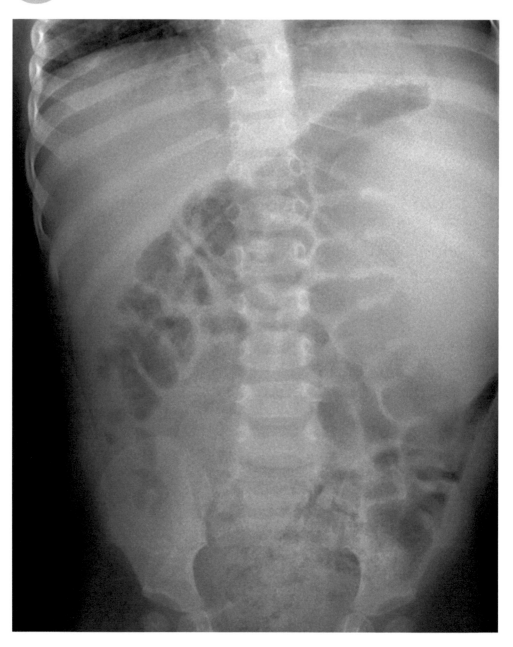

Fig. 10.5A Supine AXR.

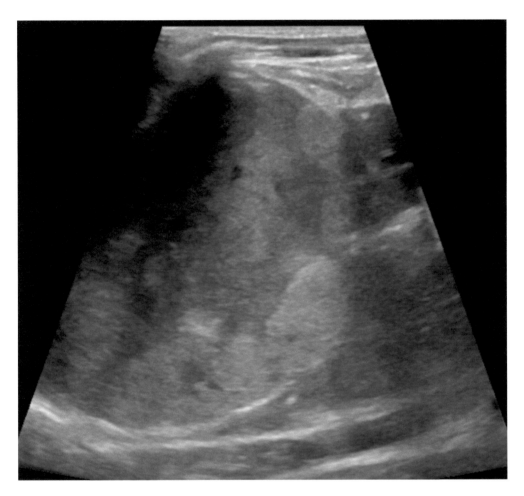

Fig. 10.5B Abdominal US image of the LUQ in longitudinal section.

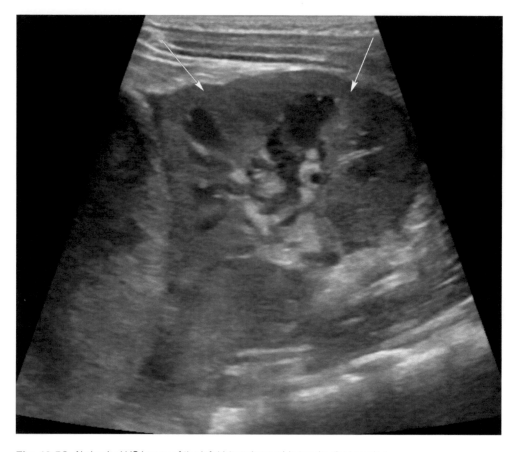

Fig. 10.5C Abdominal US image of the left kidney (arrows) in longitudinal section.

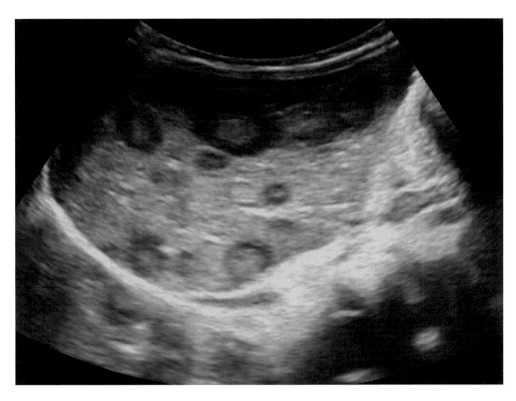

Fig. 10.5D Abdominal US image of the liver in the same child.

A 22-month-old female is taken to her GP with a suspected abdominal mass. She is irritable and has become less confident on her feet. Her growth has also faltered. On examination she is tachycardic and hypertensive. Her abdomen is distended but not tender, and a tender mass is palpable in the left loin.

She is referred to the paediatric unit and an AXR and abdominal US are arranged (**Figures 10.5A–10.5D**).

CASE 10.5: QUESTIONS

1 What does the AXR show?
2 What do the abdominal US images show?
3 What is the likely diagnosis?
4 How should this patient be managed?
5 What are the common differentials?

CASE 10.5: ANSWERS

1 What does the abdominal XR show?

The AXR shows a well-circumscribed, soft-tissue density mass in the LUQ with mass effect on the adjacent splenic flexure of colon, which is displaced inferiorly and medially (**Figure 10.5E**).

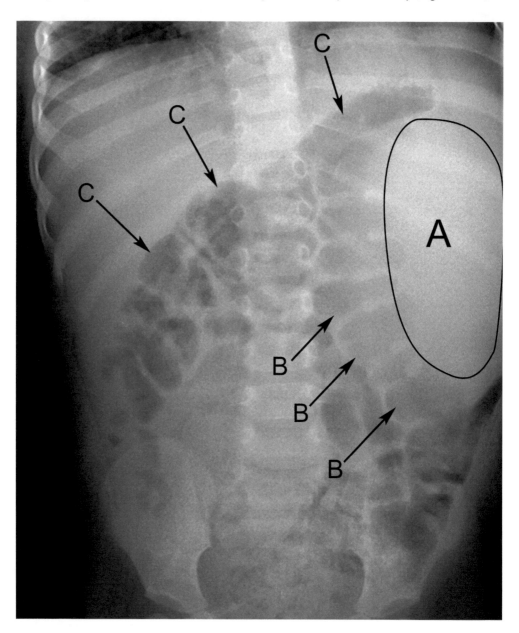

Fig. 10.5E AXR showing a soft tissue mass in the LUQ (A) with medial displacement of the descending colon (B). Transverse colon is labelled C.

2 What do the abdominal US images show?

A large, left suprarenal mass, measuring almost 8 cm in diameter is present. The echotexture is heterogeneous (light and dark). The kidney appears distinct from the mass and is displaced inferiorly (**Figure 10.5C**). The images of the liver show multiple hypoechoic (dark) 'target' lesions in keeping with metastases.

   The mass can be seen in **Figure 10.5B** and also at the left edge of the image in **Figure 10.5C**, displacing the left kidney inferiorly, to the right of the image.

3 What is the likely diagnosis?

There is a suprarenal neoplasm with liver lesions. The most likely diagnosis is adrenal neuroblastoma with liver metastases.

- Neuroblastoma is the most frequent solid neoplasm in childhood (8–10%) and the most frequent malignancy in the first year of life.
- It is the third most common paediatric malignancy (the first being CNS tumours and the second leukaemia).
- The median age of diagnosis is 22 months.
- Neuroblastoma can arise anywhere along the neural crest tissues, which give rise to the adrenal medulla and sympathetic ganglia.
- The clinical features will reflect the size and site of the mass. The majority (45%) arise from the adrenal medulla and present as an abdominal mass.
- Lesions arising from the sympathetic chain can manifest as a thoracic mass in the posterior mediastinum.
- Approximately 60% of infants will have metastatic disease at presentation.
- Metastatic spread to the bones, liver, lymph nodes, skin, and brain are common and children may present with bone and joint pain and/or hepatomegaly.
- Approximately 90% of patients will have elevated levels of hormones and may present with hypertension secondary to catecholamine secretion or watery diarrhoea owing to the production of vasoactive intestinal peptide.
- Neuroblastoma in children under 1 year often presents with hepatic, skin, and bone marrow metastases (stage IV-S disease). This paradoxically has a good prognosis and the lesions can spontaneously regress.

4 How should this patient be managed?

Neuroblastoma is treated according the stage of the tumour at diagnosis. This is based on the radiological findings, surgical resectability, and the presence of metastatic disease. The presence of the n-MYC proto-oncogene is a poor prognostic indicator (n-MYC amplification).

- Neuroblastoma is usually initially identified on US; the tumour appears heterogeneous and hypervascularised. Hypoechoic (dark) areas are common and caused by haemorrhage or necrosis. Although the primary tumour may be detected with US, CT and MRI are required for staging and to help define the local extent of the disease and tissue of origin (**Figure 10.5.F** and **10.5G**). Tumour calcification is seen on CT in 85% of cases. Neuroblastoma typically displaces the kidney without distorting the renal collecting system. It spreads locally by engulfing and encasing the large vessels.

   Metaiodobenzylguanidine (MIBG) nuclear medicine scans are used to check for distant spread of the disease. MIBG is a catecholamine precursor and is taken up by the cells producing catecholamine. In children, this uptake is specific for neuroblastoma; 30% of primary neuroblastomas do not take up MIBG.

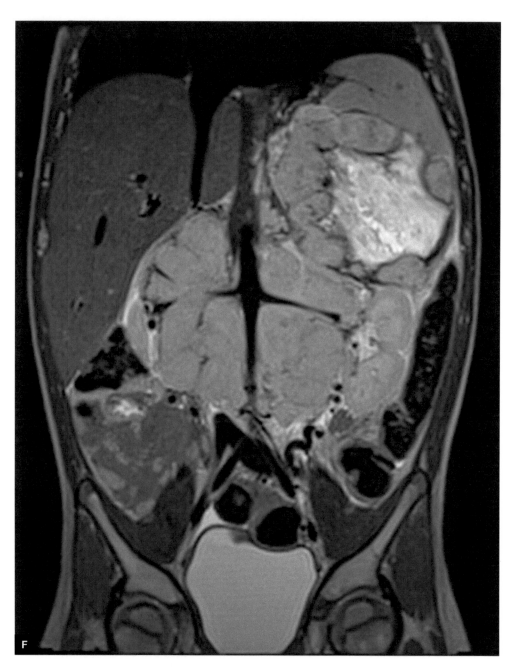

Figs. 10.5F, G Coronal T2-weighted MR images of a different child with neuroblastoma (without [**10.10F**] and with [**10.5G**] annotations). The primary tumour can be seen in the LUQ (A). The bright high signal central area represents necrosis (B). The left kidney (C) is displaced inferiorly. The tumour has spread (D) locally to engulf the aorta (E). Note the normal liver right lobe (F) and spleen (G).

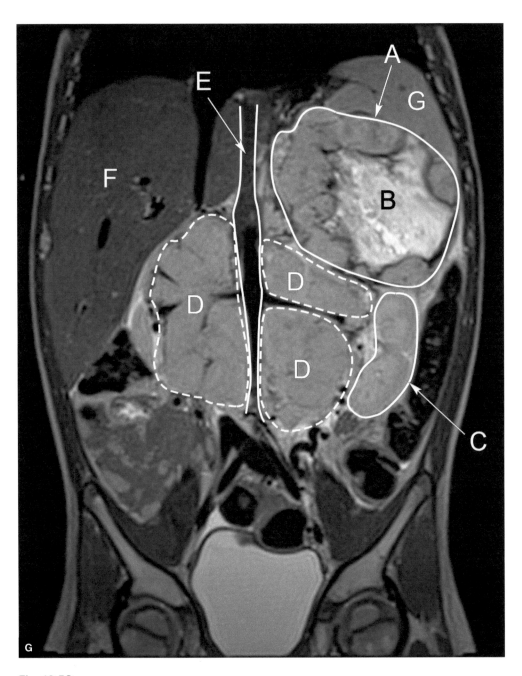

Fig. 10.5G

5 What are the common differentials?

The main differential diagnoses are Wilm's tumour and adrenal haemorrhage. Wilm's tumours arise from the kidneys and tend to displace the adjacent vessels, whereas neuroblastomas tend to surround and engulf vascular structures. Wilm's tumours produce a typical claw sign of renal parenchyma as tumour expands and splays the kidney. Another differential is adrenal haemorrhage, which is common in the neonatal period; this is characteristically avascular and will show regression over time.

LEARNING POINTS: NEUROBLASTOMA

- Neuroblastoma is the most frequent solid neoplasm in childhood (8–10%) and the most frequent malignancy in the first year of life.
- Neuroblastoma can occur anywhere along the neural crest tissue, which gives rise to the sympathetic chain, and the majority occur in the adrenal glands.
- The common differential diagnoses would include Wilm's tumour and adrenal haemorrhage.
- Approximately 60% of infants will have metastatic disease at presentation. Metastatic spread to the bones, liver, lymph nodes, skin, and brain is common.
- Neuroblastoma is treated according the stage of the tumour at diagnosis. This is based on the radiological findings, surgical resectability, and the presence of metastatic disease.

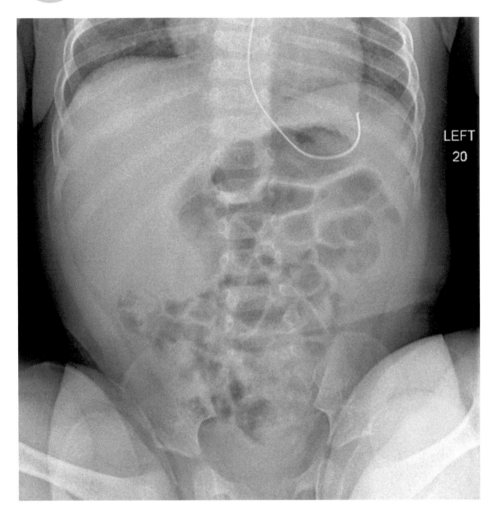

Fig. 10.6A Supine AXR.

An 8-month-old female presents to the ED with vomiting and intermittent abdominal pain. She appears to be in pain and is intermittently drawing her legs up onto her chest. She was initially irritable but now has become increasingly lethargic between episodes. Her mother is concerned as she has refused all feeds and has passed reddish stools. On examination she is pale, lethargic, and dehydrated. Her abdomen is distended and tender with a right-sided palpable mass. Initial investigations are arranged, including bloods and an AXR (**Figure 10.6A**).

CASE 10.6: QUESTIONS

1 What does the AXR show?
2 What is the most likely diagnosis?
3 What test should you arrange to confirm the diagnosis?

4 How should the patient be managed?
5 What are the potential complications of this condition?

CASE 10.6: ANSWERS

1 What does the AXR show?

Multiple central dilated bowel loops and a soft-tissue density in the RUQ are seen on AXR (**Figure 10.6B**). An NG tube is *in situ*. There is no evidence of perforation (the child will need an erect CXR in addition to confirm this).

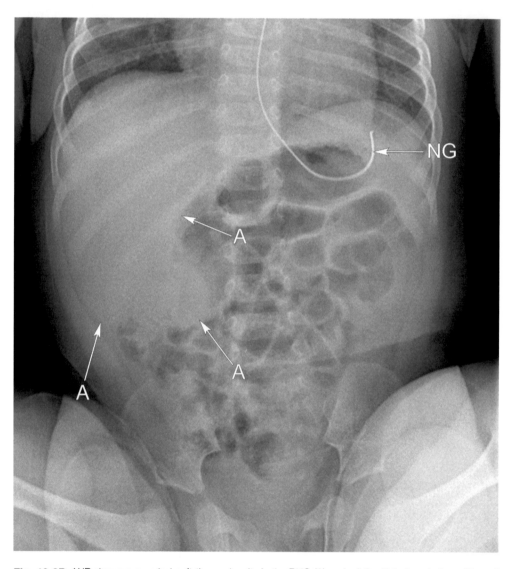

Fig. 10.6B AXR shows a rounded soft-tissue density in the RUQ (A) and mildly dilated central small bowel loops. Note the NG tube (NG) in the stomach.

2 What is the most likely diagnosis?

The history and examination findings are typical for intussusception:

- Intussusception is the telescoping of a segment of proximal bowel (known as the intussusceptum) into a distal segment (the intussuscipiens) leading to bowel obstruction.
- The bowel mesentery, which contains the lymphatics and vasculature, is drawn in alongside the intussuscepted bowel. As a consequence there is venous obstruction, which leads to swelling of the bowel wall; this further compresses the mesentery, obstructs arterial blood flow, and can cause ischaemia and necrosis of the affected segment.
- The point of invagination of the bowel is known as the 'lead point'. This most commonly occurs with ileum passing through the ileocaecal valve into caecum, referred to as an ileocaecal intussusception. However, intussusception can occur anywhere in the large or small bowel.
- Often in children no cause is found. There is some evidence to suggest that it follows viral gastroenteritis, with mesenteric nodal enlargement acting as the lead point. The majority of affected children are under 1 year of age, with a peak incidence at 5–9 months. Passage of 'redcurrant jelly', bloodstained mucus, in the stool is classical.

Intussusception in adults, however, is almost always pathological. The lead point is commonly a malignancy, such as a primary bowel cancer or lymphoma.

3 What test should you arrange to confirm the diagnosis?

In children an US scan of the abdomen is required to confirm the diagnosis (**Figures 10.6C** and **10.6D**). In transverse section, the abnormal segment of bowel produces a 'target' or 'doughnut' sign of bowel within bowel. In longitudinal section one bowel loop can be seen to invaginate into another along with the mesentery. The appearances are similar to the US appearances of a kidney, and are referred to as the 'pseudokidney' sign. US is also used to detect the presence of blood flow within the segment, the absence of which is a poor prognostic indicator.

4 How should the patient be managed?

Intussusception is a surgical emergency and a systematic ABCDE approach should be used.

- If shocked, the patient will need resuscitation with IV fluids.
- Blood should be sent for analysis including FBC, U&Es, CRP, and LFTs. A group and save and cross match are also recommended as the child may go on to have surgery.
- A urine sample should be used to screen for infection.
- A NG tube should be passed to aspirate the stomach contents.
- The child will need an urgent paediatric review and discussion with a specialist paediatric surgical team.
- Imaging is required in the form of an urgent AXR and US (also erect CXR if suggestion of perforation).
- If there are signs of peritonitis the child should proceed straight to theatre.

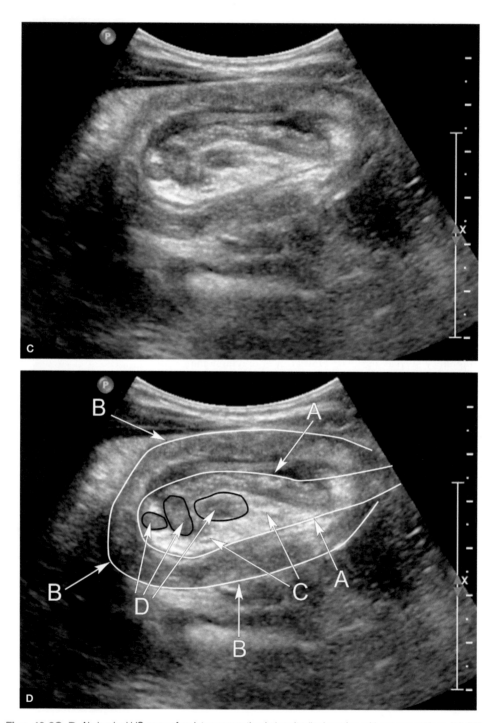

Figs. 10.6C, D Abdominal US scan of an intussusception in longitudinal section without annotations (**10.6C**) and with annotations (**10.6D**), showing the intussusceptum (A) invaginating into the intussuscipiens (B). The bright hyperechoic area in the middle is mesenteric fat (C), which has been drawn in alongside the intussuscepted bowel. In this case the lead point was enlarged reactive lymph nodes (D).

- In the majority of cases, nonoperative management with fluoroscopy or US-guided air enema reduction is the first line of treatment (**Figure 10.6E**). Air is insufflated per rectum to push the intussusceptum back to its normal position. Resolution is confirmed by visualising gas reflux back into the small intestine. If this fails, the child should be taken to theatre for laparoscopic or open reduction. An important complication of rectal air enema reduction is bowel perforation.

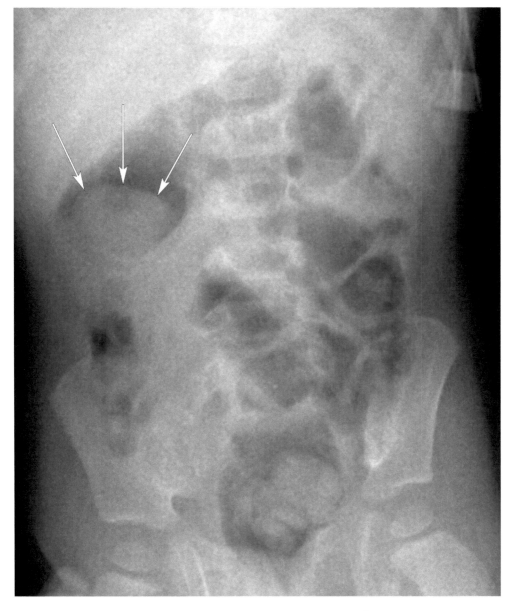

Fig. 10.6E AXR from a fluoroscopic-guided air enema reduction, showing air outlining the intussusceptum (arrows) in the hepatic flexure.

5 What are the potential complications of this condition?

If left untreated, the involved segment of bowel can undergo necrosis and subsequent perforation and peritonitis, which may be fatal.

Recurrence of intussusception is common and can generally be resolved with repeated rectal air enema reduction.

LEARNING POINTS: INTUSSUSCEPTION

- Intussusception is the invagination of proximal bowel into a more distal segment, frequently involving ileum passing into the caecum, via the ileocaecal valve.
- It often presents with severe, colicky, intermittent abdominal pain and vomiting, and characteristically 'redcurrant jelly' stool containing blood-stained mucus.
- It occurs most frequently in children under 1 year, with a peak incidence at 5–9 months.
- There are characteristic diagnostic features on AXR and abdominal US.
- Treatment is usually nonoperative with rectal air insufflation, unless there is evidence of perforation or peritonitis. Adequate resuscitation is vital before any attempt at definitive management.
- If left untreated, bowel perforation, ischaemia, and necrosis can occur, requiring laparotomy and bowel resection.

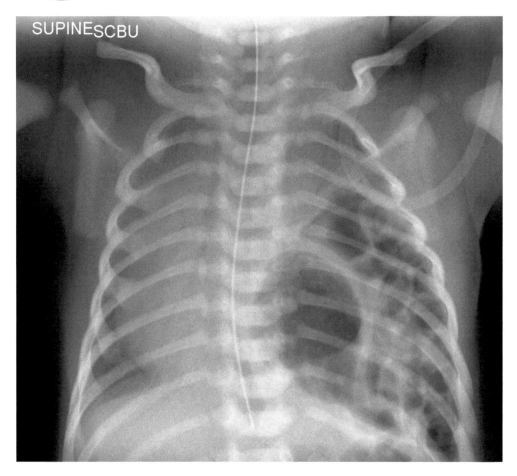

SUPINESCBU

Fig. 10.7A Supine CXR.

A term baby presents at birth with respiratory difficulty and cyanosis. The mother missed her antenatal appointments and her 20 week anomaly scan. The neonatal Senior House Officer is fast bleeped. On examination the baby has reduced air entry on the left with evidence of tracheal deviation to the contralateral side. The abdomen appears scaphoid. The child is admitted to the neonatal intensive care unit (NICU).

A CXR is obtained on admission to the unit (**Figure 10.7A**).

CASE 10.7: QUESTIONS

1 What are the key abnormalities seen on the CXR?
2 What is the most likely diagnosis and the differential diagnosis?
3 What other imaging may help to confirm the diagnosis?
4 How should this child be managed?

CASE 10.7: ANSWERS

1 What are the key abnormalities seen on the CXR?

There are bubbly lucencies in the left hemithorax, with the appearances of air-filled loops of bowel (**Figure 10.7B**).

There is mediastinal shift to the right, with right-sided cardiac and tracheal deviation. In addition, the NG tube has a right-sided convexity to it.

The left hemidiaphragm is not clearly visualised. The right hemidiaphragm images normally. Within the left hemithorax, normal lung markings are seen in the left apex only.

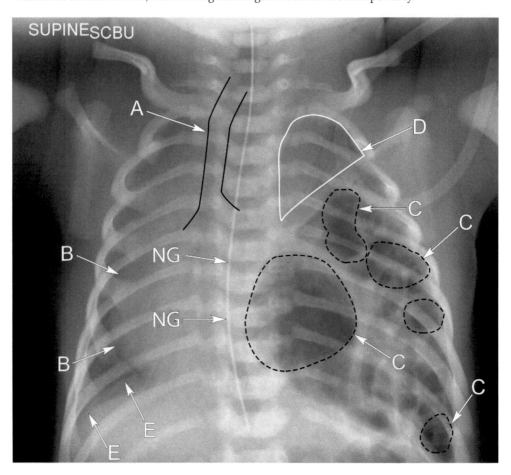

Fig. 10.7B Supine CXR. The trachea (A) and heart (RHB, B) are deviated to the right in keeping with mediastinal shift. There is also deviation of the NG tube (NG) to the right. There are multiple rounded cystic lucencies (C) in the left hemithorax. There is a small amount of normal left lung (D) in the left apex. The right hemidiaphragm (E) is well defined but the left hemidiaphragm is not delineated.

2 What is the most likely diagnosis and the differential diagnosis?

A congenital diaphragmatic hernia (CDH) is most likely. In this condition, bowel loops and other abdominal viscera herniate into the chest through a congenital defect in the diaphragm.

The lung on the side of the hernia will be underdeveloped. The morbidity and mortality associated with this condition is as a consequence of this pulmonary hypoplasia.

There are two main types of CDH in neonates:

- Bochdalek hernias: most common and occur in the posterolateral corner of the diaphragm, more commonly on the left (5:1). (**BBB** = **B**ochdalek, **B**ack-left, **B**ig)
- Morgagni hernias: much less common in neonates and occur in the anterior and medial segments of the diaphragm, more commonly on the right. These are seldom associated with lung hypoplasia and, therefore, have less morbidity. (**MMM** = **M**orgagni, **M**edial-right, **M**ini)

The differential diagnoses for cystic lung lucencies in a neonate are:

- Diaphragmatic hernia.
- Congenital lobar overinflation (previously known as congenital lobar emphysema).
- Congenital pulmonary airway malformation (previously known as congenital cystic adenomatoid malformation).
- Pulmonary sequestration.

Diaphragmatic herniation, in which abdominal viscera herniate into the thorax, is usually detected with antenatal US. It is associated with respiratory distress and cyanosis at birth. Examination will reveal reduced breath sounds on the side of the hernia and a flat or sunken ('scaphoid') abdomen because of the displaced loops of bowel.

3 What other imaging may help to confirm the diagnosis?

In most cases the CXR is diagnostic. However, if the bowel loops are filled with fluid the chest will appear opaque, making it difficult to identify individual loops. In such cases, there can be confusion with other congenital pulmonary lung malformations and US is used to show fluid-filled thoracic bowel loops. US is less sensitive, however, once the bowel loops become filled with gas. If there is ongoing uncertainty, a CT scan can help to confirm the diagnosis (**Figure 10.7C**).

4 How should this child be managed?

If the abnormality is diagnosed antenatally, then an amniocentesis is offered to detect a chromosomal abnormality. A termination may be offered if this is found, as the combination of a CDH and a chromosomal abnormality is usually fatal.

Infants should be delivered in a specialist centre where the necessary obstetric and neonatal surgical facilities are available.

On delivery, the child should be assessed with an ABCDE approach. Prolonged resuscitation with bag-valve-mask ventilation should be avoided as this will cause gaseous distension of the intestines and exacerbate the respiratory distress. The child should be intubated and ventilated as soon as possible. A large bore NG tube should be inserted to decompress the stomach. Hypoventilation owing to lung hypoplasia is the main source of morbidity and mortality, and if severe can be incompatible with life. Occasionally infants with severe ventilatory failure, who do not respond to conventional ventilator support, may be treated with extracorporeal membrane oxygenation (ECMO), a form of complete cardiopulmonary bypass.

Definitive treatment is with surgical repair, which can safely be delayed once the child demonstrates cardiopulmonary stability. The abdominal viscera are returned to the abdomen through a subcostal approach. An artificial patch may be used to repair the diaphragmatic defect. Survival rates vary between 47 and 93%.

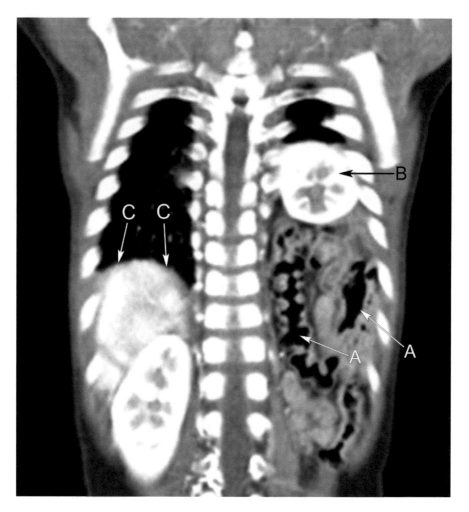

Fig. 10.7C Coronal CT image postcontrast of another neonate with CDH. Bowel loops (A) and the left kidney (B) have herniated up into the left hemithorax. The left hemidiaphragm is absent but the right (C) is clearly visualised. Note the normally positioned right kidney.

LEARNING POINTS: CONGENITAL DIAPHRAGMATIC HERNIA

- Bochdalek and Morgagni are the two main types of congenital diaphragmatic hernia.
  The Bochdalek variant is more common and tends to occur in the posterolateral left diaphragm.
- The morbidity and mortality associated with this condition are related to the degree of pulmonary hypoplasia.
- The diagnosis is usually made on antenatal US. Postnatally the diagnosis can be made on CXR, which will demonstrate bowel loops within the chest and displacement of the NG tube.
- The differential for cystic lung lesions in neonates includes: cystic pulmonary airway malformations, congenital lobar emphysema, and pulmonary sequestration.
- Children with this condition can have severe respiratory failure. Management requires ventilator support and possibly extracorporeal membrane oxygenation, prior to surgical repair.

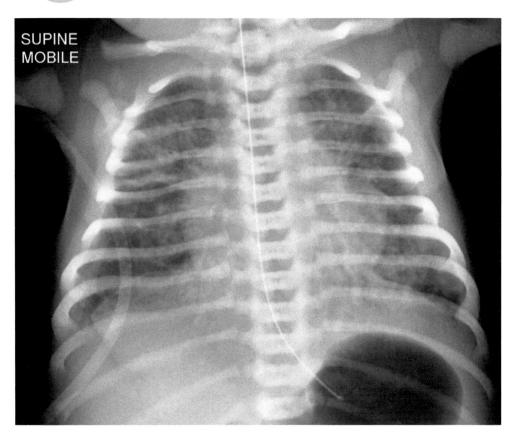

Fig.10.8A Supine CXR.

A newborn child develops respiratory distress following a prolonged delivery with meconium staining of the amniotic fluid at 42 weeks gestation. You are crash called with the paediatric registrar to the delivery room.

On examination there is nasal flaring and intercostal and subcostal recessions. An expiratory grunt is heard. Auscultation reveals widespread rhonchi and crepitations. The child is intubated and meconium is seen in the larynx. The child is then transferred to the NICU. Blood gases are taken:

| pH | 7.1 (7.35–7.45) | P_aCO_2 | 8 kPa (4.5–6) |
| P_aO_2 | 6 kPa (11–14) | BE | −15 (−3–+3) |

After stabilisation on the NICU a CXR is performed (**Figure 10.8A**).

CASE 10.8: QUESTIONS

1 What is the diagnosis?
2 How should this patient be managed?
3 What are the complications of this disorder?

4 What lines and catheters may be inserted to support this baby and what is their optimal position?

CASE 10.8: ANSWERS

1 What is the diagnosis?

The clinical and CXR findings are consistent with meconium aspiration syndrome (MAS).

Placental insufficiency or postmaturity can lead to intrauterine or intrapartum passage of meconium (the infant's first stool), aspiration, and respiratory distress. Approximately 10% of deliveries have meconium stained amniotic fluid at 38 weeks' gestation, and this rises to 22% by 42 weeks.

Inhaled meconium is extremely toxic to the newborn lungs, acting as a chemical irritant inhibiting the production of surfactant. It can also cause partial or complete bronchial obstruction, leading to peripheral lung collapse or hyperexpansion via a 'ball-valve' effect.

The CXR appearances are of asymmetric lung abnormalities (**Figure 10.8B**) with a mixed picture of patchy infiltrates, areas of collapse, and segments of hyperexpansion. Hyperexpansion of the lungs is particularly common in the early stages.

In severe cases the CXR appearances remain abnormal beyond 14 days and produce a similar pattern to bronchopulmonary dysplasia. The CXR appearance can also mimic congenital infection and all babies with MAS are commenced on empirical antibiotics after a septic screen.

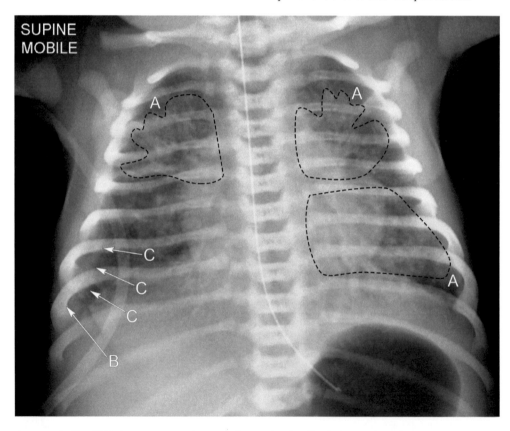

Fig. 10.8B The CXR shows asymmetric areas of consolidation (A) with bronchial wall thickening and air bronchograms. The lungs are hyperexpanded with at least 8 anterior ribs visible (anterior right 8th rib, B) above the diaphragm. There is a small right pleural effusion (C). Note the NG tube and oxygen tubing.

2 How should this patient be managed?

All babies in respiratory distress should be managed using an ABCDE approach. The management for MAS is purely supportive, allowing time for macrophage clearance of the inhaled debris. Intubation and ventilation may be required in severe cases with ECMO support. In addition, the use of exogenous surfactant has been shown to reduce the duration for respiratory support.

Hypoxia is common and oxygen is required to maintain saturations to greater than 95%. Ventilation is usually not a problem in mature infants and the P_aCO_2 is usually normal or only slightly raised.

The first blood gas taken after birth may show a marked metabolic acidaemia owing to birth asphyxia. The acidaemia may need to be corrected if the base deficit is greater than −15.

Close monitoring is required on the NICU. This may require insertion of central umbilical catheters to monitor the baby's BP and for the administration of drugs, an endotracheal tube (ETT) and a NG tube to aspirate stomach contents (**Figure 10.8C**).

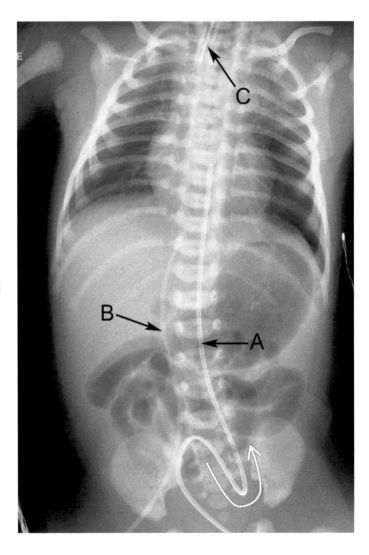

Fig. 10.8C Whole body XR of a child on the NICU. This type of XR is often used to confirm the position of the support apparatus. Note: course of the umbilical catheters. The umbilical arterial catheter (UAC, A) curls inferiorly in the umbilical artery (curved arrow) before extending upwards through the iliac artery into the aorta. The tip of the umbilical catheter must be confirmed not to be passing into an aortic branch (e.g. renal artery); the tip optimally lies either high (T6–T10) or low (L3–L5) and not in-between to avoid aortic major branches. The umbilical venous catheter (UVC, B) passes towards the liver and into the inferior vena cava (IVC) via the ductus venosus: the tip is optimally placed at the junction of the IVC with the right atrium. Note also the ETT (C).

3 What are the complications of this disorder?

Potential complications include air leaks such as pneumothorax and pneumomediastinum. These are caused by the lung hyperexpansion secondary to the ball-valve effect of partially obstructing viscous meconium, (**Figure 10.8D**).

Persistent pulmonary hypertension of the newborn (PPHN) is another complication. Babies with MAS develop hypoxia, and this can lead to pulmonary artery vasoconstriction and a raised pulmonary artery pressure, which is a feature of PPHN. In this condition the pulmonary arterial pressure rises above the systemic arterial pressure, resulting in right-to-left shunting across the ductus arteriosus and foramen ovale, similar to that seen in the fetal circulation.

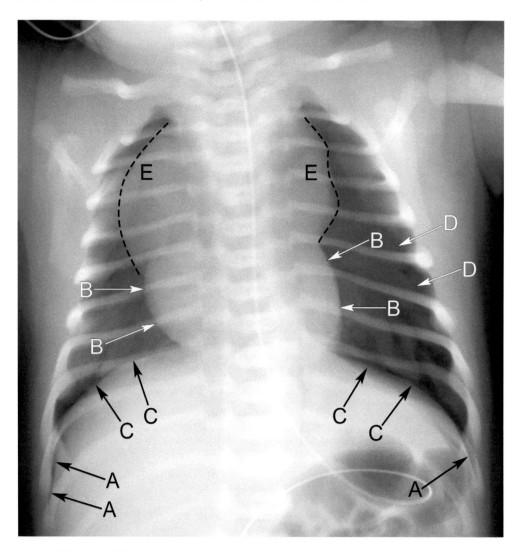

Fig. 10.8D Supine CXR with bilateral anterior pneumothoraces in a child with meconium aspiration. Signs of an anterior pneumothorax include lucent hemithoraces, a deep diaphragmatic sulcus (A), overly well-defined heart (B) and diaphragmatic (C) borders, and a visible lung edge (D) with absent vascular marking peripherally. Note: widened superior mediastinum owing to normal thymus (dotted lines, E).

The mortality from MAS is between 4 and 12%. The majority of deaths are from respiratory failure, air leaks, and PPHN.

4 What lines and catheters may be inserted to support this baby and what is their optimal position?

Lines and catheters required to support the baby include an ETT, UAC, UVC, and a NG tube.

The ETT allows ventilator support. The tube tip should be in the mid-tracheal position about 1 cm above the carina. Paradoxically, when the neck is flexed the tube travels downwards and when the neck is extended the tube travels upwards. The most common malposition is within the right main bronchus.

The UAC allows fluids and medication to be administered and can be used to monitor the arterial BP and gases. The catheter passes from the umbilical artery inferiorly into the iliac arteries before passing up into the aorta. The optimum tip position is at T6–T9 level, well away from the renal and mesenteric arteries.

The UVC also allows fluids and medication to be administered and is used for blood sampling. The catheter passes from the umbilical vein up to the left portal vein then courses through the ductus venosus into the IVC. The optimum tip position is at the right cavoatrial junction.

The NG tube can be used for enteral feeding and to aspirate stomach contents in an intubated child. The tube tip should lie in the stomach, well below the left hemidiaphragm and beyond the gastro-oesophageal junction.

LEARNING POINTS: MECONIUM ASPIRATION SYNDROME

- Meconium is the first neonatal stool and can be passed *in utero* in response to fetal hypoxic stress.
- If inhaled, meconium can obstruct the airways and produce a chemical pneumonitis causing severe, and sometimes fatal, respiratory distress known as MAS.
- The CXR findings include collapse and consolidation as well as peripheral hyperexpansion owing to air trapping.
- This condition can be complicated by air leaks (such as pneumothorax and pneumomediastinum) and persistent pulmonary hypertension.

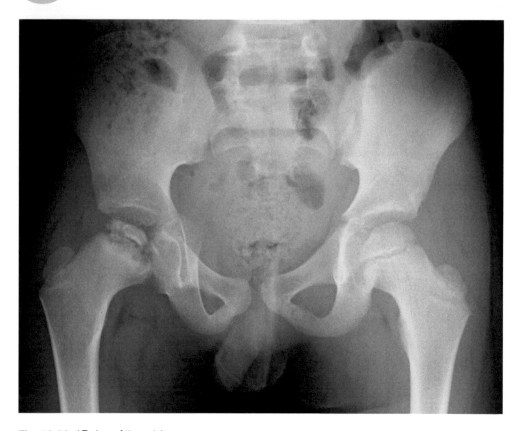

Fig. 10.9A AP view of the pelvis.

A 10-year-old male presents to his GP with a 3-month history of right hip pain and a limp. There is no history of trauma. The pain is worse on activity and improves with rest. He is otherwise well and his height and weight are between the 50th and 75th centiles. On examination of his right hip there is no erythema or swelling. He has slightly reduced range of movement but the remainder of the examination is normal. The GP refers him for an XR series (**Figure 10.9A** and **10.9B**).

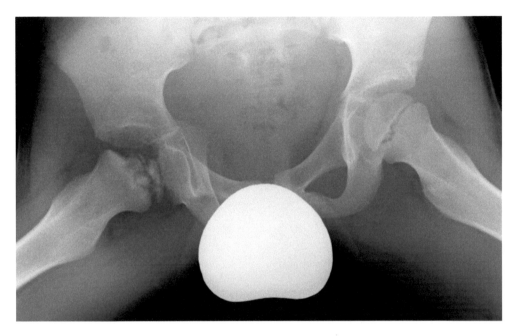

Fig. 10.9B Frog leg lateral view of the hips (gonad protection applied).

CASE 10.9: QUESTIONS

1 What do the XRs show?
2 What is the aetiology of this condition?
3 What are the differential diagnoses for an acutely painful limp in a child?
4 What further imaging would you recommend?
5 What are the management options?
6 What are the potential complications?

CASE 10.9: ANSWERS

1 What do the XRs show?

They show (**Figure 10.9C**) a small and fragmented right capital femoral epiphysis. The physis is widened and the metaphysis irregular in contour. There is an effusion in the right hip joint. These are the features of Perthes' disease. The left hip is normal.

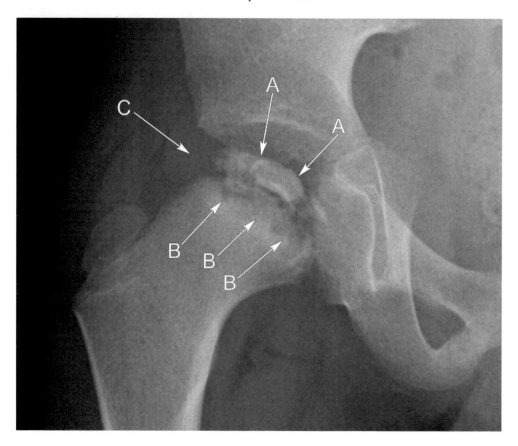

Fig. 10.9C AP magnified view showing features of Perthes' disease in the right hip. Note the necrotic, fragmented right capital femoral epiphysis (A), irregularity and widening of the metaphysis (B), and hip effusion (C).

2 What is the aetiology of this condition?

Perthes' disease is avascular necrosis of the capital femoral epiphysis. The blood supply to the femoral head is compromised leading to bone necrosis. Over time, the necrotic bone is removed and revascularisation occurs with reossification. The aetiology is unknown.

- The quality of new bone growth can be variable and this is where the various treatment options play a key role.
- The onset is insidious and is usually unilateral. It generally occurs in children aged 4–10 years and is more common in boys.

- In the early stages, the XR can be normal or may only show increased density of the capital femoral epiphysis. As the disease progresses the femoral head becomes necrotic and fragmented with irregularity of the metaphysis and an effusion.
- It is usually detected and managed in the early stages (**Figure 10.9D**), with severe deformity now being rare.

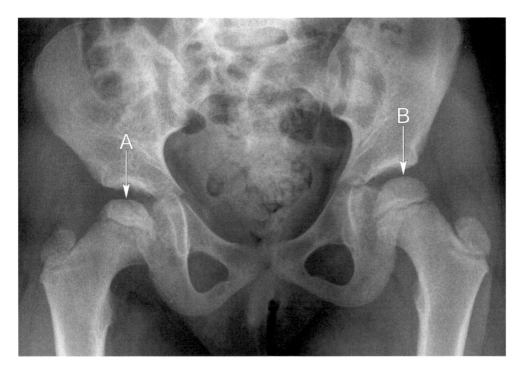

Fig. 10.9D AP view of the pelvis showing early features of Perthes' disease in the right hip. Note the increased density of the right femoral capital epiphysis (A) with some loss of height and normal appearance on the left (B).

3 What are the differential diagnoses for an acutely painful limp in a child?

The differential diagnoses are listed in *Table 10.9* (see page 514).

4 What further imaging would you recommend?

In the early stages of the disease the XR may be normal, and this partially explains why Perthes' disease may be mistaken for transient synovitis. Therefore, it is important not to be falsely reassured by normal imaging. MRI is recommended for detecting very early changes and is particularly useful where there is a normal XR despite ongoing symptoms.

5 What are the management options?

Management depends on the severity of disease at presentation. Early diagnosis and management is the key to preventing early onset OA. The main aims of treatment are to reduce pain, preserve the hip range of movement, and prevent deformity.

Table 10.9 Differential diagnosis for a child with an acutely painful limp

Differential	How this may present as a limp
Transient synovitis of the hip	Also known as irritable hip, this is the most common cause for an acute painful limp in school age children (2–12 years of age) and often follows a viral illness
Septic arthritis	Septic arthritis is an infected joint
	This can quickly lead to irreversible cartilage destruction and early onset osteoarthritis
	Blood inflammatory markers, blood cultures, and joint aspiration are required to confirm the diagnosis followed by early IV antibiotics and joint washout in theatre
	Septic arthritis usually presents with a red hot swollen painful joint and is is more common in children less than 2 years old
Slipped capital femoral epiphysis	This is posteroinferior displacement of the capital femoral epiphysis presenting with acute or gradual onset hip/knee pain and a limp
	Most common in obese adolescent boys
	Urgent surgical treatment is required to prevent avascular necrosis of the femoral head
Leukaemia	Leukaemia can present with a limp owing to bony involvement
	These children tend to appear pale and unwell
	There are usually other symptoms such as bruising and bleeding due to low platelets, and signs of infection due to the compromised immune system
Trauma related injury	A history of trauma is usually offered

- Conservative management may be sufficient in young children with early disease and only minor changes to the femoral head. This can include observation of the hip joint with serial XRs to ensure there is adequate bone regrowth. Physiotherapy and analgesia (including NSAIDs) help pain and stiffness.
- Further damage to the femoral head can be prevented by limiting high-impact activities and sometimes crutches are used to prevent any weight being put through the affected hip joint.
- Plaster casts and braces may be used to keep the hip in abduction, thereby maintaining the femoral head within the acetabulum to promote adequate healing. This is usually kept on for 4–6 weeks but may need to be repeated until healing is complete.
- Surgery is usually reserved for more severe cases, where the child is older (over 8 years old at diagnosis) or where conservative management has been unsuccessful. This usually involves osteotomy of the femur or pelvis followed by a cast to hold the hip in position while healing occurs. Physiotherapy, crutches, and analgesia again play a role.

6 What are the potential complications?

In the shorter term, complications are largely related to the degree of deformity after healing. These may include pain, stiffness, and reduced range of movement.

- Indicators of poor prognosis in the longer term include late diagnosis, older age at onset, and severe disease of the femoral head with residual deformity after healing.

- Each of these factors increases the potential for OA in adulthood, with a poorer prognosis related to the development of OA at an earlier age. This may necessitate hip joint replacement.
- With prompt diagnosis and early intervention, the prognosis is generally very good.

LEARNING POINTS: PERTHES' DISEASE

- Perthes' disease is avascular necrosis of the capital femoral epiphysis.
- It often presents with a limp and hip or knee pain, in children aged 4–10 years, and is more common in boys than girls.
- Initial XRs can appear normal leading to a misdiagnosis of transient synovitis of the hip. Further imaging is required if symptoms persist.
- The aims of treatment are to reduce pain, preserve range of movement, and prevent deformity. Treatment may be conservative or involve surgery.
- Prognosis depends on the level of residual deformity, age at diagnosis, and severity at diagnosis. The main consequence in later life is OA.

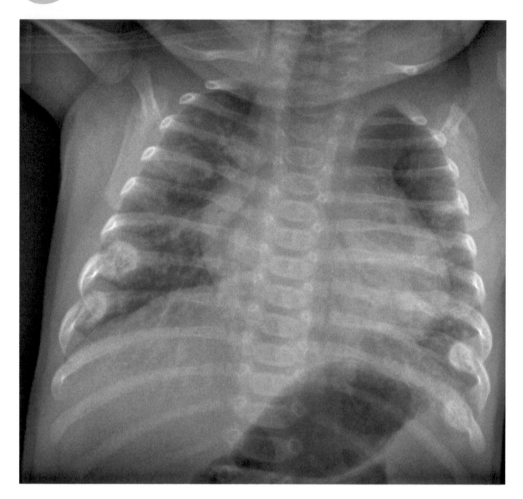

Fig. 10.10A Supine CXR.

A 3-month-old male is taken to the ED with drowsiness and lethargy. His breathing is laboured and he is floppy. His parents give a history of him becoming quiet after rolling off a couch and onto the carpeted floor. There is no relevant past medical or family history; however, the family is known to social services owing to a history of paternal substance abuse.

On examination the child is drowsy and lethargic with a bulging anterior fontanelle. The right leg appears swollen and red. There are skin bruises overlying his chest.

A CXR and an XR of the right lower leg are obtained (**Figures 10.10A** and **10.10B**).

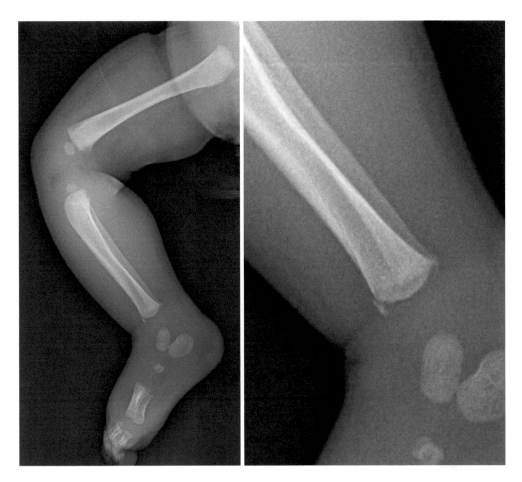

Fig. 10.10B XR of the right lower leg. The left image is a lateral view; the right image is a magnified lateral view of the ankle/lower leg.

CASE 10.10: QUESTIONS

1 What do the XRs show?
2 What are your concerns regarding this child?
3 How should the child be managed initially?
4 What further investigations should be performed?

CASE 10.10: ANSWERS

1 What do the XRs show?

The CXR (**Figure 10.10C**) shows multiple bilateral posterior and lateral rib fractures with exuberant soft and hard callus formation. The lower leg XR shows a corner fracture of the distal tibial metaphysis (**Figure 10.10D**).

- The precise dating of fractures is not possible. Estimates can be made, however, based on the pattern of XR changes (*Table 10.10A*).

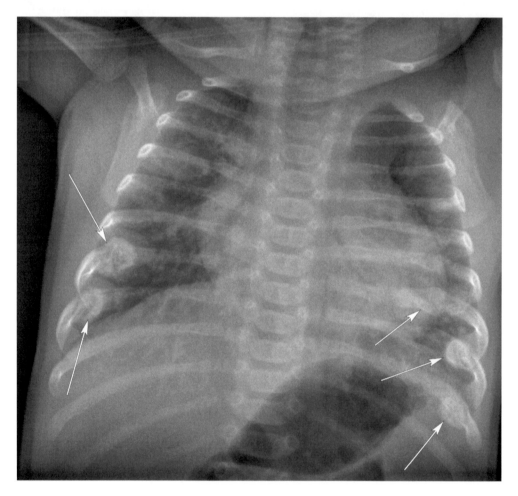

Fig. 10.10C CXR showing posterior rib fractures on both sides of the chest (arrows). Soft and hard callus formation is present indicating subacute fractures of differing ages.

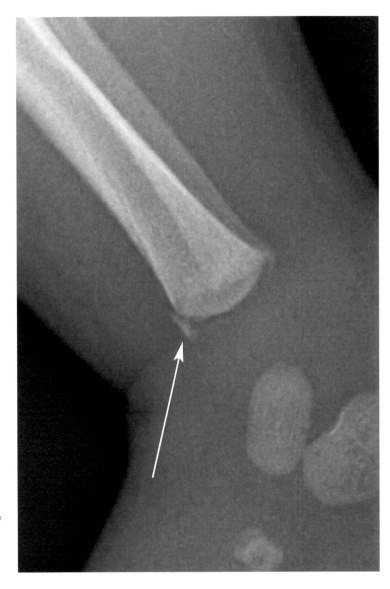

Fig. 10.10D XR of the right lower leg showing a triangular fragment of bone at the corner of the distal metaphysis of the right tibia (arrowed). This is known as a metaphyseal corner fracture.

Table 10.10A Radiographic changes in childhood fractures

Radiological features	Early	Peak	Late
Soft-tissue resolution	2–5 days	4–10 days	10–21 days
Periosteal new bone	4–10 days	10–14 days	14–21 days
Loss of the fracture line definition	10–14 days	14–21 days	42–90 days
Soft callus	10–14 days	14–21 days	2 years
Hard callus	14–21 days	21–42 days	
Remodelling	3 months	1 year	

2 What are your concerns regarding this child?

The XR findings of multiple fractures of different ages, at different sites, is suspicious for nonaccidental injury (NAI). In particular, metaphyseal corner fractures and posterior rib fractures have a high specificity for NAI. The clinician should be further alerted by the injuries not correlating with the given history and the additional social concerns.

- Rib fractures in infants are almost always secondary to abuse. Up to 82% of rib fractures in children <1 year of age are caused by abuse. The classic location is within the posterior ribs at the articulation with the transverse process. Accidental rib fractures are extremely rare, even in the presence of major trauma. The incidence of rib fractures in children with proven NAI is 5–27%. Fractures are caused by compression of the chest while the baby is being shaken.
- Metaphyseal corner fractures are also known as bucket handle fractures. These fractures are highly specific for NAI. They are most commonly seen in nonambulatory infants under 18 months of age. The most frequent locations are around the feet and ankles. The fractures are caused by twisting of the limb or from acceleration/deceleration forces applied to the limb as a result of shaking. Other fractures that are associated with NAI are listed in *Table 10.10B*.

Table 10.10B Fractures associated with NAI

High specificity	Metaphyseal corner fractures
	Rib fractures
	Scapular fractures
	Sternal fractures
	Spinous process fractures
Moderate specificity	Multiple fractures
	Fractures of differing ages
	Finger fractures in nonmobile children
	Vertebral body fractures
	Epiphyseal separation
	Complex skull fractures
Low specificity	Midclavicular fractures
	Simple linear skull fractures
	Long bone diaphyseal fractures
	Greenstick fractures

3 How should the child be managed initially?

The child should be stabilised and resuscitated with an ABCDE approach. This may entail the need for invasive ventilation, particularly in the context of an associated head injury and reduced conscious level. The child may be in haemodynamic shock if there is internal haemorrhage and will require monitoring of his BP with fluid resuscitation.

The paediatric team should be alerted immediately. A detailed clinical history and examination is required to gather information of the mechanism of injury and to look for any other signs of physical abuse. Measures should be taken to ensure the wellbeing of the child. The lead clinician with a responsibility for child safeguarding should be informed and child protection procedures initiated. The child should be admitted to hospital both for treatment and as a place of safety. The social care team and police will need to be informed as there may be siblings who are also at risk.

4 What further investigations should be performed?

The child will need further investigation with a CT brain scan and an XR skeletal survey.

- CT is the first-line neuroimaging used to exclude traumatic brain injury (**Figure 10.10E**). An MRI may also be used to help date any identified intracranial haemorrhage.
- XR skeletal surveys are used to exclude further fractures anywhere else in the skeleton. A repeat skeletal survey is also performed after 2 weeks to detect any previously occult fractures by the identification of callus formation. Occasionally, a nuclear medicine bone scan is used to detect occult fractures before callus has had a chance to form.
- Ophthalmological assessment is also recommended to look for retinal haemorrhages, which are also associated with NAI.

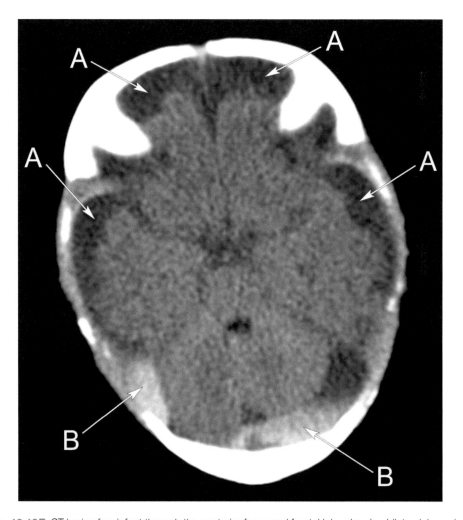

Fig. 10.10E CT brain of an infant through the posterior fossa and frontal lobe showing bilateral, large, low density, chronic, subdural haematomas surrounding both cerebral hemispheres (A). There are also two large, high density, posterior fossa collections in keeping with acute subdural haemorrhage (B).

The two main mechanisms of intracranial haemorrhage in NAI are impact injuries from a direct blow or from a shaking injury with acceleration and deceleration forces on the brain. Direct trauma will result in a skull fracture and contusion to the underlying brain. A shaking injury is characterised by subdural haemorrhages, often of different ages (**Figure 10.10E**). There is a high association with parenchymal ischaemic damage owing to hypoxia. Retinal injury in the presence of a subdural haemorrhage is very suggestive of an acceleration/deceleration mechanism of NAI. The term 'shaken baby syndrome' describes the association of subdural haemorrhage, massive cerebral oedema, fractured ribs, and metaphyseal injury in the absence of external signs of head injury.

LEARNING POINTS: NONACCIDENTAL INJURY

- Rib fractures and metaphyseal corner injuries have a high specificity for NAI.
- NAI should be suspected in the context of unexplained trauma, particularly in a nonambulatory child.
- Brain injury from NAI may be result from direct impact or from the acceleration/deceleration forces produced by shaking.
- The term 'shaken baby syndrome' refers to the association of subdural haemorrhages, rib fractures, and metaphyseal corner injuries in the absence of external signs of head injury.
- You must promptly communicate any abnormal findings or concerns about NAI to the senior responsible clinician. If a Social Services referral is not made and you still have concerns, it is your duty to contact the designated doctor for child protection within the Trust.

Case 10.11

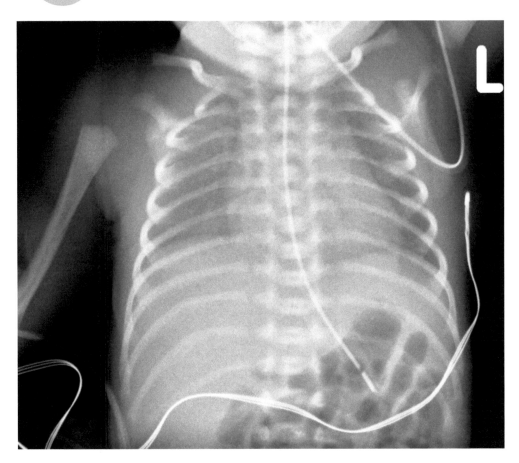

Fig. 10.11A Supine neonatal CXR.

A woman goes into spontaneous labour at 28 weeks gestation. You are called with the neonatal registrar to attend the delivery. The baby shows immediate signs of respiratory distress with cyanosis and expiratory grunting. Oxygen is administered via a bag, valve, and mask, and the child is transferred to the NICU for respiratory support.

While on the unit, the baby's respiratory status deteriorates and necessitates intubation and ventilation. Arterial blood gases and a CXR are obtained (**Figure 10.11A**).

pH	7.20 (7.35–7.45)	P_aCO_2	8 kPa (4.5–6 kPa)
P_aO_2	4 kPa (11–14 kPa)	HCO_3	35 mmol/L (18–25 mmol/L)

CASE 10.11: QUESTIONS

1 What is the diagnosis?
2 What are the three main radiographic features?

3 What is the underlying pathophysiology?
4 What are the short- and long-term complications?

CASE 10.11: ANSWERS

1 What is the diagnosis?

The diagnosis is respiratory distress syndrome (RDS). The blood gases show hypoxia, which is universal in this condition, and the degree of hypoxia correlates well with the severity. In most cases the P_aCO_2 will be raised in keeping with a respiratory acidosis.

2 What are the three main radiographic features?

The main CXR features of RDS are (**Figure 10.11B**):

- Small lung volumes.
- Air bronchograms.
- Fine granular (reticular nodular) parenchymal lung pattern.

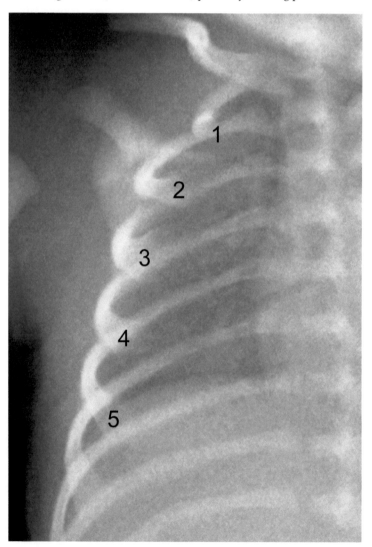

Fig. 10.11B Magnified view of the neonatal CXR (from **Figure 10.11A**). Diffuse granular lung markings with a 'ground glass' appearance are present. There is lung volume loss with only 5 anterior ribs demonstrated (1–5).

The CXR features vary according to the severity of the condition:

- Mild disease: lung markings are uniform, diffuse, linear, and granular. They are often described as having a 'ground glass' pattern. This describes mild diffuse opacification that is not enough to obscure the pulmonary vasculature.
- Moderate disease: the opacification of the lungs is denser and coarser with the presence of air bronchograms (**Figures 10.11C** and **10.11D**).
- Severe disease: complete opacification of both lungs. This manifests as a total 'white out' on the CXR.

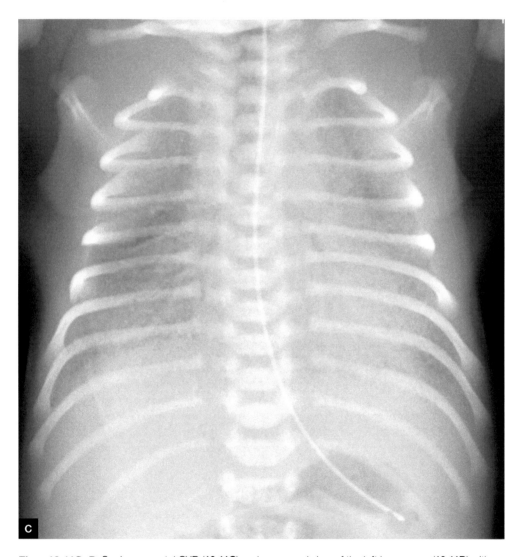

C

Figs. 10.11C, D Supine neonatal CXR (**10.11C**) and a cropped view of the left lower zone (**10.11D**) with signs of moderate-severe RDS. There is bilateral volume loss and lung opacification. As the lungs become denser and consolidated, air bronchograms appear (arrows).

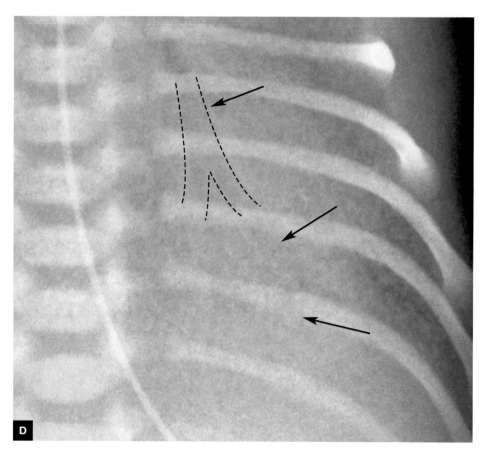

Fig. 10.11D

3 What is the underlying pathophysiology?

RDS is primarily a disease of prematurity. Half of all babies born before 30 weeks of gestation develop RDS compared with 2% of those born after 35 weeks. The underlying pathophysiology is the absence of lung surfactant, manufactured by type II alveolar pneumocytes, from around week 24 of gestation. Surfactant acts to lower the surface tension of the alveoli, preventing their collapse on expiration. Without surfactant the alveoli collapse and epithelial cells undergo necrosis.

Treatment is, therefore, based on respiratory support of the immature and fragile lungs and administration of synthetic surfactant.

4 What are the short- and long-term complications?

Short-term complications include:

- Air leak syndromes (pneumothorax, pneumomediastinum, and pulmonary interstitial emphysema) owing to barotrauma (**Figures 10.11E** and **10.11F**).
- Persistent patent ductus arteriosus (owing to reduced oxygen stimulus).
- Oxygen toxicity (from treatment).
- Pulmonary haemorrhage.
- Recurrent pulmonary infection.

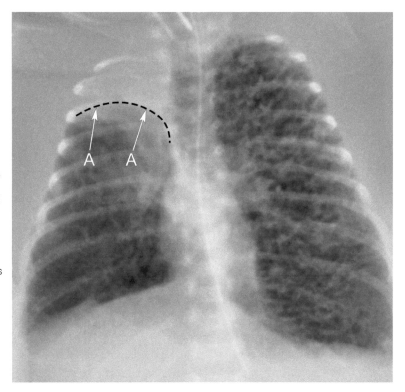

Fig. 10.11E Supine neonatal CXR with pulmonary interstitial emphysema in the left lung, predominantly perihilar, secondary to previous ventilation. Gas leaks out of the small airways and tracks in a radial pattern towards the hilum. The condition gives a cystic 'bubbly' appearance. Note also the right upper lobe collapse (A).

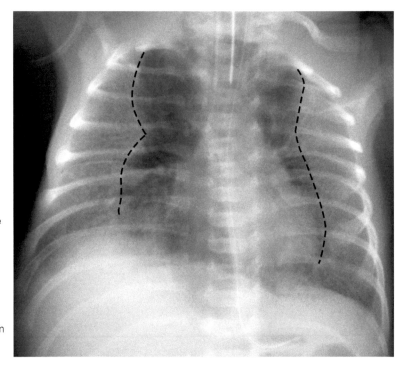

Fig. 10.11F Supine neonatal CXR with a marked bilateral zone of lucency outlining the heart and mediastinal structures (dotted lines). The findings are in keeping with pneumomediastinum on a background of RDS.

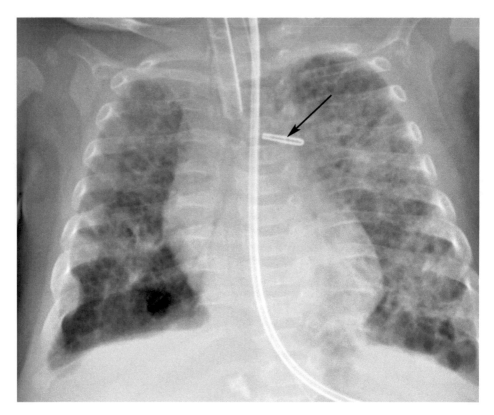

Fig. 10.11G Supine neonatal CXR with bilateral coarse reticular lung markings with cyst-like areas of hyperexpansion. The findings are typical of bronchopulmonary dysplasia. Note also the correctly positioned ETT and NG tube, also the clipped ductus arteriosus (arrow).

Long-term complications include: bronchopulmonary dysplasia (BPD), also know as chronic lung disease of prematurity (CLD).

Infants who have a prolonged oxygen requirement beyond 28 days (or a corrected gestational age of 36 weeks) are described as having BPD/CLD. The lung damage is a manifestation of pressure and volume trauma from artificial ventilation. The CXR characteristically shows coarse interstitial densities, caused by fibrosis and scarring, interspersed with cyst-like areas, which reflect hyperexpansion, (**Figure 10.11G**).

> **LEARNING POINTS: RESPIRATORY DISTRESS SYNDROME**
>
> ▪ RDS is primarily a disease of premature infants caused by the lack of endogenous surfactant, without which the alveoli collapse and undergo necrosis.
> ▪ Treatment of respiratory distress is based on respiratory support of the immature lungs and administration of synthetic surfactant.
> ▪ The three main CXR characteristics are small lung volumes, air bronchograms, and a fine granular (reticular nodular) pattern.
> ▪ Air leak syndromes are a common short-term complication caused by alveolar rupture.
> ▪ As a result of chronic ventilator support the lungs can undergo pressure and volume trauma leading to BPD.

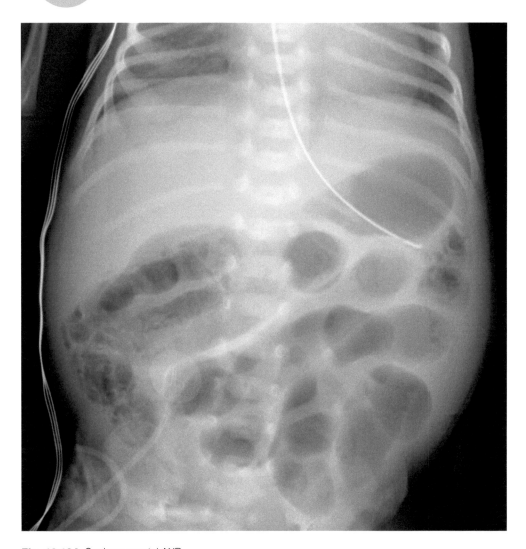

Fig. 10.12A Supine neonatal AXR.

A premature infant born at 24 weeks gestation begins to develop feed intolerance 3 days after birth while on the NICU. There is bile stained vomiting and increasing volume of NG tube aspirates. The abdomen is tender and distended. Feeding is stopped; however, the infant continues to remain unstable with apnoeas, tachycardia, tachypnoea, and shock. An arterial blood gas confirms a metabolic acidosis and an AXR is performed (**Figure 10.12A**).

CASE 10.12: QUESTIONS

1 What does the AXR show?
2 What is the diagnosis?

3 What are the complications of this condition?
4 How is the condition treated?

CASE 10.12: ANSWERS

1 What does the AXR show?

Multiple dilated bowel loops and intramural gas (pneumatosis intestinalis) are visible (**Figure 10.12B**). There is no evidence of pneumoperitoneum to indicate bowel wall perforation, or of any portal venous gas. The NG tube is adequately sited.

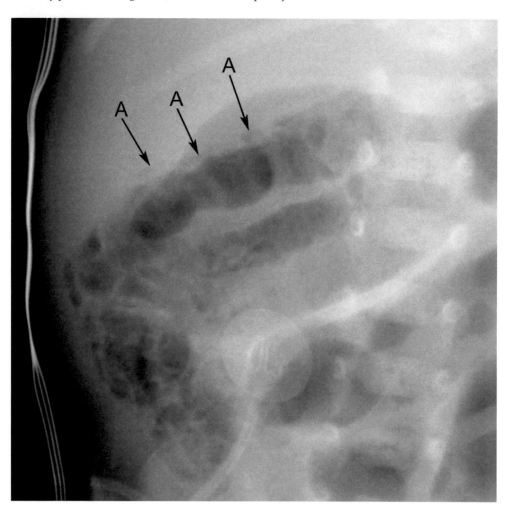

Fig. 10.12B Magnified view of the same neonatal AXR as in **Figure 10.12A** showing gas within the bowel wall (arrows, A) known as pneumatosis intestinalis.

2 What is the diagnosis?

In this clinical context the imaging appearances are pathognomonic for necrotising enterocolitis (NEC). This is a severe enterocolitis, which can affect any part of the large or small bowel. The commonest sites are the terminal ileum, caecum, and ascending colon. Inflammation starts at the mucosal surface and progresses to transmural necrosis and perforation. Bowel discolouration, distension, and pneumatosis, (submucosal or subserosal gas) are common findings at surgery.

Although a combination of ischaemic and infective aetiologies has been proposed, NEC is usually considered idiopathic and multifactorial (*Table 10.12A*).

Table 10.12A Risk factors for NEC

Prematurity
Intrauterine growth restriction
Perinatal asphyxia
Umbilical catheterisation
Hypoxia
Patent ductus arteriosus
Nonhuman milk feeds
Rapid introduction of enteral feeding
Polycythemia
Exchange transfusion
Cyanotic congenital heart disease

Neonates with NEC initially demonstrate nonspecific signs such as temperature instability and increased gastric aspirates. As the disease progresses there is increasing abdominal distension with bloody stools and vomiting. In severe cases the abdominal wall will appear erythematous and there may even be palpable bowel loops. The blood gases will usually show a metabolic acidosis, indicative of shock. There may be hypoxia representing respiratory failure owing to apnoea or diaphragmatic splinting, and this may indicate the need for respiratory support.

AXR is mandatory to confirm the diagnosis. The radiographic findings are listed in *Table 10.12B*.

Table 10.12B AXR features of NEC

- **Dilated bowel loops** – often asymmetrical in distribution. May be fixed over serial AXRs
- **Bowel wall thickening** – due to oedema, often with thumb printing pattern
- **Separation of bowel loops** – due to the accumulation of intraperitoneal fluid
- **Intramural gas (pneumatosis)** – bubble-like lucencies, which can mimic stool (**Figures 10.12B, 10.12D**)
- **Portal venous gas** – intramural gas is absorbed into the mesenteric veins and into the portal venous system. It manifests as linear branching lucencies within the liver (**Figure 10.12C**)
- **Pneumoperitoneum secondary to perforation** – air on both sides of the bowel (Rigler's sign) or air outlining the falciform ligament (football sign)

3 What are the complications of this condition?

The natural history of NEC is of transmural bowel necrosis leading to perforation and peritonitis. There is a 30% mortality associated with this condition.

It is not always possible to determine free gas on a supine AXR; indeed, only 50–75% of patients with proven perforation will have visible free gas. If perforation is suspected then a horizontal shoot-through XR, with the patient lying on their left side, will increase the chance of

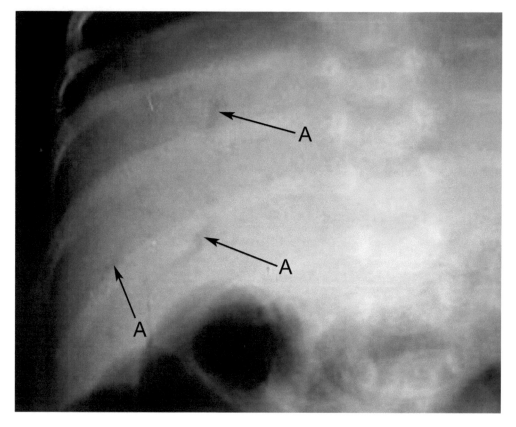

Fig. 10.12C Magnified view of another neonatal AXR showing linear lucencies across the liver (arrows, A) indicative of portal venous gas.

detecting free gas gathering alongside the liver. Note: an erect CXR will not be possible in a ventilated neonate.

4 How is the condition treated?

This is a neonatal emergency and the patient should initially be treated with an ABCDE approach. This may require assisted ventilation if there is respiratory distress. A NG tube should be inserted if not already in place. With suspension of enteral nutrition, parenteral nutrition should be commenced. Antibiotic treatment is given empirically to treat any underlying infection.

Further management can be divided into medical and surgical. The aim of medical management is to allow the gut to rest and to treat any underlying infection with broad-spectrum antibiotics.

Surgery is indicated in the following scenarios:

- Intestinal perforation.
- Formation of a mass.
- Failure to respond to medical management.

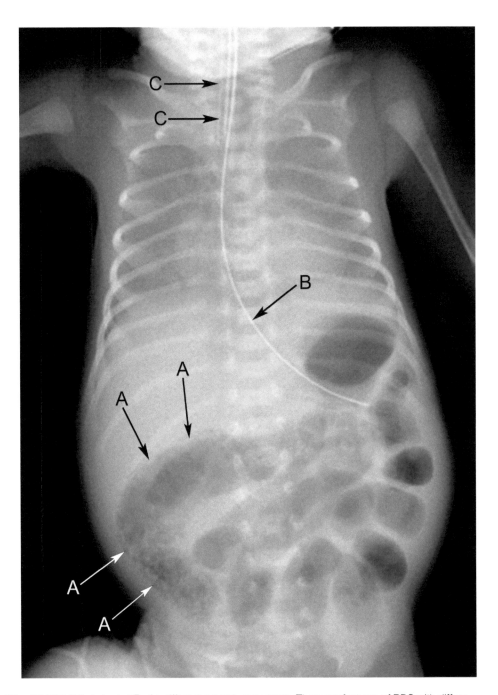

Fig. 10.12D Whole body XR of a different premature neonate. There are features of RDS with diffuse bilateral ground glass lung opacification. Also evidence of NEC with distended bowel loops, a mottled bowel gas pattern, and pneumatosis (A). No evidence of pneumoperitoneum. Satisfactory nasogastric (B) and endotracheal (C) tube positions.

Surgery involves the removal of necrotic bowel, usually with the creation of a stoma. Overall, 10–40% of surviving patients go on to develop intestinal strictures, which may require further surgery. Another complication is malabsorption owing to extensive gut resection, a condition known as short gut syndrome.

> **LEARNING POINTS: NECROTISING ENTEROCOLITIS**
>
> - NEC is a multifactorial disease associated with prematurity and low birthweight.
> - The clinical features are nonspecific with temperature instability and increased NG aspirates. As the disease progresses there is increasing abdominal distension.
> - AXR features include dilated bowel loops, bowel wall thickening, separation of bowel loops, intramural gas, portal venous gas, and pneumoperitoneum.
> - NEC is a neonatal emergency owing to its high mortality. If it is complicated by perforation, urgent surgery is indicated.

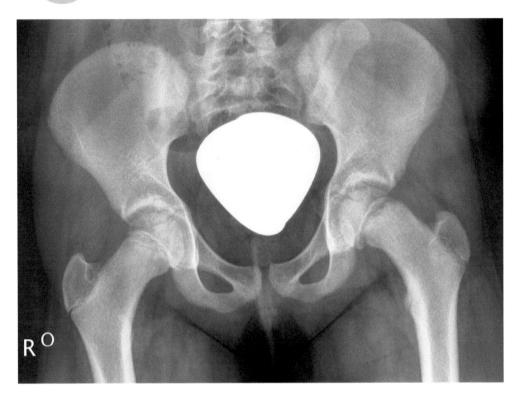

Fig. 10.13A AP view of the pelvis (female gonad protection applied).

A 14-year-old female presents to her GP with a limp and left hip pain. It started when she fell over at school a few weeks earlier but the limp has not improved and the pain is worsening. On examination, she has a raised BMI and her mother reports she has recently undergone a growth spurt. She has restricted and painful abduction and internal rotation of the left hip. The remainder of the examination is normal. Her GP arranges an XR.

CASE 10.13: QUESTIONS

1 What abnormalities can you see in **Figure 10.13A**?
2 What other XR view should you request?
3 What are the main clinical features of this condition?
4 What treatment is required?
5 What are the possible complications of this condition?

CASE 10.13: ANSWERS

1 What abnormalities can you see in Figure 10.13A?

The AP view of the pelvis shows slippage of the left capital femoral epiphysis (**Figure 10.13B**). The epiphysis appears relatively dense, the physis is widened, and there is disruption of Shenton's line.

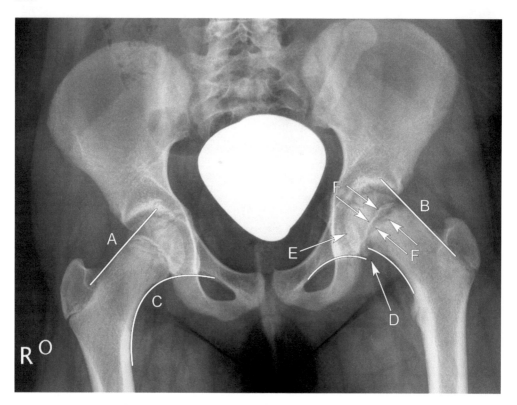

Fig. 10.13B AP view of the pelvis demonstrating on the right side the normal alignment of the superior border of the femoral neck, which cuts through the lateral aspect of the femoral capital epiphysis. This is known as Klein's line (A). On the left, however, the epiphysis has slipped and this line (B) no longer traverses the femoral capital epiphysis. Also note that Shenton's line (C), which follows the contour of the superior pubic ramus and inferomedial border of the femoral neck, is disrupted on the left (D). The left femoral capital epiphysis has slipped posteromedially, disrupting the smooth contour (E). The physis is widened on the left (F). Note also the white circle in the bottom (patient's right side) of the XR – this is the equivalent of a 'red dot' and is placed by the radiographer if pathology is suspected. Take note of these as they can guide you and ask the radiographer what concerned them if you are unsure.

2 What other XR view should you request?

It is important to also request a frog leg lateral view in children with hip pain (**Figure 10.13C**). This view gives better visualisation of the medial aspect of the hip joint, the growth plate, and femoral neck. This view is particularly useful where the suspected diagnosis is either slipped capital femoral epiphysis (SCFE) or Perthes' disease.

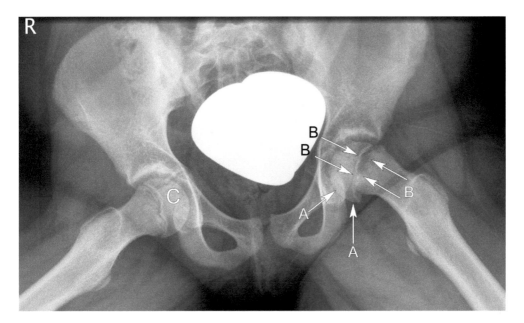

Fig. 10.13C Frog leg lateral view of the pelvis. There is posteromedial slip of the left superior capital femoral epiphysis (A) with widening of the physis (B). Note the gonadal shield used to protect the female reproductive organs from radiation exposure. Normal right capital femoral epiphysis (C).

3 What are the main clinical features of this condition?

SCFE (or slipped upper femoral epiphysis, SUFE) is posterior and medial displacement of the femoral head at the growth plate (physis). There is weakening of the physis, which leads to slippage of the femoral head.

- It typically occurs in overweight adolescent boys. The exact cause is unknown but identified risk factors include a positive family history, raised BMI, certain endocrine disorders including hypothyroidism, and renal osteodystrophy.
- The typical age of onset is 12–15 years. Presentation in children less than 10 years of age, particularly if they are of normal weight or short stature, may suggest an underlying endocrine abnormality.
- SCFE usually presents insidiously over several weeks to months and often during a growth spurt. Occasionally it can be triggered by minor trauma.
- It presents with intermittent hip or knee pain, which is worse with activity. There may be a limp owing to the inability to weight bear on the affected side and reduced passive external rotation of the leg (the leg appears outwardly turned).
- In the majority of patients only one hip joint is affected at presentation, although it presents with bilateral disease in 20% of cases. Up to 40% of patients with a unilateral diagnosis will go on to develop the problem in the opposite hip.

4 What treatment is required?

Management for SCFE is always surgical and should happen within 24 hours of diagnosis to reduce the risk of complications. The surgery required depends on the degree of the slippage of

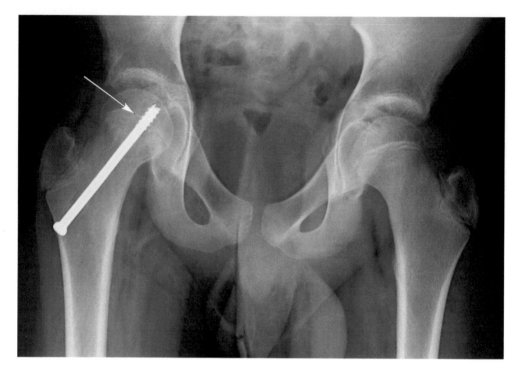

Fig. 10.13D AP view of the pelvis showing an example of *in-situ* fixation in a child with SCFE in their right hip. The screw can be seen crossing the nearly fused physis (arrow).

the femoral head. Generally the treatment required is *in-situ* fixation with a cannulated screw, which crosses the growth plate (**Figure 10.13D**). This maintains the position of the femoral head and prevents further slippage. If the SCFE is unstable with severe slippage, open reduction may be required to manipulate the femoral head back into its correct position before fixing it in place.

- Physiotherapy and adequate analgesia are an important part of postoperative recovery. The child is kept partial weight bearing on crutches for 6–8 weeks until pain free with full strength. Most patients make a good recovery, returning to a normal level of function, but may be advised to avoid high-impact sports until their growth plate has closed. They will be followed up with XRs until their growth plate has fused to ensure no further slippage of the femoral head and to check for involvement of the opposite hip.
- Owing to the risk of involvement in the other hip, prophylactic surgery may be offered. This would depend on the individual's risk. For example, if the child was young at presentation with endocrine abnormalities they would be at a higher risk of disease in the opposite hip. However, an overweight child presenting in their teens, with no other risk factors, may purely be monitored with XR follow-up to check for disease in the opposite hip.
- These children should be referred to a paediatrician for investigation of an underlying cause particularly if the presentation is atypical, i.e. the child is not overweight and younger than the usual age of presentation (<10 years). Investigations for endocrine abnormalities, such as thyroid dysfunction and panhypopituitarism, should be considered in these circumstances.

5 What are the possible complications of this condition?

Complications can occur if left untreated.

- The earlier a diagnosis of SCFE is made, the better the outcome for the child.
- If left untreated, SCFE will lead to increasing pain and deformity with reduced range of movement in the hip. Avascular necrosis of the femoral head could occur if the blood supply to the femoral head becomes disrupted; this is more likely with unstable SCFEs, which have more significant slippage. If avascular necrosis has occurred, the child may eventually need a total hip replacement.
- With *in-situ* fixation, there is the possibility that the child may outgrow their screw and require a revision surgery.
- Most children do well with prompt surgery. Those children with more severe slippage and deformity are more likely to develop problems, such as avascular necrosis, as well as OA in later life.

LEARNING POINTS: SLIPPED CAPITAL FEMORAL EPIPHYSIS

- SCFE is posterior and inferomedial displacement of the femoral head around the growth plate (physis).
- It frequently occurs in children aged 12–15 years; it is more common in boys and if the child is overweight.
- There are certain predisposing conditions such as renal osteodystrophy and some metabolic endocrine conditions.
- Diagnosis is with XR, including frog lateral view of the hips, where displacement of the epiphysis is seen on the affected side(s).
- Management is surgical with *in-situ* fixation of the hip. If left untreated, avascular necrosis of the femoral head may occur and this may cause problems in later life.

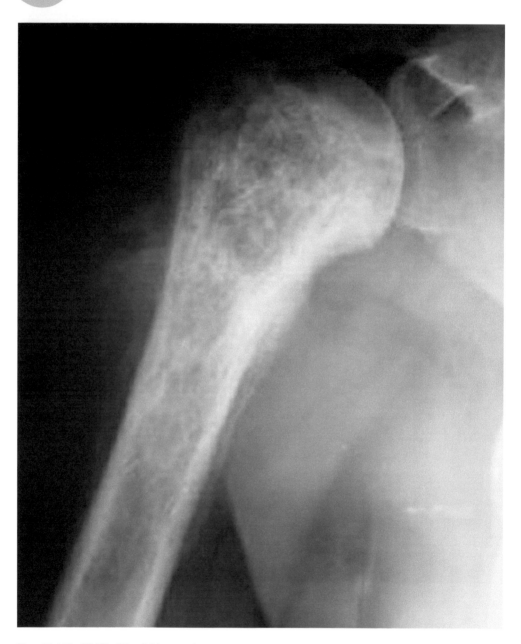

Fig. 10.14A AP XR of the right upper humerus.

A 15-year-old male presents to his GP with 3 months of progressive pain and swelling in his right shoulder. He is mildly pyrexial with a temperature of 37.5°. The shoulder is swollen and painful, and there is a palpable soft-tissue mass.

The GP, concerned about osteomyelitis, refers the child urgently for an orthopaedic opinion. In the hospital, blood tests and an XR of the right shoulder are requested (**Figure 10.14A**).

The bloods reveal a mild anaemia with a Hb of 9 g/dL (12–16 g/dL) and a leukocytosis with a WCC of 16×10^9/L ($4.5–13.5 \times 10^9$/L). The ESR is raised at 50 mm/hr (0–10 mm/hr).

CASE 10.14: QUESTIONS

1 Describe the XR appearances.

2 What are the key differential diagnoses?

3 What is the most likely diagnosis?

4 How should this patient be managed?

CASE 10.14: ANSWERS

1 Describe the XR appearances.

The upper humerus has an abnormal permeative texture with small rounded lucencies particularly in the metaphysis (**Figure 10.14B**). The destruction has a broad zone of transition such that it is difficult to determine the boundary between the abnormal and normal bone. There is also a periosteal reaction. These are features of an aggressive destructive process.

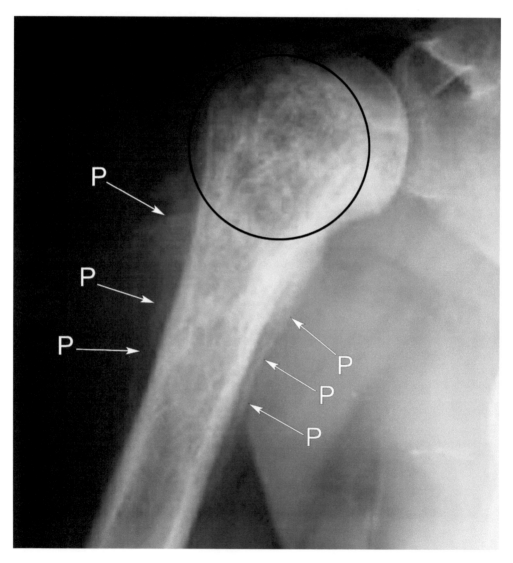

Fig. 10.14B XR of the right shoulder with an aggressive destructive lesion in the humeral metaphysis (circled region) with a permeative or 'moth-eaten' appearance extending into the humeral shaft. Note the periosteal reaction (P) and broad zone of transition.

2 What are the key differential diagnoses?

The differential for these aggressive, destructive appearances includes neoplastic and infective causes (*Table 10.14*).

- Periosteal reactions are caused by local damage to the periosteum (the connective tissue membrane around bone). There are benign and aggressive patterns of reaction that help differentiate the likely cause. The most common causes are trauma, infection, and malignancy.
- In slow, chronic, inflammatory processes, the periosteum has time to remodel and lay down new bone. The periosteal reaction is wave-like and thickened.
- In rapid, aggressive processes (as in this case), new bone is laid down in a disorganised manner before the periosteum has time to consolidate. The periosteal reaction is irregular and can be amorphous, multi-lamellated (onion-skin appearance) or sunburst. Codman's triangle describes a triangular area of periosteal new bone created when a tumour raises periosteum from the bone.

Table 10.14 The differential for 'moth-eaten bone' pattern in a child

Neoplastic	Neuroblastoma metastases
	Leukaemia
	Ewing's sarcoma
	Lymphoma
	Osteosarcoma
Infective	Acute osteomyelitis

3 What is the most likely diagnosis?

The diagnosis in this case is Ewing's sarcoma, a highly malignant primary bone tumour. This belongs to a family of small blue round cell tumours, which also includes lymphoma, rhadomyo-sarcoma, and primitive neuroectodermal tumours. It is the second most common bone tumour in children after osteosarcoma (osteosarcoma 60%; Ewing's 30%) and has a peak incidence at 10–15 years of age.

Ewing's can cause pain, swelling, and limitation of movement, which is sometimes incorrectly ascribed to a sports injury. There may be systemic symptoms and signs such as lassitude and fever, and a leukocytosis and raised ESR are common. These features can mimic osteomyelitis, which has similarly aggressive appearances on XR.

4 How should this patient be managed?

This is a rare tumour and should be managed with a multidisciplinary approach in a specialist bone tumour centre where the relevant orthopaedic, oncology, and diagnostic expertise is gathered.

The child should have an MRI scan to evaluate the intraosseous extent of the disease and also the soft-tissue component, which is typically extensive (**Figure 10.14C**).

A CT scan of the chest, abdomen, and pelvis is performed to assess for distant metastatic spread. A radioisotope bone scan can also help to identify bone metastases.

Core biopsy of the lesion is necessary and should be undertaken at the specialist unit for histological confirmation, and carefully planned to avoid compromising the potential for limb-salvage surgery.

Treatment involves chemotherapy and resection of the tumour with limb-sparing surgery if possible.

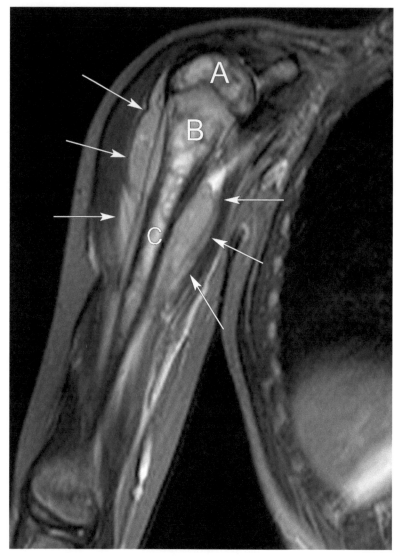

Fig. 10.14C MR T2 fat saturated coronal image of the right shoulder in the same child. Note: the extent of the soft-tissue component of the tumour (arrows) surrounding the bone, and high signal involvement of the proximal humeral epiphysis (A), metaphysis (B), and diaphysis (C).

LEARNING POINTS: EWING'S SARCOMA

- Ewing's sarcoma is the second most common bone tumour in children, after osteosarcoma, and has a peak age of incidence at 10–15 years. Urgent referral to a specialist bone tumour unit is essential.
- The radiological features of an aggressive bone lesion include:
  - Cortical destruction.
  - A broad zone of transition.
  - Irregular, amorphous, multilamellated or sunburst periosteal reaction.
- MRI can evaluate the intraosseous and significant extraosseous components of the disease.
- Chemotherapy followed by limb-sparing surgery is the mainstay of treatment.
- Osteomyelitis can have a similar appearance and should always be considered and excluded.

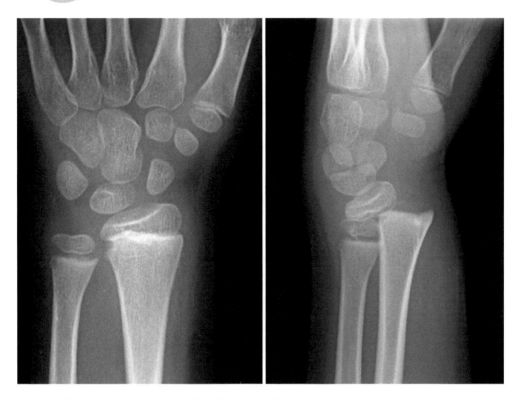

Fig. 10.15A XR of the left wrist with AP (left) and lateral (right) views.

A 9-year-old female presents to accident and emergency after falling off a trampoline and landing on her outstretched left arm. She cried immediately and now complains of pain in her left wrist and arm. On examination, her wrist is tender and she is reluctant to move it. The overlying skin is intact. Her remaining examination is normal. An XR is arranged (**Figure 10.15A**).

CASE 10.15: QUESTIONS

1 Explain the importance of obtaining more than one XR view in suspected bone trauma.
2 Describe the XR abnormality.
3 What is the physis and how are physeal fractures classified?
4 What complications can arise as a result of this type of injury?
5 Name the common fracture types in children.

CASE 10.15: ANSWERS

1 Explain the importance of obtaining more than one XR view in suspected bone trauma.

When obtaining an XR of a suspected bone fracture it is important to review at least two orthogonal plane views at 90° to one other. Generally, AP and lateral are adequate. Some bones and joints require a third view for further assessment, usually an oblique view, and examples of these include the metacarpal bones and the paediatric elbow.

It is difficult for very young children to localise their pain. For this reason, it is important to examine the joints above and below the suspected site of injury. For example, a child with pain in their forearm should have both their wrist and elbow examined. Additional XRs of these joints may be necessary.

2 Describe the XR abnormality.

The XR shows a fracture-dislocation of the left distal radial epiphysis (**Figure 10.15B**). The fracture line passes straight through the growth plate and has caused the epiphysis to dislocate dorsally (posteriorly). This pattern of fracture through the growth plate is known as Salter–Harris (SH) type 1.

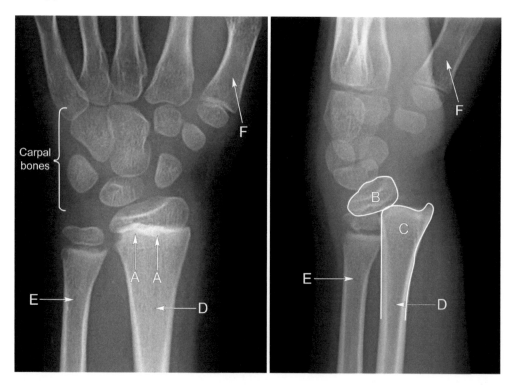

Fig. 10.15B AP (left) and lateral (right) views of left wrist, showing a fracture-dislocation of the left distal radial epiphysis. On the AP projection, this manifests as overlap of the epiphysis and metaphysis at the growth plate (A). On the lateral projection, the radial epiphysis (B) and carpus bones have slipped dorsally off the radial metaphysis (C). Note the normal radial shaft (D), ulna (E), and 1st metacarpal (thumb, F).

3 What is the physis and how are physeal fractures classified?

The physis is the growth plate in developing bones and it is seen between the metaphysis and the epiphysis. Tubular bones grow via a process of endochondral bone formation whereby cells migrate from the physis towards the metaphysis, simultaneously pushing the growth plate in the opposite direction and leading to bone growth. As the cells migrate they mature and calcify laying down new bone.

The physis forms a line of weakness in the immature bone and is prone to fracture. The physis is involved in as many as 18% of paediatric long bone fractures. Physeal injuries are grouped according to the SH classification, of which there are 5 types. **Figures 10.15C–10.15G** are illustrations of the SH classification (Types I–V), with real examples.

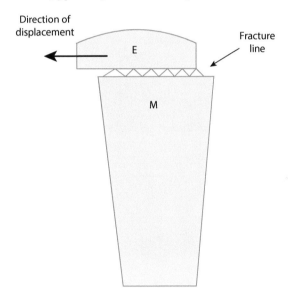

Fig. 10.15C Type 1 fractures involve the physis only (as in the patient at the start of this case); the epiphysis (E) slips in relation to metaphysis (M).

TOP TIP

A useful mnemonic to remember the Salter–Harris classification is SALTR

S lipped	Type I
A bove the growth plate	Type II
BeLow the growth plate	Type III
T hrough the growth plate	Type IV
R ammed growth plate	Type V

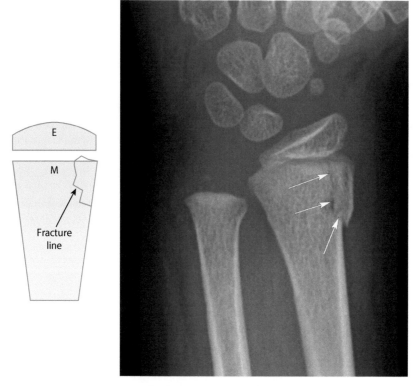

Fig. 10.15D
Type II fractures involve the metaphysis (M) and the physis (growth plate). This example demonstrates a fracture of the distal radius (small arrows). These are the most common type of physeal injury.

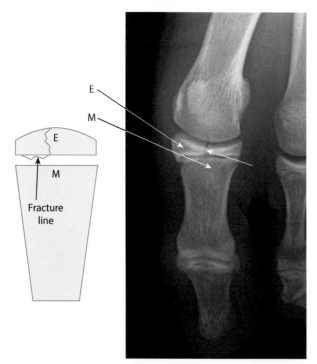

Fig. 10.15E Type III fractures involve the growth plate and the epiphysis (E). This is an XR of the proximal phalanx of a big toe (inverted); the epiphyseal fracture is arrowed. These injuries have a greater risk of growth arrest. Metaphysis (M).

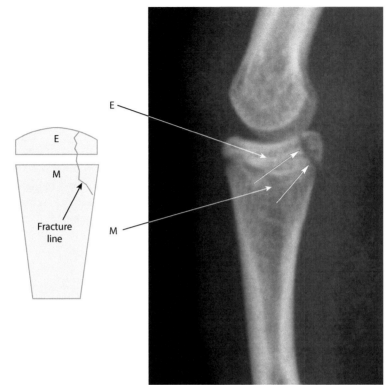

Fig. 10.15F Type IV fractures extend from the metaphysis (M) through the growth plate and the epiphysis (E). This example shows a fracture (white arrows) through the growth plate of a finger (inverted). These injuries also have a higher tendency to growth arrest.

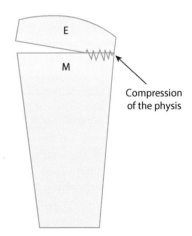

Fig. 10.15G Type V fractures are compression fractures of the physis owing to an axial crush injury. These are rare and difficult to detect. They often only become apparent after growth arrest. Metaphysis (M), epiphysis (E).

4 What complications can arise as a result of this type of injury?

The most important complication of a SH fracture is growth disturbance owing to premature fusion of the growth plate. This includes both growth acceleration and retardation, and can lead to limb length discrepancies and angular deformation. The complications that arise from these depend on the location, plane of injury, SH type, fracture severity, and the age of the child. Growth disturbance tends to be more severe with higher grades of SH injury. Older children in their teens tend to have fewer complications because of their reduced growth potential.

- Most SH fractures can be managed conservatively with closed reduction and application of a cast. More severe fractures, particularly those with joint involvement, may require surgical fixation. The complications that can arise as a result of these fractures may require further management as the child grows. SH type V fractures are very difficult to detect and may have very subtle XR changes. They tend to present months or years after the injury with problems such as leg length discrepancy or gait disturbance. In these cases, MRI can play an important role in the initial diagnosis.

5 Name the common fracture types in children.

Paediatric bones are elastic and have a greater propensity to bend and bow before fracturing. This produces certain patterns of fractures, which are unique to the paediatric age group. These include greenstick, torus, and plastic bowing fractures (**Figures 10.15H–10.15J**).

- These fractures are incomplete, in that the fracture involves one cortex and does not extend through the entire diameter of the bone. These fracture types are commonly seen in the diaphysis of the radius and ulna of the forearm. The mechanism of fracture is from an angular or longitudinal force exerted on the forearm, for example from a FOOSH.
- A greenstick fracture results from an angular force on the bone. The bone bends and results in a break in the cortex on the convex site of the bone, while the opposite cortex remains intact. The appearances are likened to bending an immature tree branch, hence 'greenstick' (**Figure 10.15H**).
- Sometimes the immature bone may just bend without fracturing. This is known as a plastic bowing fracture (**Figure 10.15H**). There is no visible fracture line on XR but microfractures are seen under the microscope. The diagnosis is easy when an adjacent bone in the arm or leg is fractured. If there are no associated fractures and there is diagnostic uncertainty, comparison with the same bone on the other side may be necessary. Also, repeating the XR after 10–14 days to look for callus formation may help to confirm the diagnosis.
- Buckle fractures are also known as torus fractures. The cortex at the site of injury buckles rather than fractures. The cortex can bulge in or out on the side of compression. The fracture may appear as a subtle bump or undulation of the cortex (**Figure 10.15I**). They are commonly seen in the distal metaphyses of the radius, ulna, tibia, fibula, metacarpals, and phalanges.

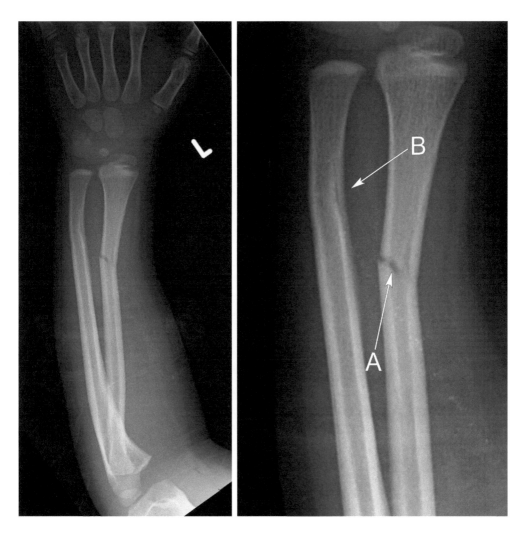

Fig. 10.15H Left forearm XR, with magnified view (right) of the distal forearm, showing a greenstick fracture of the radius (A) and a plastic bowing fracture of the ulna (B).

- Toddler's fractures are spiral or oblique fractures of the distal tibia without displacement (**Figure 10.15J**). They occur in young ambulatory children (from 9 months to 3 years of age) and result from a rotational force on the limb caused by falling and twisting on the leg. The periosteum remains intact and the bone is stable. The lack of displacement in such fractures means that they are easily missed on XR and an additional oblique view may be required if there is a strong clinical suspicion of injury. A repeat XR at 10–14 days after the injury will demonstrate a periosteal reaction. These fractures heal well with a plaster cast.

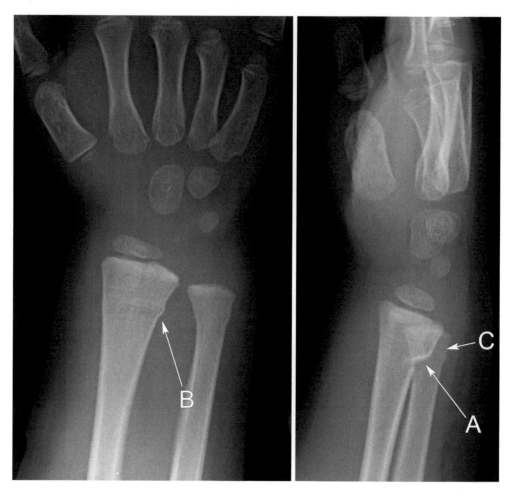

Fig. 10.15I Wrist XR with AP (left) and lateral (right) views showing a buckle fracture of the distal radius. Note the angular deformity of the radius on the lateral projection with buckling (A) of the cortex rather than a simple fracture line. The outward bulge seen on the AP projection is also referred to as a torus fracture (B). There is also a subtle torus fracture of the distal ulna (C).

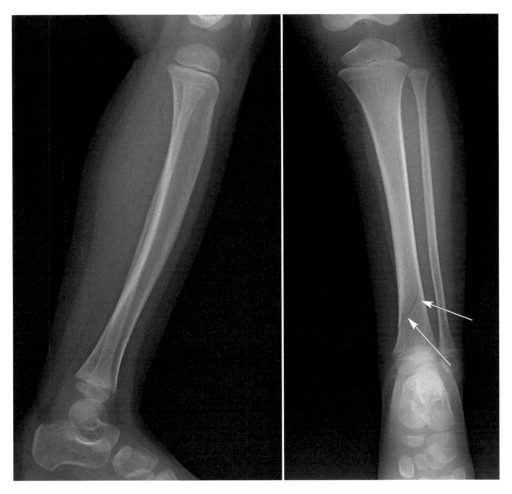

Fig. 10.15J Lower leg XRs, AP (right) and lateral (left) views, showing an oblique Toddler's fracture of the distal tibia (arrows). Note the lack of displacement. The fracture is not seen on the lateral projection, further demonstrating the importance of reviewing two orthogonal views.

LEARNING POINTS: PAEDIATRIC FRACTURES

- At least two orthogonal views are required to fully assess a fracture on an XR.
- The growth plate or physis is the site of new bone formation and bone growth.
- The physis forms a line of weakness in the immature bone.
- Physeal fractures are organised according to the Salter–Harris classification.
- The paediatric skeleton is malleable, and the bones can bend and buckle with trauma rather than completely fracture.

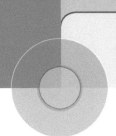

Bibliography

Banerjee AK (2006) *Radiology Made Easy*. Cambridge: Cambridge University Press.

Barrett T, Shaida N, Shaw A, Dixon AK (2010) *Radiology for Undergraduate Finals and Foundation Years: Key Topics and Question Types*. Oxford: Radcliffe Publishing.

Begg JD (2006) *Abdominal X-rays Made Easy*, 2nd edn. Edinburgh: Elsevier Health Sciences.

Chan O (ed.) (2013) *ABC of Emergency Radiology*, 3rd edn. Oxford: Wiley-Blackwell.

Chowdrey R, Wilson I, Rofe C, Lloyd-Jones G (2010) *Radiology at a Glance*. Chichester: John Wiley.

Clarke C (2015) *Abdominal X-rays for Medical Students*. Chichester: Wiley-Blackwell.

Daffner RH (2007) *Clinical Radiology: The Essentials*, 3rd edn. Baltimore: Wolters Kluwer/ Lippincott Williams & Wilkins.

Darby MJ, Barron DA, Hyland RE (2012) *Oxford Handbook of Medical Imaging*. Oxford: Oxford University Press.

Davies SG (2013) *Chapman & Nakielny's Aids to Radiological Differential Diagnosis*, 6th edn. Edinburgh: Saunders Ltd.

de Lacey G, Morely S, Berman L (2008) *The Chest X-ray. A Survival Guide*, 2nd edn. Edinburgh: Elsevier Health Sciences.

Grainger RG, Adam A, Dixon AK, Allison DJ (2007) *Grainger and Allison's Diagnostic Radiology: A Textbook of Medical Imaging: Volumes 1–2*, 4th edn. London: Churchill Livingstone.

Howlett DC, Ayers B (2004) *The Hands-on Guide to Imaging*. Oxford: Blackwell Publishing.

Howlett DC, Gainsborough N (eds.) (2013) *100 Cases for Medical Data Interpretation*. Boca Raton: Hodder Education.

Hussain SM, Latif SAA, Hall AD (2010) *Rapid Review of Radiology*. London: Manson Publishing.

Lisle DA (2007) *Imaging for Students*. London: Hodder Arnold.

Mettler FA (2013) *Essentials of Radiology*, 2nd edn. Philadelphia: Elsevier Health Sciences.

Moeller TB, Reif E (1999) *Pocket Atlas of Radiographic Anatomy*, 2nd edn. Stuttgart: Thieme Publishing Group.

Patel PR (2010) *Lecture Notes, Radiology*. Chichester: Wiley-Blackwell.

Qureshi Z (2012) *The Unofficial Guide to Passing OSCEs*, 3rd edn. London: Zesham Qureshi.

Raby N, Berman L, de Lacey G (2005) *Accident and Emergency Radiology. A Survival Guide*, 2nd edn. Edinburgh: Elsevier Health Sciences.

Renton P, Butler P (2004) *Medical Imaging: An Illustrated Colour Text*. Edinburgh: Elsevier Churchill Livingstone.

Rodrigues M, Qureshi Z (eds.) (2014) *The Unofficial Guide to Radiology: Chest, Abdominal and Orthopaedic X-rays, plus CTs, MRIs and Other Important Modalities. Core Radiology Curriculum Covered: 100 Annotated X-rays (including how to present them), 300 Multiple Choice Questions (with detailed explanations)*. London: Zeshan Qureshi.

Semelka RC, Birchard KR, Busireddy KR (2015) *Critical Observations in Radiology for Medical Students*. Chichester: Wiley-Blackwell.

Shaw AS, Godfrey EM, Singh A (2009) *Radiology: Clinical Cases Uncovered*. Chichester: Wiley-Blackwell.

Ter Meulen D, Kelly B, Bickle IC (2008) *Imaging*. Philadelphia: Mosby/Elsevier.

Wasan R, Grundy A, Beese R, Wasan R (2004) *Radiology Casebook for Medical Students*, 2nd edn. London: Pastest.

Weill FS, Manco-Johnson ML (1997) *Imaging of Abdominal and Pelvic Anatomy*. London: Churchill Livingstone.

List of cases

List of cases

Index

Note: Page numbers in **bold** refer to figures; those in *italic* refer to tables or boxes.